Developed by experts.
Backed by science.

MENOPAUSE

What Your **Ob-Gyn** Wants You to Know

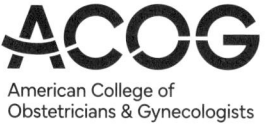

American College of
Obstetricians & Gynecologists

Menopause: What Your Ob-Gyn Wants You to Know was developed by a panel of experts working with staff of the American College of Obstetricians & Gynecologists (ACOG).

Editorial Board

Nanette F. Santoro, MD, Chair
Esther Eisenberg, MD, MPH, Vice Chair
Cheryl B. Iglesia, MD, FACS
Andrew M. Kaunitz, MD, MSCP
Charles C. Kilpatrick, MD, MEd
Gloria A. Richard-Davis, MD, MBA, MSCP
Mary L. Rosser, MD, PhD, MSCP
Carrie Ann Terrell, MD

ACOG Staff

Sandra E. Brooks, MD, MBA, Chief Executive Officer
Christopher M. Zahn, MD, Chief of Clinical Practice and Health Equity and Quality
Jennifer Walsh, Chief Operating Officer
Martha Hawley-Bertsch, Director, Product Management
Jennifer Hicks, MS, Director, Editorial Development
William Howard, MA, ELS, Copyeditor/Proofreader
Amy Goldenberg, PhD, Managing Editor, Publications
Taskin Monjur, Product Manager, Clinical and Patient Resources
Elizabeth Frey, Project Manager, Products
Hosnia N. Jami, Graphic Designer
Samantha Lee, Senior Manager, Marketing and Creative Design

The contributions of the following people are gratefully acknowledged:

Lucy M. Berrington, MS, Writer
Robin Marwick, CPE, ELS, Editor
Andrea Schmidt, Book Design
Kathleen Dyson, Typesetting and Layout
Lightbox Visual Communications Inc., Illustration

Cataloging-in-Publication data are available from the Library of Congress for this book.

ISBN 9781948258630 (trade paperback) | ISBN 9781948258647 (ebook)

Printed in the United States of America

Copyright 2026 by the American College of Obstetricians & Gynecologists, 409 12th Street SW, Washington, DC 20024-2188. All rights reserved. No part of this publication may be reproduced, stored in a retrieval system, posted on the internet, or transmitted in any form or by any means, electronic, mechanical, photocopying, recording, or otherwise, without prior written permission from the publisher. Any use of this publication to train generative artificial intelligence (AI) technologies, or as part of a generative AI language model (LLM) to generate text or responses to prompts, is expressly prohibited. Unauthorized use of this publication for AI training or development is strictly prohibited. The College reserves all rights to license uses of this work for generative AI training and development or as part of an LLM platform.

Designed as an informational resource for patients, *Menopause: What Your Ob-Gyn Wants You to Know* sets forth current information and opinions on subjects related to women's health and menopause care. *Menopause: What Your Ob-Gyn Wants You to Know* is a resource for informational purposes only. This resource does not constitute advice from your physician or health care professional, and it is not intended to replace the advice or counsel of a physician or health care professional. You should consult with, and rely only on the advice of, physicians or health care professionals familiar with your particular condition. While *Menopause: What Your Ob-Gyn Wants You to Know* makes every effort to provide information that is accurate and timely, the publisher cannot make any guarantees or warranties in that regard. The information does not dictate an exclusive course of treatment or procedure to be followed and should not be construed as excluding other acceptable methods of practice. Variations, taking into account the needs of the individual patient, resources, and limitations unique to the institution or type of practice, may be appropriate. The mention of a product, device, or drug in this publication does not constitute or guarantee endorsement of the quality or value of such product, device, or drug or of the claims made for it by the manufacturer.

1 2 3 4 5 / 0 9 8 7 6

CONTENTS

Introduction ix

Part I: Menopause Basics

Chapter 1: Understanding the Menopause Transition 3
    The Timing of the Menopause Transition 3
    What Can Affect Timing 4
    Perimenopause Comes First 5
    Menopause on Your Mind 6
    Your Hormones and Menopause 7
    Sometimes Menopause Shows Up Much Earlier 8
    Your Healthy Lifestyle in Menopause and Beyond 9
    Navigating Menopause: Your Best Resources 10
    Resources 10

Chapter 2: Understanding Perimenopause 13
    Tracking the Early Signs 13
    When Bleeding Changes Raise a Red Flag 14
    Other Symptoms of Perimenopause 15
    Other Causes of Abnormal Bleeding 19
    Talking With Your Ob-Gyn 21
    Resources 22

Chapter 3: Understanding Early and
Premature Menopause 23
    Causes of Premature and Early Menopause 23
    Causes of Medical and Surgical Menopause 26
    What Premature and Early Menopause Mean for Fertility 29
    Other Concerns When Menopause Comes Too Soon 29
    Treatment for Premature and Early Menopause 30
    What Happens in Primary Ovarian Insufficiency 30
    Resources 31

Chapter 4: Menopause Signs and Symptoms ... 33
Five Ways to Have a Better Menopause ... 33
Symptoms and How They Feel ... 35
Talking With Your Ob-Gyn ... 41
Resources ... 41

Chapter 5: Choosing Your Menopause Care Team ... 43
Ob-Gyns Who Provide Menopause Care ... 43
How to Find an Ob-Gyn ... 45
Other Doctors and Health Care Professionals ... 47
Taking Charge of Your Care ... 50
Resources ... 51

Part II: Detailing Signs and Symptoms

Chapter 6: Hot Flashes and Night Sweats ... 55
Vasomotor Symptoms: The Basics ... 55
Who Gets Hot Flashes and Night Sweats ... 57
Hot Flash Triggers ... 59
Managing Hot Flashes and Night Sweats ... 60
Medical Treatment for Hot Flashes ... 62
Talking With Your Ob-Gyn ... 65
Resources ... 65

Chapter 7: Abnormal Bleeding ... 67
Why Bleeding Changes in Perimenopause ... 67
When Bleeding Should Be Evaluated ... 68
Conditions That Can Cause Abnormal Bleeding in Perimenopause ... 69
Testing for Abnormal Bleeding in Perimenopause ... 70
Medications for Abnormal Bleeding in Perimenopause ... 72
Procedures to Treat Abnormal Bleeding in Perimenopause ... 74
Before and After Your Procedure ... 76
Bleeding After Menopause ... 77
Resources ... 78

Chapter 8: Mood and Memory ... 79
Am I Just Feeling Down or Is It Depression? ... 80
Is This Nervous Energy or Is It an Anxiety Disorder? ... 81
Treatment for Depression and Anxiety ... 82
Is This Brain Fog or Am I Just Tired? ... 85

Is This Brain Fog or ADHD?..85
Is This Brain Fog or Early Dementia?..86
Resources..87

Chapter 9: Sleep Problems..89
What Happens to Sleep in Perimenopause...89
Key Steps for Improving Your Sleep...91
What Happens With Sleep Disorders..96
Treatments for Sleep Disorders...97
When to Talk With Your Doctor..98
Resources..99

Chapter 10: Sexual Health..101
Sexual Health in Midlife..102
Treatments for Sexual Problems..104
When to Talk With Your Ob-Gyn...108
When to Talk With a Partner...109
When You Have a New Partner...110
Resources...111

Chapter 11: Vaginal and Vulvar Conditions..113
Changing Hormone Levels...113
Talking About Discomfort..115
Treatments for Vaginal Dryness..116
Other Disorders of the Vulva..118
Self-Care for Vulvar Conditions...121
What Menopause May Mean for Chronic Pelvic Pain.................................122
Resources...124

Chapter 12: Urinary Incontinence...125
Types of Urine Leakage..125
Why Urinary Problems Are Happening Now..127
What You and Your Ob-Gyn Can Do...128
Approaches to Try First...129
Devices and Physical Therapy..130
Medications...131
Nerve Stimulation Treatments..132
Surgical Treatments...132
Managing Accidental Bowel Leakage...134
Talking With Your Ob-Gyn..135
Resources...136

Chapter 13: Pelvic Organ Prolapse 137
   Symptoms of Pelvic Organ Prolapse 138
   Causes of Prolapse 138
   Types of Prolapse 139
   Talking With Your Ob-Gyn 141
   Nonsurgical Treatments for Prolapse 142
   Surgery for Prolapse 143
   How Prolapse Surgery Is Done 144
   Risks and Recovery 146
   Resources 148

Chapter 14: Weight and Menopause 149
   Midlife Changes and Weight Gain 150
   Managing Fitness and Weight in Midlife 151
   When to Talk With Your Ob-Gyn 155
   Other Medications for Weight Loss 156
   Surgery for Weight Loss 157
   Resources 158

Chapter 15: Bone Health 161
   How Bone Is Formed 161
   What Increases the Risk of Bone Loss 164
   How Bone Loss Is Diagnosed 165
   When and How to Treat Bone Loss 166
   Lifestyle and Bone Loss 169
   Resources 171

Part III: Management of Symptoms

Chapter 16: Lifestyle Changes and Alternative Approaches 175
   Self-Care as a Starting Point 175
   Nonprescription Products and Supplements 181
   Evaluating Product Claims 185
   When What You're Trying Isn't Working 185
   Resources 186

Chapter 17: Hormone Therapies....187

Hormone Therapy: History and Controversy....188
How Systemic Therapy Works....188
Benefits of Systemic Hormone Therapy....190
Side Effects and Risks of Systemic Therapy....191
How Long to Stay on Hormone Therapy....193
Local Hormone Therapy....193
Side Effects of Local Hormone Therapy....194
Talking With Your Ob-Gyn....196
Resources....196

Chapter 18: Estrogen-Free Medical Therapies....197

Medications for Hot Flashes and Night Sweats....198
Medications for Vaginal Symptoms....201
When to Talk About Estrogen-Free Medications....202
Talking With Your Ob-Gyn....203
Resources....203

Part IV: Staying Healthy in Menopause and Beyond

Chapter 19: Heart Disease and Diabetes....207

What to Know About Heart Disease....208
Who's at Highest Risk of CVD....210
A Guide to High Blood Pressure....210
A Guide to Triglycerides and Cholesterol....212
What to Know About Diabetes....212
Who's at Highest Risk of Diabetes....215
Lifestyle Changes and Reducing Risk....215
Options for Medication....218
Resources....219

Chapter 20: Managing Stress....221

When Stress Is a Health Issue....222
Managing Stress in Different Environments....224
Science-Based Self-Care Strategies....226
Talking With Your Ob-Gyn....228
Working With a Counselor....229
Resources....230

Chapter 21: Screenings and Vaccinations After Menopause 233
    Annual Wellness Visits After Menopause. 233
    Breast Cancer Screening 236
    Other Health Screenings. 238
    Vaccination for Midlife and Beyond. 242
    Resources. 244

Part V: Resources

For More Reading. 249
Terms You Should Know. 261

Index 277

INTRODUCTION

A quick scan of social media tells the story: Menopause is frustrating for many women, and plenty of them want to talk about it. There's no shortage of people offering advice, both anecdotal and accurate. But there's rarely a resource that combines evidence-based information and medical experience to explain every aspect of the menopause transition.

Until now. This book, *Menopause: What Your Ob-Gyn Wants You to Know*, comes from the experts at the American College of Obstetricians & Gynecologists (ACOG). For more than 70 years, ACOG has written the medical guidelines that obstetrician–gynecologists (ob-gyns) use when taking care of women. You can trust that the information you read here is supported by research, science, and the everyday experience of ob-gyns who have cared for millions of women in midlife.

Why Use This Book?

First, *Menopause: What Your Ob-Gyn Wants You to Know* draws on a wealth of ACOG guidance, trusted scientific studies, verified research data, and proven treatment options. It contains everything ob-gyns know about the menopause transition today, including ways you can thrive during this time of life.

Second, the book presents medical information in a straightforward, easy-to-understand way. *Menopause: What Your Ob-Gyn Wants You to Know* explains

- what's going on in your body and why
- what's normal for menopause and how to be alert to possible signs of disease
- what types of self-care and medications may make the biggest difference
- what menopause means for your health—now and in the future
- how to partner with your ob-gyn to find care that works for you

And third, this book recognizes that menopause brings complex emotions. Research shows that while it's a natural process, everyone experiences the menopause transition differently. So throughout the chapters, you'll find stories from real women on how they've managed their symptoms, common menopause questions with answers from ob-gyns, and resources you can use to learn more.

How Is This Book Organized?

You'll notice that Part I covers menopause basics, including how the menopause transition is defined, what triggers perimenopause, how menopausal symptoms may feel if you experience them, and how to choose the team that will care for you during your menopause transition.

In Part II, you'll find detailed chapters on the most common symptoms, including hot flashes and night sweats, changes in menstrual periods, mood and memory challenges, weight concerns, sleep problems, and vaginal changes. There are also chapters on related topics, including sexual function, urinary incontinence, pelvic organ problems, and bone loss.

Part III takes on questions around treatment, including hormone therapy, estrogen-free medications, self-care, and over-the-counter remedies. The focus is on finding the treatment that fits with your symptoms, your medical history, and your preferences for your care.

Part IV addresses staying healthy in menopause and beyond with chapters on heart health and diabetes, stress management, and postmenopausal screenings and vaccination. And at the back, Part V offers a "For More Reading" section that lists some of the most current and important research on menopause care.

In short, you hold in your hands a factual, comprehensive guide that helps you take control of your menopause experience and the care you receive in midlife.

What Else Should I Know?

There's still more to learn about the menopause transition, including exactly what causes some of the most bothersome symptoms. But based on what ob-gyns know now, there's a growing focus on delivering personalized, science-backed solutions. Your care should be a collaborative effort that leads to better health and well-being, and *Menopause: What Your Ob-Gyn Wants You to Know* can put you in the driver's seat. ACOG hopes this book becomes a reassuring and empowering resource as you navigate your menopause transition.

More to Explore Online

Looking for more on menopause care? Go to acog.org/MyMenopause for the latest from the leading experts in women's health care. Online you'll find

- top menopause questions answered by ACOG ob-gyns
- more menopause stories from women and ob-gyns
- an A-Z directory of health topics—covering perimenopause, menopause, and many other women's health concerns

Part I
MENOPAUSE BASICS

CHAPTER 1

Understanding the Menopause Transition

Around the time Lena turned 50, she started having hot flashes a couple of times a day and sometimes at night. "I also developed sleep problems and vaginal irritation," she says. "I've taken different types of hormone medications that have helped with the hot flashes. Now I also use a vaginal estrogen cream and take a low-dose antidepressant to help me sleep better." Lena says if she had it to do over, she would look for solutions more aggressively, going to an ob-gyn in addition to talking with her primary doctor. "Many women just don't talk about menopause. It can be hard, and I think it's important to talk to each other and with your ob-gyn."

It's here, the time in life you knew was coming: *menopause*. Maybe you've dreaded the thought of hot flashes and other symptoms, or maybe you've looked forward to no longer having *menstrual periods*. In any case, menopause is a natural process. It's the transition between your reproductive years and the rest of your life—an integral part of you and your story.

Most people have certain ideas about what menopause is and what it involves. Generally, though, menopause is not well understood. Many women experience menopause without major discomfort—yet daunting stories are common. It's true that menopause, like any life transition, can come with surprises and challenges. But it's important to know that there are many ways to treat menopausal symptoms that can improve your comfort, well-being, and quality of life.

It's also true that everyone experiences the *menopause transition* differently. Research tells us that how you experience menopause is not just about what's changing in your body. It's also about cultural influences and your own perceptions and expectations—the same factors that shape other major life experiences. There's a lot going on, and not all of it is easily visible.

The Timing of the Menopause Transition

Menopause is the time in your life when you stop having monthly periods. It marks the end of your reproductive years. In the United States, the average age that women go through menopause is 51. Any age between 45 and 55 is considered normal. For some women, menopause can arrive even earlier if they have a health condition or certain medical treatments. Chapter 3, "Understanding Early and Premature Menopause," explains more about this.

In medical terms, menopause is defined as your last menstrual period, but that's not the way people commonly think and talk about it. In conversation, "menopause" often refers to a life stage or the years when you have symptoms, which often continue after the last period. No matter how you use the word, these things are true:

- Over time, the *ovaries* naturally make less *estrogen*, a **hormone** that helps control the **menstrual cycle**.
- There's usually a change in menstrual periods during the few years before they stop altogether.
- Along the way, you may have certain symptoms, such as **hot flashes**, disturbed sleep, brain fog, mood swings, vaginal dryness, and changes to your skin and hair.

In this book, we'll use the term "menopause transition" to refer to this whole stage of life, from the time of your first symptoms to the few years after your last period, when you are clearly **postmenopausal**.

But let's return for a moment to the technical definition of menopause: your last menstrual period. How do you know if it's your last period? Well, by waiting a year and not having another. This is the inconvenient reality: Menopause is confirmed in hindsight. That uncertainty can make it harder to know what's going on with your body, what's normal for you, what to expect, and what types of health care might ease your way through.

What Can Affect Timing

Although the average age of the last period is 51, the timing varies. The timing matters, partly because it affects whether a woman can still get pregnant, and also because timing can help predict certain health risks, including heart disease and **bone loss**. Here are some things researchers know about the timing of menopause:

- Family history—When your mother or grandmother reached menopause may give you a clue about the timing of yours. Certain **genes** have been identified that may play a role in timing. (But even if the timing is similar, you may not have the same symptoms.)
- Early life stressors—Difficult experiences in early childhood, such as poor nutrition, delayed growth, and poverty, may contribute to an earlier menopause. It's possible that chronic stress over a lifetime may shorten the reproductive years.
- *Intimate partner violence*—Violence inflicted by spouses and partners is linked to an earlier menopause.

- Race and ethnicity—Some research shows that Black women reach menopause months earlier than White women. Researchers think this may be related to increased stress associated with discrimination in society and the health care system. Experiencing persistent racism can increase stress over a lifetime and affect overall health. Also, Black women are more likely to have a *hysterectomy* than women of other races and ethnicities, which can affect the timing of menopause.

- Smoking—Women who smoke may go through menopause up to 2 years earlier than nonsmokers.

- Menstrual history—Women whose menstrual cycles were fewer than 26 days from ages 20 to 35 may experience menopause more than a year earlier than women with longer cycles.

It's also important to know that the age when you had your first period does not predict the timing of your last period. And *birth control* does not influence the timing of menopause. That said, some birth control methods can make periods lighter or stop them altogether. This can mask the signs and symptoms of *perimenopause*, making it more difficult to know where you are in the transition.

Perimenopause Comes First

There's a lot happening in your body before your final period. The run-up to that last period is called perimenopause. Typically, perimenopause starts in the late 40s, though it's possible for symptoms to start earlier. And perimenopause lasts several years. Four to 8 years is common, but some women are in perimenopause for a decade or more.

You will likely notice signs of your body adjusting. The signs may be subtle at first, like a period coming earlier or later than usual. Over time, and as your estrogen levels remain consistently low, you may notice other changes, including more obvious changes in period timing, and bleeding that is heavier or lighter than usual. You may also skip periods.

> **How do I know if my symptoms are "normal"?**
>
> It's typical for your first symptoms of perimenopause to be changes in menstrual bleeding. It's also typical for hot flashes to come next, followed by or along with other symptoms. As you get closer to your last period, all symptoms may be more obvious and bothersome. The most important thing is that you talk with your ob-gyn, especially about bleeding changes. Though these changes are often normal, your ob-gyn will want to be sure they aren't a sign of a medical problem.
>
> –DR. NANETTE SANTORO

Some women have only a few mild symptoms in perimenopause. Others have multiple symptoms that can be severe. It's important to understand what's normal to experience during this transition. Read Chapter 2, "Understanding Perimenopause," and Chapter 4, "Menopause Signs and Symptoms," to learn more.

Menopause on Your Mind

The menopause transition can bring up complex emotions. You may welcome the freedom: no more decisions about birth control, no more shopping for tampons. Or you may be sad that your childbearing years are ending. You may feel free *and* sad.

Your thoughts may go well beyond this, however. Your perspective on menopause may be tied to how you experience growing older: your shifting roles and responsibilities, your relationships and sexuality, your health and wellness, your career and interests, your family dynamics, your life goals. In other words, when you think about menopause, you're likely thinking about more than menopause.

You may also notice that the way you experience menopause is influenced by how menopause is talked about within your family or community. Perhaps, in your community, menopause is seen as just another hazard of getting older. Maybe menopause is associated with celebration and respect. Perhaps it barely gets a mention. You can read more about this in the box "How and Why Menopause Varies Across Cultures."

How and Why Menopause Varies Across Cultures

One interesting aspect of the menopause transition is how much it is influenced by cultural attitudes and practices—the ways in which ethnic and community experiences affect individual experiences.

One clue to this is the wide variation in the ways women talk about menopause. If menopause were simply about hormonal changes, women across the world would experience it the same way. Instead, studies in different countries and communities have found big differences in menopause experiences, including the timing and physical symptoms. For example, in the United States, hot flashes are the most frequently reported symptom among White, Hispanic, and Black women. Asian American women, though, are more likely to report backache, muscle stiffness, and joint pain than hot flashes.

Studies also reveal differences in attitudes based on racial background. Black women tend to have a more positive view of menopause and aging than White and Asian American women. Hispanic women tend to have positive attitudes as well, but for this group, menopause is more often seen as disruptive and associated with irritability and depression. But it's also important to note that each person's experience is different and may not align with the experiences of other people in their racial or ethnic group.

(continued)

How and Why Menopause Varies Across Cultures (continued)

We do not understand why menopause can feel so different for different groups. There are some reasons for this: People of color are not represented enough in studies on menopause. It's possible that women's descriptions of menopause reflect differences in language, education, and so on, even though their bodily changes are the same. Another possibility is that biology and culture interact in ways we don't yet understand.

We do know that around the world, the end of the childbearing years is linked to different attitudes and beliefs. These tie in with how communities think about aging, older women, and their place in society. Some of these attitudes and beliefs are positive. Some research suggests that in societies that celebrate wisdom and experience, menopausal symptoms may be less bothersome. In contrast, in societies where menopause is tied to disease and the decline of sexual interest, menopause symptoms may bring more distress.

What does this all mean for you? Community and family beliefs can transfer to you, affecting how you see yourself and how you feel in your body. These beliefs may influence how you feel about your own menopause and the decisions you make about it. Keep this in mind as you move through your transition and talk with your ob-gyn. Talking about how you want things to be can be a first step toward a better and healthier menopause experience.

Some of the things you may hear about menopause are uninformed and could use a fact check. This book is designed to talk about the facts and help move past stereotypes. But ultimately, there is no right or wrong way to feel about your menopause experience.

Your Hormones and Menopause

The same hormones that supported **menstruation** throughout your life now affect how and when you go through the menopause transition. During your reproductive years, your body relies heavily on two hormones: estrogen and **progesterone**. Throughout a typical menstrual cycle—one that's not controlled by hormonal birth control—the levels of these hormones rise and fall in a regular pattern. These hormonal shifts help control the release of eggs and prepare your **uterus** for a possible pregnancy. If no pregnancy occurs, these hormones help control your periods. The box "Hormones Explained: What Estrogen and Progesterone Do in the Body" has more details on these hormones.

During the menopause transition, your body no longer makes much estrogen and progesterone. The levels of these hormones decline. This decline can lead to the symptoms that come to mind when you think about menopause, like hot flashes, vaginal irritation or dryness, changes in your sex drive, sleep, or mood

> **Hormones Explained: What Estrogen and Progesterone Do in the Body**
>
> Up until the menopause transition, the hormones estrogen and progesterone are constant companions that help regulate your menstrual cycle. In women who are cycling naturally, each month these hormones signal your uterus to build up a blood-rich lining called the **endometrium**. Meanwhile, another hormone sends a signal to an egg, causing it to mature in a **follicle** in one of your ovaries.
>
> When an egg is ready, it is released from the follicle and moves through a **fallopian tube** and down to the uterus. If the egg is fertilized by **sperm**, a pregnancy may result. If it doesn't, the cycle starts all over again. It's a highly coordinated process that continues throughout the reproductive years.
>
> Estrogen and progesterone do other things, too. Estrogen helps keep the **vagina** lubricated and flexible. It's involved in the health of the heart, blood vessels, urinary tract, skin, pelvic muscles, brain, and more. Meanwhile, progesterone is essential for the body to be able to carry a pregnancy and allows regular menstrual cycles to occur. This is why the slow decline in these hormones over time affects so many parts of the body.

shifts. For some women, menopausal symptoms can be bothersome. You can find symptom details in Chapter 4, "Menopause Signs and Symptoms."

This book discusses many lifestyle changes and medical treatments that can support you through menopause. One of these is called **hormone therapy**. It's available in different forms, and many women feel better when they take medications containing estrogen and progesterone. For some women, it is a safe and valuable tool for managing the menopause transition. You can find information on hormone therapy in Chapter 17, "Hormone Therapies."

Still, hormone therapy is not right for everyone and should be discussed with your *obstetrician–gynecologist (ob-gyn)*. Whether to go on hormone therapy is an individual decision and depends in part on your health status and medical history. Fortunately, there are other effective ways that menopausal symptoms can be treated for those who don't want or cannot take hormone therapy. You can find information on nonhormonal treatments in Chapter 18, "Estrogen-Free Medical Therapies."

Sometimes Menopause Shows Up Much Earlier

You may have heard that some women have their last period much earlier than is typical. When the last period happens before 40, it's called ***premature menopause***. When it happens between 40 and 45, it's called early menopause.

The signs of premature or early menopause are like those of perimenopause when it happens at a more typical age. Periods may become irregular, with changes in vaginal bleeding. Hot flashes, sleep problems, vaginal changes, dry skin, difficulty concentrating, or mood shifts all may be part of the picture, too. Chapter 3, "Understanding Early and Premature Menopause," explains why menopause comes much sooner for some women and how to talk with your ob-gyn if you think it's happening to you.

> **Do I need to have testing of my hormone levels?**
>
> You probably don't need hormone testing. Your ob-gyn should be able to tell if you are in perimenopause based on your age, your symptoms, and any changes you have in your periods. But if you are younger than 45 and have changes in menstrual bleeding, you may be offered a blood test to check your hormone levels, and especially if you are younger than 40. Your ob-gyn can review the results to see if you are experiencing premature or early menopause.
>
> –DR. GLORIA RÍCHARD-DAVIS

If your menopause is premature or early, there's a chance you may have more severe symptoms than average. You may feel greater sadness about losing your fertility. Be alert for signs of **depression** and anxiety, especially if you've had them before. In addition, because you face more years without exposure to natural estrogen, your risk of serious medical problems may be higher than average if you don't take hormone therapy. These risks can be managed with the help of your ob-gyn.

Your Healthy Lifestyle in Menopause and Beyond

During and after the menopause transition, some health conditions become more important. For example, the hormones produced by the ovaries before menopause protect against heart disease and other serious illnesses. After menopause, and with further aging, much of this protection is lost. Midlife is also the time when other risk factors for chronic disease become more common—such as high **cholesterol** and **high blood pressure**. This is why managing your risk for heart attack, **stroke**, bone loss, and dementia is so important now and going forward. You can read more on some of these conditions in Chapter 15, "Bone Health," and Chapter 19, "Heart Disease and Diabetes."

Other things are also important to watch for during perimenopause and after your last period, including changes in mental health. Plus, this is the time in life when eating a balanced diet and getting enough exercise can help set you up for good health in your later years. You'll find chapters on these topics in this book.

Another aspect of staying healthy is your annual checkup with your ob-gyn. It's important to continue your annual visits through and beyond the menopause transition. Your ob-gyn can help you keep track of when to have screenings for *cervical cancer* and breast cancer and can refer you for colon cancer screenings. They can also help identify whether you are at risk for anxiety or depression, *diabetes*, heart disease, or *osteoporosis*. And they can help you keep track of *vaccines* or booster shots you may need over the years. Chapter 21, "Screenings and Vaccinations After Menopause," addresses all of these topics.

Navigating Menopause: Your Best Resources

Understanding what's happening in your body, and having a resource for accurate health information, are especially important now. Think of this book as your guide to the menopause transition and one of your best resources. It was developed by ob-gyns, doctors who are dedicated to helping women thrive throughout their lives, including during the menopause transition and well beyond.

Everything you read here is based on scientific research and the most up-to-date medical practice. This book will be straight with you about what is known about menopause and explain

- what's going on in your body and why
- what's normal for menopause and how to be alert to possible signs of disease
- what types of self-care and medications may make the biggest difference
- what menopause means for your health—now and in the future—and how to maintain and improve your health and quality of life
- how to work with your ob-gyn and other health care professionals and find care that works for you

That last point brings us to your other best resource: your own ob-gyn. In Chapter 5, "Choosing Your Menopause Care Team," we'll cover why ob-gyns are well qualified to support you through menopause and how to find an ob-gyn if you don't have one already. We'll also talk about how you can be an active decision-maker in your medical care. Your care should be a collaborative effort that leads to better health and well-being. You and your ob-gyn should make decisions together. And remember, no matter where you are in your menopause transition, it's possible to navigate this change with confidence.

RESOURCES

Menopause
womenshealth.gov/menopause
Website from the Office on Women's Health with information on menopause symptoms, treatments, premature and early menopause, overall health, and sexuality.

Menopause Education for Patients
menopause.org/patient-education

Website from The Menopause Society with frequently asked questions, videos, a glossary, and other resources.

Menopause Preparedness Toolkit: A Woman's Empowerment Guide
swhr.org/swhr_resource/menopause-preparedness-toolkit-a-womans-empowerment-guide/

Resource from the Society for Women's Health Research that discusses different experiences of menopause around the world, stigma around menopause, navigating health insurance and medical care, and wellness tips.

My Menopause
acog.org/MyMenopause

Web resource from ACOG with information on the menopause transition, signs and symptoms, treatments, and self-care. Includes the latest information from the experts in ob-gyn care, menopause stories from real women, expert columns on how to manage symptoms, Q&A articles, videos, and more.

CHAPTER 2

Understanding Perimenopause

Lisa's menopause experience was very different from her mother's. "In her late 40s, my mom just stopped having periods," she says. "That was it. No symptoms." Lisa thought that her transition to menopause would be as easy, but in her early 50s, her periods and sleep changed. She started feeling depressed and got hot flashes. "Then my period stopped for about 7 months, and I thought, 'Yes! This is coming to an end!' Unfortunately, since then, I am still getting periods and I've had a year and a half of just plain discomfort." Lisa talked with her ob-gyn to confirm perimenopause and says she'll take things as they come. "I'm going to ride this wave and keep discussing with my ob-gyn. Everybody has their own menopause path."

P erimenopause is the body's passage from regular *menstrual periods* to your final period. It's the first part of your *menopause transition*. Typically, perimenopause starts in the 40s, though it's possible for symptoms to start earlier. And perimenopause lasts several years. Four to 8 years is common, but some women are in this phase of life for a decade or more.

Some women do not experience any symptoms or have only a few mild symptoms. Others have multiple symptoms that can be severe. Each woman experiences menopause differently. It's important to understand what symptoms are typical during perimenopause.

Staying connected to yourself and alert to changes in your body and emotions is key. Remember that perimenopause is natural—and a reminder to live healthfully and look forward. If you're not feeling ready to embrace it right now, that's OK. But it's still good to learn about what may be ahead.

Tracking the Early Signs

For those who still have a *uterus*, the first thing that happens in perimenopause is a change in menstrual periods. A change can mean different things for different women.

At first the changes may be subtle, like a shorter cycle or fewer days of bleeding. As perimenopause goes on, the period flow may be lighter or heavier, or you may have spotting instead of a period. Later in perimenopause, you may skip a period one month and have a normal period the next month. This is all related to the decline in ovarian *follicles*, where *eggs* grow and mature, and the variations in *estrogen* and *progesterone* that come with it.

Although changes in menstrual bleeding are normal during this time, some bleeding changes may signal a problem. This is why you should talk with your *obstetrician–gynecologist (ob-gyn)* about any bleeding that is different from what you're used to. It's a good idea to keep a diary and track your period and any other symptoms you notice during your days of bleeding. You can use anything to track your bleeding change—a phone app, a notebook, the Abnormal Bleeding Diary at the ACOG website (see the Resources section). You and your ob-gyn will have an easier discussion if you keep a record and can talk about details at your office visit.

> **How can I talk with my ob-gyn about what I'm experiencing?**
>
> First, remember that every detail you share helps your ob-gyn understand what you're going through. Second, plan what you want to talk about. Write down in advance the concerns and questions you have. Third, know that your ob-gyn has had many conversations with women about all aspects of menopause. It's unlikely that anything you share will surprise them. And finally, you can open the door to any topic by simply saying, "Can we talk about something that's bothering me?" When you open up to your ob-gyn, they can provide the best possible care.
>
> –DR. MARY ROSSER

Early in perimenopause you may also start to have *hot flashes*, rushes of heat that have you fanning yourself with whatever's at hand. Night sweats are nighttime hot flashes and may interrupt your sleep. You may find your mood shifting, sometimes with symptoms like sadness or irritability, which can be worse with lack of sleep. Irritation of the *vagina* and *vulva* are also typical around this time. Remember that most women have only some of these symptoms, and symptoms can be mild, moderate, or severe. You can read more in Chapter 4, "Menopause Signs and Symptoms."

Many changes during these years are normal and mild. If they rarely bother you, they probably won't require action. Some changes are normal but uncomfortable, and they may even interfere with your daily functioning. These can be addressed in different ways. And other changes may be a sign of a medical condition that needs attention. Later in this chapter we'll cover how to work with your ob-gyn during perimenopause and ensure you get the right care for you.

When Bleeding Changes Raise a Red Flag

Many women know what's usual for them when it comes to monthly bleeding, and they'll likely know when things don't seem right. All bleeding changes are called *abnormal uterine bleeding*, but sometimes the changes can be more than just shorter cycles or skipped periods. Some changes in bleeding can be unsettling and affect your quality of life, including

- bleeding that soaks through one or more tampons or pads every hour, or is so heavy you have to double up on pads
- bleeding that lasts more than 7 days
- flooding or gushing when you stand up
- passing blood clots the size of a quarter or larger
- menstrual cycles that are longer than 35 days or shorter than 21 days
- irregular periods in which cycle length varies by more than 7 to 9 days
- bleeding or spotting after *sexual intercourse*

This type of bleeding can be frightening. It's important to see your ob-gyn if you have this type of bleeding for two cycles or more. Together you can make a plan to learn why it's happening and discuss treatment, if needed.

If abnormal bleeding happens often for at least 6 months, it is a chronic condition. Certain medical conditions can cause abnormal bleeding. You can find more details on irregular bleeding, causes, and treatments in Chapter 7, "Abnormal Bleeding."

Sudden, unusual episodes of abnormal bleeding can also happen in perimenopause. This is called acute abnormal uterine bleeding. If you are changing pads or tampons every hour for more than 2 hours in a row, and you also have chest pain, have shortness of breath, and are lightheaded or dizzy, seek emergency medical care right away.

Other Symptoms of Perimenopause

As you learn more about perimenopause, you'll notice that the symptoms may overlap with and influence each other. Night sweats can disrupt your sleep. Poor sleep can drag down your mood. A low mood can make you more likely to experience hot flashes, night sweats, and poor sleep. This cycle can be frustrating and impact your quality of life.

On the other hand, it's a reminder that the body and mind are intertwined. In this context, doing what you can to take care of yourself is all the more important. Easing a particular symptom may have ripple effects that help you feel better in other ways, too. For example, if you experience vaginal dryness and treat it, you'll likely find sex more pleasurable, with potential benefits for your mood, sleep, and relationship.

In Part II of this book, we'll explore the following symptoms in more detail. In Part III, we'll cover ways to manage and treat them.

Hot Flashes

Also called hot flushes, hot flashes are perhaps the best-known symptom of menopause. Hot flashes are sudden feelings of heat in the face, neck, and chest lasting up to 5 minutes. They can cause sweats, chills, clamminess, or anxiety. When these flashes happen at night, they're called night sweats.

The experience of hot flashes and night sweats varies. If you get hot flashes in perimenopause, you may notice them before you start skipping periods or around the same time. They may be mild or intense and happen daily or a few times a day. Hot flashes may interfere with your sleep, and for some, they may go on from several months to several years. In a large U.S. study, about 2 in 5 women in early perimenopause reported hot flashes. Some women continue to have hot flashes for years after their final period, although for most they subside or go away completely.

We don't fully understand why women in the menopause transition have such varied experiences of hot flashes. Some women are more likely than others to get them. We know that hot flashes may be related to your race and ethnicity, certain life experiences, emotional health, whether you smoke, and whether you have *obesity*, among other factors. Any time you feel the heat rising, remember that you have options for managing and treating this symptom. Read Chapter 6, "Hot Flashes and Night Sweats," for more discussion.

Sleep Changes

For some women, sleep problems begin or become more disruptive in early perimenopause and are worst during late perimenopause. One third to one half of women have more trouble sleeping as they move through perimenopause. Some women report trouble falling asleep or trouble staying asleep (*insomnia*). They wake up during the night or wake earlier than usual.

This sleep disruption is often related to night sweats. You might find yourself throwing off the covers or changing into fresh pajamas. More severe hot flashes are linked to insomnia. Your sleep may also be disrupted by other symptoms of perimenopause, like urinating more often than usual at night.

Other health conditions that affect sleep can become more common in midlife. These include anxiety, *depression*, or other mood disorders. More women are diagnosed with *obstructive sleep apnea* during these years, a condition that causes brief pauses in breathing during sleep. Chronic health conditions, such as arthritis and *metabolic syndrome*, may also affect sleep quality. So can some medications. It's important to talk with a doctor so your symptoms can be evaluated. Sleep disruption during the menopause transition is probably not directly linked to *hormone* levels. But it is linked to night sweats, which are influenced by hormones.

> **I'm anxious about so many things changing in my body at once. How can I manage?**
>
> It's natural to feel anxious about what you're feeling. Sometimes just knowing that your symptoms are typical of this stage of life can be calming. Your ob-gyn can help with this, especially if you keep track of your symptoms and talk about them at an office visit. But if you feel your anxiety getting worse over time, or the anxiety comes with worry that is hard to control, make an appointment to talk with your ob-gyn. These symptoms can be a sign of an anxiety disorder, which can be treated.
>
> —DR. ESTHER EISENBERG

Not getting enough sleep, or not getting good-quality sleep, can make everything feel harder. That includes coping with change—and your perimenopause is change. Getting better sleep can make a huge difference in how you feel physically and emotionally. If you're struggling with sleep, lifestyle changes can help. Medication may be an option, too. Reach out to your ob-gyn for support. Read Chapter 9, "Sleep Problems," for more discussion.

Vaginal and Vulvar Changes

During and after the menopause transition, many women notice changes to their vagina and vulva. Surveys suggest that more than 35 percent of women report vaginal and vulvar changes. The vulva and vagina can start to feel dry, irritated, and itchy. A burning feeling is also common. Vaginal infections can occur more often.

These symptoms are caused by hormonal changes in the body. As your estrogen level declines, the tissues in your genital area can become thinner, less flexible, and more easily injured. Your vagina starts to lose the interior ridges that allowed it to stretch, and its natural lubrication may decrease. These changes can lead to general discomfort or pain during sex.

But perimenopause does not have to define your sexual health. Plenty of women find that their desire, arousal, sexual activity, and physical and emotional satisfaction remain steady. That's because hormones appear to be less important in this regard than your previous level of sexual activity, your feelings for your partner, and your emotional well-being.

Treatments are available if vaginal or vulvar symptoms affect your physical comfort and quality of life. This is especially valuable because vaginal and vulvar symptoms may not improve when you are *postmenopausal*. Read Chapter 11, "Vaginal and Vulvar Conditions," for a discussion of things that may help, including over-the-counter products and prescription medications.

Urinary Changes

During perimenopause, many women notice they need to urinate more frequently. They may leak urine, especially when coughing, sneezing, or lifting heavy objects. They may also get *urinary tract infections (UTIs)*. That's when the urge to urinate comes with a burning or stinging sensation and perhaps fever or nausea.

As your estrogen level declines, the *urethra*—the tube through which urine leaves the *bladder*—can become dry, inflamed, or irritated. In addition, your *pelvic floor* may lose strength. This is the set of muscles and connective tissues that support your bladder, uterus, vagina, and *bowels*. These bodily changes may mean you need to urinate more frequently. You may experience urine leakage (*urinary incontinence*).

Urinary symptoms can interfere with your daily life. You may feel self-conscious or start avoiding certain activities. If you have urinary symptoms, you do not need to suffer in silence. Make an appointment with your ob-gyn to talk about treatment options. Together you may discuss some of the treatments found in Chapter 12, "Urinary Incontinence."

Mood and Memory Changes

Feeling anxious, down, or forgetful like never before can also be related to perimenopause. Commonly, women experience mood changes that can feel like *premenstrual syndrome (PMS)*. You might be low on energy, distracted, irritable, or tearful. This can happen even at times that do not seem to be related to the menstrual cycle (in whatever form it's currently taking).

Depressive symptoms are common during perimenopause and reported by 1 in 4 women. Symptoms include crying more than usual, feeling empty, or losing interest in activities that used to feel good. In women who were anxious before perimenopause, anxiety tends to continue. Anxiety can make muscles tense or cause nausea or sweating. Some women may also have trouble retaining information or focusing—a symptom sometimes described as "brain fog."

The connection between your menopause status, mood, and memory is complex. Declining estrogen levels seem to directly affect mood and memory. Reduced "working memory" is the most common issue noted by perimenopausal women, and, in many cases, it improves once the menopause transition is over. Other menopausal symptoms do, too, like those hot flashes or visits to the bathroom that disrupt sleep. Any disruption in sleep can raise the risk of depression and foggy thinking.

Mood changes can be worse when you are managing other concerns in midlife—a demanding job, financial pressure, communication with a partner, health concerns, or family care, whether that's aging parents or children. Any midlife challenges can make it harder to take care of yourself. But without care, the struggles can weigh heavier. If you've had problems with depression or anxiety before, be on guard for signs of mood changes during your run-up to menopause. If symptoms last for more than 2 weeks, make an appointment with your ob-gyn. Chapter 8, "Mood and Memory," walks through how to talk about what you're feeling.

Other Causes of Abnormal Bleeding

In Chapter 1, we talked about abnormal menstrual bleeding and seeing your ob-gyn when you notice changes in your monthly cycle. Tracking your periods and symptoms will help you with the conversation. You'll want to tell your ob-gyn if your bleeding is light, medium, or heavy and how long your cycles are. If your symptoms aren't typical for perimenopause, your ob-gyn may recommend testing for other conditions.

Pregnancy

If you are sexually active and haven't had a period in a few months, it's worth taking a pregnancy test. The chances of pregnancy decline as you get older, but it's possible to get pregnant during perimenopause if you aren't using **birth control**. If an at-home pregnancy test is positive, make an appointment with your ob-gyn.

Birth Control

Some forms of birth control can affect bleeding patterns. For example, with the copper ***intrauterine device (IUD)***, bleeding may increase at first and periods may be more painful. Hormonal IUDs may cause frequent spotting, more days of bleeding, and heavier bleeding in the first few months of use. Sometimes the hormonal IUD causes bleeding to stop completely.

Using birth control pills or the ***vaginal ring*** with no breaks can stop menstrual periods entirely, but sometimes it can cause breakthrough bleeding. If you recently started a new form of birth control, talk with your ob-gyn about any bleeding changes.

Uterine Conditions

Several conditions of the uterus can cause abnormal bleeding during perimenopause. Some of these conditions are not usually dangerous, but they may cause discomfort or pain in addition to bleeding changes. You can read more about these conditions in Chapter 7, "Abnormal Bleeding."

- *Polyps*—These growths arise from the inside of the uterus or the ***cervix***. They can cause irregular or heavy menstrual bleeding. Polyps on the cervix may cause bleeding after sex. Polyps almost always are ***benign*** (not cancer), but some can become cancerous over time. This is rare.

- *Fibroids*—These growths develop from the muscle tissue of the uterus. They can cause longer, more frequent, or heavy menstrual bleeding, more pain during periods, and bleeding between periods. Fibroids do not cause cancer, and only very rarely are fibroid-like growths found to be cancerous.

- *Adenomyosis*—In this condition, the *endometrium*—the tissue that lines the uterus—grows into the muscle wall of the uterus. This can cause heavy menstrual bleeding, back pain with periods, and menstrual pain that gets worse with age.

- *Endometriosis*—In this condition, the type of tissue that forms the lining of the uterus is also found in other parts of the *pelvis*. When hormones change, this tissue breaks down and bleeds, the same way the lining of the uterus breaks down and bleeds during a period. Endometriosis causes pain in addition to heavy menstrual bleeding. It is most often diagnosed in women in their 30s and 40s.

- Endometrial atrophy—In this condition, low estrogen causes the uterine lining to become too thin. As the lining thins, a woman may have abnormal bleeding. It happens most often in postmenopausal women, but sometimes women in perimenopause develop endometrial atrophy.

- *Endometrial hyperplasia*—In this condition, the lining of the uterus grows and gets too thick. In some cases, it can lead to cancer. It is most often caused when a woman has too much estrogen and not enough progesterone. Endometrial hyperplasia, if left untreated, may progress in some cases to *endometrial cancer*. Early treatment may reduce the risk of endometrial cancer.

- Endometrial cancer—This type of cancer begins in the lining of the uterus. It is sometimes called uterine cancer. This is the most common type of cancer of the female reproductive system. Most cases occur in women in their 60s, but it can happen at an earlier age. Bleeding is the most common sign. When diagnosed early, most cases can be treated successfully.

Bleeding Disorders

Heavy or irregular periods are sometimes a symptom of a bleeding disorder. A bleeding disorder means your blood may not be clotting properly. Problems with certain proteins in the blood, called clotting factors, or small cells in the blood, called platelets, can lead to a bleeding disorder.

While many people are born with bleeding disorders, others can develop them later in life. Make an appointment with your ob-gyn if you have any of the abnormal bleeding signs listed earlier in this chapter. The treatment for bleeding disorders depends on the type. Some medications work by replacing the clotting factor in the blood. Birth control pills can often help reduce heavy menstrual bleeding.

Medications

Some medications can cause or worsen heavy menstrual bleeding. Talk with your ob-gyn if you have heavy bleeding and use

- aspirin, warfarin, heparin, and other medicines used to prevent blood clots
- *nonsteroidal anti-inflammatory drugs (NSAIDs)*, such as ibuprofen and naproxen
- certain supplements, such as vitamin E, fish oil, ginkgo, ginseng, and motherwort

Conditions That Cause Bleeding to Stop

In perimenopause, the absence of periods may be a sign of a medical condition that's not related to hormonal shifts. If you do not have a period for 3 months or longer and are not pregnant, contact your ob-gyn. Some reasons periods can stop besides menopause include

- rapid weight loss or being underweight
- eating disorders
- chronic stress
- problems with the *pituitary gland* or *thyroid gland*
- *polycystic ovary syndrome (PCOS)*
- *primary ovarian insufficiency (POI)*
- other chronic medical conditions, such as *kidney* failure or *inflammatory bowel disease (IBD)*

Talking With Your Ob-Gyn

Whether you're dealing with menstrual changes or any other symptoms of perimenopause, talk with your ob-gyn. During an office visit, your ob-gyn may review your medical history and any medications you take. If bleeding is your main concern, your ob-gyn may do a *pelvic exam* or *ultrasound exam* or recommend tests to find out the cause of bleeding problems. If other symptoms are bothering you, together you can talk about lifestyle changes, over-the-counter products, or prescription medications that may help. Your office visit is a time to advocate for yourself and work with your ob-gyn to understand and find solutions. You can read more about working together in Chapter 5, "Choosing Your Menopause Care Team."

RESOURCES

Abnormal Bleeding Diary
acog.org/AbnormalBleeding

Online, printable form from ACOG that you can use to record bleeding changes and share with your ob-gyn.

Abnormal Uterine Bleeding
medlineplus.gov/ency/article/000903.htm

Article from the National Library of Medicine on causes, testing, and treatments for abnormal menstrual bleeding.

Get Your Well-Woman Visit Every Year
health.gov/myhealthfinder/healthy-living/sexual-health/get-your-well-woman-visit-every-year

A website from the Office of Disease Prevention and Health Promotion that covers what to expect at an annual doctor's visit, including the physical exam, health goals, family health history, screenings, and tips on staying healthy.

Women and Bleeding Disorders
bleeding.org/bleeding-disorders-a-z/overview/women-and-bleeding-disorders

Information on bleeding disorders from the National Bleeding Disorders Foundation.

My Menopause
acog.org/MyMenopause

Web resource from ACOG with information on the menopause transition, signs and symptoms, treatments, and self-care. Includes the latest information from the experts in ob-gyn care, menopause stories from real women, expert columns on how to manage symptoms, Q&A articles, videos, and more.

CHAPTER 3

Understanding Early and Premature Menopause

At 33, Leah was a mother of a 5-year-old and trying to control an autoimmune condition. Part of her treatment included high-dose chemotherapy. Several weeks later, Leah started experiencing intense hot flashes, sleep problems, and other symptoms—the beginning of premature menopause. Her gynecologic care provider prescribed low-dose birth control pills to help manage her symptoms and reduce her future risk of heart disease, stroke, and bone loss. She tried different types of pills and is still trying to figure out the best dose to manage her hot flashes. Leah has also come to terms with the early end to her childbearing years. "It's important to know that it's OK to struggle with losing your fertility," she says. "I'm fortunate that I have an incredible son."

Some women experience *menopause* sooner than expected, having their last period before age 45, and sometimes even earlier. When the last period happens before 40, it's called *premature menopause*. When the last period happens between 40 and 45, it's called early menopause. Like natural menopause that typically happens after a woman reaches her 50s, premature and early menopause put an end to a woman's ability to get pregnant naturally. (Note, though, that *egg* donation could help a woman get pregnant after premature or early menopause.) Another condition, *primary ovarian insufficiency (POI)*, can look like premature or early menopause, but it is not true menopause. You can read more about POI later in the chapter.

The symptoms of premature and early menopause are similar to those of natural menopause. They include changes in *menstrual periods*, *hot flashes*, night sweats, and more. If you are experiencing any of these things earlier than you expected, talk with your *obstetrician–gynecologist (ob-gyn)*. If you are diagnosed with premature or early menopause, it's important to understand what it means for your long-term health and how treatment might help.

Causes of Premature and Early Menopause

Part of the frustration around premature and early menopause is that the cause is often unknown. That said, we do know some of the factors that contribute to earlier onset of menopause. These factors may be linked to *genes*, behavior, the environment, or certain diseases.

Family History and Genetics

The timing of your menopause is partly determined by your genes. If your mother or grandmother experienced early menopause, your likelihood of early menopause is five to six times higher than someone whose relatives did not. (Similarly, if your mother or grandmother had a late natural menopause, you may, too.)

It's possible that genetic factors affect menopause timing, especially when menopause comes earlier than is typical. In the future, gene testing may be able to predict the chance of premature or early menopause. This could help women make decisions about when to try to get pregnant or when to freeze their eggs. That said, genes explain only part of the timing of menopause.

Smoking

Cigarette smoking is the behavior that most clearly affects the timing of the last period. Cigarette smoke is known to affect the levels of reproductive *hormones*. It may directly speed up aging of the *ovaries*. Research also shows that the more women smoke, the higher their chance of early menopause. Here are some details from one U.S. study:

- Current heavy smokers—Women who currently smoked heavily were almost twice as likely as nonsmokers to experience early menopause. In some cases, menopause occurred before 40. These women had smoked a pack a day for 20 or more years.

- Former heavy smokers—Women who had previously smoked heavily and then quit also had a higher-than-average risk of early menopause. These women had smoked a pack a day for 10 years. Those who quit smoking in their 30s had a lower risk of early menopause than those who smoked into their 40s.

- Former light smokers—Women who had smoked lightly in the past—meaning, smoked fewer than five cigarettes a day and quit by age 35—did not have a greater risk of early menopause.

Chemical Exposure

Certain chemicals found in everyday life can block or interfere with hormone activity. They are called endocrine-disrupting chemicals (EDCs). EDCs can be found almost everywhere but especially in plastics, pesticides, flame retardants, and many more everyday products. Some of these chemicals are no longer in production but remain in the environment.

Some EDCs build up in the body and are linked to reproductive health disorders, including ovarian problems and premature or early menopause. In a large U.S. study, women with high concentrations of EDCs in their blood or urine had their last period 2 to 4 years earlier than those with low concentrations.

Diabetes

Diabetes is a disease in which the body does not make enough *insulin* or does not use it as it should. Insulin is a hormone that helps balance the amount of *glucose* in your blood. Normally, your body changes most of the food you eat into glucose, the body's main source of energy. Glucose is then carried to the body's cells with the help of insulin.

If your body does not make enough insulin, or the insulin does not work as it should, glucose cannot be used by the body's cells. Instead, it stays and builds up in the blood. This makes your blood glucose level too high, which happens with diabetes. Some evidence suggests that women diagnosed with diabetes in their 30s may experience earlier menopause. More research is needed to understand how diabetes affects ovarian aging.

Chronic Fatigue Syndrome

As many as 2.5 million Americans may have *chronic fatigue syndrome (CFS)*, though most have not been diagnosed. This condition is best known for causing profound fatigue that does not improve with rest. It also comes with memory problems, difficulty concentrating, pain, and reproductive health issues.

Women are 2 to 4 times as likely as men to develop CFS. Reproductive symptoms may include abnormal periods, pelvic pain not necessarily linked to periods, *endometriosis*, *cysts* on the ovaries, uterine *fibroids*, and early menopause.

This syndrome may be triggered by an infection. Some research also suggests CFS is more common in women who have had *hysterectomies*, especially if the surgery happened at a younger age. In some women, CFS may be linked to declining levels of *estrogen* and *progesterone*.

Fibromyalgia

This condition is similar to CFS. It causes pain, fatigue, sleep difficulties, and joint and muscle stiffness. It affects about 4 million Americans, and the vast majority are women. Fibromyalgia is also linked to early menopause and hysterectomy. In addition, fibromyalgia symptoms may get worse during the *menopause transition*. The condition may be caused by infection or by physical or emotional trauma.

Human Immunodeficiency Virus

Human immunodeficiency virus (HIV) is the virus that causes *acquired immunodeficiency syndrome (AIDS)*. Once HIV is in the body, it attacks the *immune system*. As the immune system weakens, it is less able to fight disease and serious infections. These include **pneumonia**, **tuberculosis**, certain types of cancer, and other life-threatening infections.

Among women with HIV, the last period occurs about 5 years earlier than in women without HIV. The reasons are not clear, but changes in periods and hormones are common among women with HIV. If you have HIV, your periods can stop even when your levels of reproductive hormones are normal. It's possible, then, that "early menopause" in HIV may not be true menopause. In any case, the prolonged absence of periods places women with HIV at similar risk of heart disease and *bone loss* as those who experience early menopause.

Mumps

Mumps is an illness caused by a virus. One sign is swelling of the saliva glands on either side of the face. The illness is not common in the United States, thanks to a *vaccine* that's usually given in childhood. But sometimes there are outbreaks, and it can spread easily among people who have not had the vaccine.

In rare cases, mumps can cause swelling of the ovaries. This is called mumps oophoritis. This can disturb ovarian function and affect *fertility*. Some cases of premature or early menopause have been linked to mumps.

Causes of Medical and Surgical Menopause

For some women, certain medical and surgical treatments may cause early menopause. These treatments can stop the ovaries from working before menopause would normally happen.

Chemotherapy and Radiation

Chemotherapy uses medications that stop the growth of cancer cells. **Radiation therapy** uses high-energy radiation to kill cancer cells. Both therapies can also damage normal cells in the body. Sometimes, chemotherapy or radiation therapy can cause a loss of ovarian function. This loss may be temporary or permanent.

If you have either of these therapies, their effects on your reproductive health may depend on

- the type of chemotherapy you receive
- the age at which you have chemotherapy
- the strength and number of doses of chemotherapy or radiation you receive
- which part of your body is treated with radiation—radiation to your **pelvis**, spine, whole body, or whole brain can raise the risk of ovarian damage

- whether you first have a procedure to temporarily relocate the ovaries outside the field of radiation before radiation therapy to the pelvis
- whether you have one or both treatments—having both chemotherapy and radiation therapy raises the risk of reducing ovarian function

For some women undergoing chemotherapy and radiation, *ovulation* and periods stop and then restart later. The younger an adult you are, the more likely it is that your ovarian function and periods will go back to normal. But *infertility* can be an issue for those who had radiation to the pelvis before *puberty*.

Cancer Medications

Some types of breast cancer can be treated with medication that reduces or block hormones. This can slow the growth of cancer cells. Using these medications before natural menopause can trigger an earlier menopause.

Common breast cancer medications include *tamoxifen*, which attaches to estrogen receptors in a tumor. This blocks estrogen from getting into the tumor and consequently can block tumor cells from growing. Tamoxifen may also be used to prevent breast cancer in women who are at high risk. Another type of medication, *aromatase inhibitors*, lowers levels of estrogen in the body. These medications and others can cause menopausal symptoms in some women.

> **I'm under 40 and starting cancer treatment soon. How do I know if egg freezing is right for me?**
>
> Great question. Cancer treatment can affect future fertility for women still in their childbearing years. If you know you want to have a child or more children in the future, talk with an ob-gyn who specializes in reproductive endocrinology and infertility (REI) before you start treatment. You'll learn about the potential risks of the medications used to stimulate ovulation and the surgical procedure to retrieve the eggs. It's also important to know that there's no guarantee frozen eggs will produce a healthy, full-term baby. These questions can be explored with an REI specialist.
>
> –DR. ESTHER EISENBERG

Surgery to Remove the Ovaries

If you have surgery to remove your ovaries, ovulation and periods will stop. If only one ovary is removed, ovulation and periods may continue, but the last period may happen 1 to 2 years earlier than it otherwise would have. Taking out the ovaries may be recommended for some medical conditions, including

- abscess in the *fallopian tube* and ovary
- *benign* growths or cysts
- endometriosis
- *ovarian cancer* (or prevention of ovarian cancer in women at high risk)
- ovarian torsion (a twisted ovary)
- *pelvic inflammatory disease*

When the ovaries are removed, ovarian hormone production stops and the protective effects of estrogen are lost, which raises the risk of serious health conditions. Women who have had this surgery may experience more sudden and severe menopausal symptoms. For these reasons, they are likely to need long-term *hormone therapy*. You can read about this therapy in Chapter 17, "Hormone Therapies."

Surgery to Remove the Uterus

If you have surgery to remove the *uterus* but your ovaries remain, your menopause transition will not start right away. But it may happen earlier than if you still had your uterus.

Surgery to remove all or part of the uterus is called hysterectomy. Depending on the reason for the surgery, the *cervix*, ovaries, fallopian tubes, and upper part of the *vagina* could be removed, too. Hysterectomy is the second most common surgery in U.S. women, after *cesarean birth*. Removal of the uterus may be recommended for some medical conditions, including

- *adenomyosis* (when the tissue lining the uterus grows into the muscle wall)
- cancer (or precancer) of the uterus, cervix, ovary, or *endometrium* (lining of the uterus)
- endometriosis
- uterine fibroids
- *uterine prolapse* (when the uterus slips into the vagina)

Research has shown that hysterectomies are more common among Black women than White women. There's a higher rate of hysterectomy in Southern states compared with Midwestern states and among those who smoke, are older, and have a higher weight. Hispanic women and those living in the Northeast are less likely to have hysterectomies. All of these data point to a need for better research into the health and environmental factors that affect the timing of menopause.

What Premature and Early Menopause Mean for Fertility

These days, many people choose to delay starting a family until careers and life partnerships are established, often in the 30s or even 40s. By that time, fertility is already declining. The chances of getting pregnant decline gradually from around 30 and more quickly from 40. For women at high risk of early menopause, fertility is likely to decline sooner, and pregnancy may require fertility treatment or may not be possible.

Currently, there are no reliable methods for predicting age at menopause—at least, not in time to help plan a family. If you notice early symptoms of menopause and want to get pregnant, talk with your ob-gyn right away. (Read Chapter 4, "Menopause Signs and Symptoms.") Tests can help learn if the changes are early menopause and if pregnancy is still possible. This includes testing of the levels of *anti-müllerian hormone (AMH)* and *follicle-stimulating hormone (FSH)*.

If AMH and FSH levels indicate that menopause may come early, there may still be ways to get pregnant. One option is *in vitro fertilization (IVF)* with donor eggs. With this option, your male partner's *sperm* would be used to fertilize eggs donated from another woman. A resulting embryo would be transferred to your uterus after you have taken hormones to help your body prepare for a pregnancy.

A procedure called *oocyte cryopreservation*—"freezing your eggs"—may be used to retrieve and store your eggs. This may be recommended for women who will be having cancer treatment or who want to delay childbearing until later in life. Several eggs are removed from the ovaries and frozen. Later, when the timing is right for you, the unfertilized eggs are thawed and used in IVF. The procedure requires that a woman take hormonal medications to stimulate the ovaries to make many eggs at one time. There's a time commitment, and egg freezing may be expensive. Some states have mandated coverage by insurance when there is a cancer diagnosis. Check with your insurance and state laws to be sure.

Other Concerns When Menopause Comes Too Soon

In addition to fertility concerns, there are health problems that come with premature or early menopause. These include more severe symptoms overall, including worse hot flashes, sleep problems, and other issues than you would have at the average age of menopause. This is especially true with menopause that's caused by a medical treatment, which can cause sudden, difficult symptoms.

There are also long-term health risks. With premature or early menopause, you lose the protective effects of your reproductive hormones sooner. Going forward, you face a higher risk of bone loss, *depression*, heart disease, *stroke*, diabetes, and death from other causes.

Treatments can improve your health and quality of life. Your ob-gyn will work with you to manage the symptoms and health risks. The good news—yes, there is some—is that premature and early menopause may lower the risk of some hormone-dependent cancers.

It's also important to know that a diagnosis of premature or early menopause can bring on sadness, grief, and a sense of feeling all alone. Talking with a counselor can help manage the emotions and decisions that can come with a life-changing diagnosis.

Treatment for Premature and Early Menopause

The treatment for premature or early menopause often involves hormone therapy or combined hormonal *birth control* methods. These treatments can help manage your risk of heart disease, stroke, and bone loss.

Hormone-based medication can also help relieve symptoms related to low estrogen levels, like vaginal dryness and urinary changes. Treatments without hormones can help relieve certain symptoms, too. In Part III of this book, we'll discuss treatments for menopausal symptoms in more detail. In Part IV, we'll talk about staying healthy through the menopause transition and beyond.

Talk with your ob-gyn about what treatment may work best for you based on your symptoms and your personal and family medical history. If you decide to take hormone therapy, you and your ob-gyn should talk every year about whether to continue it. Each year, this decision will depend on your symptoms, risks, and benefits. For women with premature or early menopause, treatment should continue until at least 51, the average age of the final period. Some women may need longer therapy if their symptoms go on for a long time.

> **Do I really need to take hormone therapy if I have early menopause?**
>
> Usually. In some cases, women with early menopause may be at risk of loss of bone density or other health problems. The risks and benefits of hormone therapy depend on many factors. Together you and your ob-gyn can talk about your health history, family history, and ongoing health needs.
>
> –DR. CARRIE ANN TERRELL

What Happens in Primary Ovarian Insufficiency

Primary ovarian insufficiency is not menopause, but it can cause symptoms similar to those of menopause in women younger than 40, and sometimes even in teens. With POI, ovarian function and hormone levels are severely disrupted. The ovarian *follicles*, where the eggs grow and mature, do not work properly. Typically, estrogen levels are lower than normal, and periods come less often or stop altogether. Genetics and *autoimmune disorders* may cause POI, but more research is needed to understand the condition.

Women with POI are at high risk of infertility. But this condition is unpredictable. Some women with POI can still *ovulate* and have periods, and as many as 1 in 5 can get pregnant without medical help. This is why POI is not considered true menopause.

Although POI is not the same as premature or early menopause, it comes with similar symptoms. These may include hot flashes, sleep problems, vaginal dryness, urinary changes, and mood shifts. Anxiety and depression can also be part of the picture. If you have POI, you are facing extra years of young and middle adulthood without the health benefits of natural estrogen. It's important to work with your ob-gyn to reduce your risk of cardiovascular disease, bone loss, and other conditions. You may share some health needs with women in the menopause transition, but your ob-gyn should manage your care individually.

Treatment for POI usually involves taking estrogen and progesterone. The chance of pregnancy is low with POI, but it can still happen. If you want to avoid pregnancy, talk with your ob-gyn about birth control methods, such as pills or the *intrauterine device (IUD)*. Alternatively, if you want to try for a pregnancy, don't delay. Your ob-gyn can refer you to a reproductive endocrinology and infertility specialist, or REI, for guidance. Chapter 5, "Choosing Your Menopause Care Team," has details on how REIs are trained.

RESOURCES

Early or Premature Menopause
womenshealth.gov/menopause/early-or-premature-menopause
Resource page on these conditions from the Office on Women's Health.

Primary Ovarian Insufficiency (POI)
nichd.nih.gov/health/topics/poi
An overview of POI from the *Eunice Kennedy Shriver* National Institute of Child Health and Human Development.

Primary Ovarian Insufficiency Resources
nichd.nih.gov/health/topics/poi/more_information/resources
Website from the National Institute of Child Health and Human Development that offers links to resources on POI, chromosomal causes, assisted reproduction, and health.

My Menopause
acog.org/MyMenopause

Web resource from ACOG with information on the menopause transition, signs and symptoms, treatments, and self-care. Includes the latest information from the experts in ob-gyn care, menopause stories from real women, expert columns on how to manage symptoms, Q&A articles, videos, and more.

CHAPTER 4

Menopause Signs and Symptoms

"Menopause has taken an emotional toll because of all of the ups and downs," says Anita, who is in her mid-50s. "I've had irregular bleeding, sleep problems, anxiety, hot flashes, and night sweats. It's all unpredictable and frustrating. I've learned that sometimes you have to try different solutions and decide what steps make you feel the best."

A challenge of the *menopause transition* is that you can't know in advance what it will mean for you physically and emotionally. Each person is unique, and each person will have a unique transition. As you read this chapter, remember that not everyone has all the symptoms discussed here.

Often, *menopause* is easier than people expect. For example, in a U.S. survey of more than 1,000 women who had *hot flashes*, night sweats, and sleep problems, most said their symptoms had little to no impact on daily life. But in the same study, 1 in 10 said their symptoms were so uncomfortable that it was hard to function every day. Many said that difficult symptoms had a negative impact on their lives.

Studies from other countries show that when you're not prepared for menopause, it's more disruptive. Australian researchers have described women's lack of readiness for menopause as "shocking." British women have said in surveys that they were angered by how poorly prepared they were. In a U.S. survey, some women said that not knowing what was "normal" in menopause was one reason they didn't seek health care earlier.

So it's clear that being educated about menopause can significantly improve quality of life and the care you get. But it can be difficult to find the facts. Social media and the internet are full of information, but it's hard to know what's true and which sources are credible. That's one reason this book exists. Everything you read here is based in scientific research and the experience of *obstetrician–gynecologists (ob-gyns)* who have collectively cared for and supported millions of women through the menopause transition.

Five Ways to Have a Better Menopause

We know that menopausal symptoms can erode physical or emotional comfort. They can affect relationships, social experiences, work life, and sexual well-being.

But we also know that being prepared and thinking about the kind of experience you want to have can help enormously. These five approaches can help you take control of this stage in your life.

1. **Learn about the menopause transition.** It's important to understand what's happening in your body, especially if you're coping with multiple symptoms. Learning about menopause is linked to more positive attitudes and expectations—and positive attitudes and expectations are linked to a less intrusive experience of menopause. In contrast, lack of knowledge makes symptoms harder to navigate. Often, women don't know if their symptoms are connected to the menopause transition, are not aware that effective treatments are available, or don't know how and when to talk with their ob-gyns about symptoms.

2. **Consider how you think about menopause.** The ways you think and talk about menopause shape your experience of it. Studies in multiple countries and communities have found that women who think of menopause positively are less affected by its symptoms. This doesn't mean you can banish your menopausal symptoms by sheer willpower, but it does mean you can shift your perspective (yes, night sweats are bad right now, but I'm exploring treatments that can make a big difference). Positive self-talk can be powerful.

3. **Be open to accessing health care.** If you're experiencing menopausal symptoms that lower your quality of life, talk with your ob-gyn. Women who find symptom relief with the help of their ob-gyns often say they regret not seeking health care sooner. Remember that symptoms are often connected. Treating hot flashes, for example, may also improve your sleep, mood, and memory. If you don't have an ob-gyn, check the Resources at the end of this chapter for a web link on how to find one.

4. **Talk about menopause with your family and friends.** The more you talk about menopause, the more you normalize it. It helps to be reminded that you're not alone and that your symptoms are normal. If you're having a hard time, try to find (or create) a menopause support group. Your partner, family members, and friends will benefit from learning about menopause, too.

5. **If you're struggling, know that it will get better.** In another U.S. survey, *postmenopausal* women generally were more positive about the transition than women who were in *perimenopause*. This may be because women in perimenopause tend to have more symptoms as their **hormones** shift. The takeaway: For most, symptoms improve and even go away over time.

Symptoms and How They Feel

Here's a breakdown of what many women experience during the menopause transition. If you read something that sounds familiar, you can find more details and treatment approaches in dedicated chapters.

Bleeding Changes

Was last month's period shorter or lighter than usual? Did you go longer between periods than you used to?

Of all the symptoms, changes in bleeding patterns usually come first when you enter perimenopause. The signs may be subtle at first, like a period coming a little earlier or later than usual. Over time, you may see more obvious changes in period timing, and bleeding that is heavier or lighter than usual. You may also skip periods.

For many women, the end of monthly periods is one of the most welcome aspects of menopause. But before then, you're dealing with a cycle that doesn't know which way is up. Your premenstrual symptoms, if you get them, may be less predictable, too. Not knowing when you'll get your period and how it could affect your mood and energy can make planning your days more difficult.

Be sure to discuss bleeding changes with your ob-gyn. This sign of perimenopause can sometimes mask another condition or disease, as discussed in Chapter 7, "Abnormal Bleeding." Talking with your ob-gyn may help assure you that your bleeding changes are typical for perimenopause. And if they aren't, your ob-gyn can determine what's going on and how best to approach it.

> **My symptoms seem severe. Should I worry?**
>
> Many women ask this question. The changes brought on by perimenopause can make you wonder if your experience is worse than what others go through. It's true that frequent and intense hot flashes can impair function during the day and cause you to awaken feeling hot and sweaty at night. When we don't get a good night's sleep, our mood, memory, and everyday functioning can decline, and we just don't feel well overall. Fortunately, ob-gyns have seen all of these things before. Talking with an ob-gyn is the best step to learning if your symptoms are typical and what treatment options are available.
>
> –DR. ANDREW KAUNITZ

Hot Flashes (Hot Flushes)

Have you been standing in front of your open refrigerator? Tossing sweaters aside, turning down the heater, or canceling your comforter?

Hot flashes are the most commonly reported symptom of the menopause transition. They're described as a feeling of heat that rises across the upper body, shoulders, neck, and head. A hot flash may come with sweating, a reddening face, and feeling chilly or clammy. It may bring a sense of anxiety or make your heart beat faster. Each episode can last between 3 and 10 minutes.

In the United States, almost 8 in 10 women in the menopause transition get hot flashes. Usually, hot flashes occur at least once a day. About 1 in 10 women who have hot flashes get more than seven a day during some part of their menopause transition.

Hot flashes also tend to be the symptom that most affects daily life. This is partly because hot flashes can contribute to other symptoms. If you get hot flashes at night—often called night sweats—they can disrupt your sleep. When night sweats disrupt the deepest part of sleep, it can lead to moodiness and sap your energy. Lack of energy can then affect your interest in activities you used to enjoy, including sex, as well as your ability to concentrate on work and family.

If you get hot flashes, they may continue for several years or more. Everyone is different, but studies show that Black women tend to have hot flashes the longest, for 10 years or more. Hispanic women report hot flashes for about 9 years. White women report hot flashes for about 6 years, and Asian women can have them for about 5 years or less. The good news is that hot flashes generally respond well to *hormone therapy* or hormone-free medications. To learn more, read Chapter 6, "Hot Flashes and Night Sweats."

Vaginal and Vulvar Changes

Maybe you have new sensations of itchiness or dryness in your *vagina* or on your *vulva*. Maybe these areas are sore or irritated. Or you may just notice that *sexual intercourse* has become uncomfortable or even painful.

Along with hot flashes, changes to the vagina and vulva are the symptoms most closely associated with hormonal shifts. Unlike hot flashes, which tend to be most frequent and severe in perimenopausal and recently postmenopausal women, vaginal and vulvar changes tend to happen years after menopause. About 4 in 10 women who have been through the transition report vaginal or vulvar symptoms, most commonly vaginal dryness. Some have more frequent vaginal infections with symptoms like discharge with odor, itching, irritation, or pain when urinating. These symptoms are directly related to having less *estrogen* in the body. Vaginal tissues are highly sensitive to estrogen, so the decline in estrogen that comes with the menopause transition can trigger these symptoms.

Vaginal and vulvar changes can affect how you feel about yourself, your relationship, and sex. Sex can become uncomfortable or painful. When vaginal tissue is thinner and less elastic than it used to be, intercourse can tear delicate tissue. This can cause bleeding or spotting with sex.

You may hear these symptoms described as the ***genitourinary syndrome of menopause (GSM)***. This syndrome may also include sexual health issues, ***bladder*** problems, and frequent ***urinary tract infections (UTIs)***. Fortunately, treatment can address these symptoms. To learn more, read Chapter 11, "Vaginal and Vulvar Conditions."

Urinary and Pelvic Floor Symptoms

Are you noticing sudden urges to urinate, trying to hold it while you dash to the bathroom? You're not alone. ***Urgency urinary incontinence*** becomes more common starting in perimenopause.

More than half of women who have been through the menopause transition experience some urine leakage. In the postmenopausal years, about 1 in 4 women has urgency urinary incontinence. This is a sudden need to go, sometimes with unintended loss of urine. Others have ***stress urinary incontinence***. That's when you leak while coughing, sneezing, working out, or lifting something heavy. Getting up often at night to urinate, called ***nocturia***, can also be an issue for some people.

Some women also experience ***accidental bowel leakage***. This can feel like a sudden urge to pass stool, leaking stool, or involuntarily passing gas. It is sometimes called fecal incontinence.

> **How can I talk about symptoms that upset me?**
>
> We know that some people are uncomfortable talking about genital, urinary, or sexual issues. Remember that ob-gyns have conversations like this every day. It's fine to say, "I'm not used to talking about my vagina," or "This conversation is hard for me, but I'd like your help with my bladder problems." Your voice is key. When your ob-gyn knows your concerns, they can help identify solutions that are likely to work for you.
>
> —DR. GLORIA RÍCHARD-DAVIS

These symptoms are all signs of weakening in the ***pelvic floor***. That's the set of muscles and connective tissues that support the bladder, ***uterus***, vagina, and ***rectum***. During or after the menopause transition, some women experience a ***pelvic organ prolapse***, when the uterus, bladder, or rectum drops below the ***pelvis*** and may begin to protrude from the vagina. Pelvic floor exercises can help with some forms of prolapse. To learn more, read Chapter 13, "Pelvic Organ Prolapse."

If you have bladder or bowel problems, you know they can affect your ability to function every day. Any type of incontinence can make people shy away from socializing or exercising. You may be afraid to stray far from a bathroom, and your mental health might suffer. Left untreated, urinary and pelvic floor problems can drag on or get worse. Treating these conditions can help you stay healthy, confident, and active during midlife and beyond. There are nonsurgical and surgical treatment options, so you don't need to suffer in silence. You can learn more about this in Chapter 12, "Urinary Incontinence."

Sexual Health Changes

Maybe sex has become uncomfortable or painful. Maybe you're shopping for vaginal lubricants or moisturizers for the first time. Maybe you're not feeling desire anymore, and you've told your partner it's not about them.

Sexual expression is important to many people throughout life. But during the menopause transition, issues with sexual function become more common. If this happens to you, you may feel reduced desire or arousal. You might have more difficulty reaching *orgasm*. Vaginal dryness may lead to discomfort or pain during sex or bleeding or spotting after. Pelvic floor weakening also contributes to sexual issues.

Sexual changes can chip away at your sexual satisfaction, confidence, and intimacy with a partner. Women who are afraid of pain or tissue tearing during intercourse may, understandably, avoid physical or romantic contact. Painful sex can lead to avoiding intimacy altogether. Some women hesitate to tell their partners or doctors about what they're going through.

For midlife women experiencing sexual concerns, talking with your ob-gyn is a great way to find answers. Depending on the problem, therapy, over-the-counter medications, and prescription treatments may all be options that can help. If you're anxious or uncomfortable about discussing sex with your ob-gyn, remember that they talk about sex every day with women of all ages. Write down your concerns before you see your ob-gyn and bring up your questions early in your visit. To learn more, read Chapter 10, "Sexual Health."

Mood and Anxiety Issues

Have you been worrying more than usual over things large and small? Have you found yourself swerving toward panic or snapping at family members? Mood changes and anxiety are common during the menopause transition, though not everyone is affected. Those who are affected are at risk of developing *depression*.

Anxiety symptoms include persistent worrying or dread to a level that interferes with daily life. This may come with restlessness, difficulty concentrating, tiring easily, irritability, aches and pains, and sleep problems. Some people with anxiety also have panic attacks with a racing heart, sweating, trembling, and a feeling that something bad is going to happen.

Depression symptoms include ongoing sadness or "emptiness," hopelessness, loss of interest in activities that used to bring pleasure, difficulty concentrating or making decisions, aches and pains, and sleep problems. People with depression may withdraw socially, use alcohol or drugs, or be unable to function at work and with family or friends.

Many women who report mood and anxiety problems during the menopause transition have had depression or anxiety in the past. Less commonly, women who have no history of these issues develop significant symptoms during these years.

Menopause, mood, and anxiety are connected in complex ways that we don't fully understand yet. It's likely that changing hormone levels contribute directly to these symptoms. During perimenopause, hot flashes are linked to a higher likelihood of anxiety. Women who report hot flashes are more likely to become depressed than those who don't. But other things are going on, too. Mood changes and anxiety in midlife are also influenced by aging, stress, and sleep problems.

Most women find that their mood shifts ease in the years after menopause. Even if it's needed now, treatment for anxiety and depression may not need to continue long-term. Later in this book, we'll cover what to do about mood changes and anxiety. Read Chapter 8, "Mood and Memory," to learn more.

Learning and Memory Changes

Do you find yourself looking for your phone or keys more often? Have you blanked on a name lately, lost focus in meetings, or felt overwhelmed just looking at your calendar?

"Brain fog" is a familiar complaint during the menopause transition. The term refers to issues with certain cognitive functions: the ability to learn, remember, organize, think, reason, solve problems, pay attention, and make decisions. In a large U.S. study, 2 in 3 women reported memory issues during the menopause transition.

Research suggests that declining production of estrogen affects regions of the brain related to memory. It's likely that in early midlife, issues with memory are more closely related to where you are in the menopause transition than how old you are. Other aspects of menopause, like sleep problems, also contribute to brain fog. Fortunately, annoying issues like difficulty remembering words or names improve after the menopause transition is over and a woman is postmenopausal.

Stress in midlife places people at higher risk of cognitive problems. Many women face demanding family changes. Children may need increasing attention. If you have living parents, they may be relying on you for everyday support. You may also be wrestling with concerns and decisions related to your work, finances, homes, and future retirement. Any of these issues can make it harder to concentrate.

Health issues can also contribute. Untreated anxiety or depression can cause brain fog and physical health problems. And this time in life is particularly stressful for many women.

For some, the cognitive changes of menopause have long-term implications. Of adults 65 and older who have Alzheimer disease, 2 in 3 are women. Some evidence suggests that there may be a link between women's menopause experience and their risk of dementia decades later. Keep in mind, though, that 4 in 5 postmenopausal women do *not* develop dementia. In Chapter 8, "Mood and Memory," we'll cover ways to help keep the brain healthy through midlife and beyond.

Sleep Problems

Are you waking more at night? Feeling tired when the alarm clock chimes in the morning? Catching a couple of hours of sleep here and there?

If you tended to sleep well before perimenopause, you may find that continues. But about half of women experience increased sleep disturbance during perimenopause. Most commonly, women in the menopause transition have insomnia. This can include difficulty falling or staying asleep, sleep that isn't restful, and not enough sleep.

Sleep problems can quickly lower your quality of life. Without enough good-quality sleep, your body and mind are less able to recover from illness, stress, or fatigue. Long-term lack of good sleep can also lead to health problems, including heart disease and lowered immune response. Women who are sleep-deprived also tend to snack more and find they are gaining weight. And being awake at night makes you more vulnerable to mood swings. Irritability and anger, in turn, may affect your relationships with your family, friends, and co-workers.

There's also the issue of **obstructive sleep apnea**. People with this condition may snore, gasp, or have brief pauses in breathing while sleeping. Because they do not sleep well at night, they may be drowsy during the day. This condition becomes more common in midlife.

Women in their 60s tend to sleep longer and spend less time awake at night compared to how they slept in their menopause transition years. But sleep problems can persist beyond menopause. Making sleep a priority can help now. Yes, that's easier said than done. You may not be able to control your sleep to the extent you'd wish, but you can make some gains. In Chapter 9, "Sleep Problems," we'll cover lifestyle changes and treatment options for improving sleep.

Skin and Hair Changes

Are you noticing lines on your face and loose skin on your neck? Is your hair thinning or shedding in ways you didn't expect?

Skin and hair changes are common during midlife. For some women, the changes may be alarming enough to affect quality of life. Wrinkles and a widening hair part may make you self-conscious and less confident. Feeling visibly defined by your age may reinforce any distress or anxiety you have about growing older. But skin and hair changes do not get as much attention as other menopause symptoms.

Reproductive hormones are involved in the structure of the skin and in hair growth and texture. Estrogen helps the body make **collagen**, the substance that supports the skin, hair, bones, and other tissues. So it's not surprising that as estrogen levels decline during the menopause transition, women lose collagen, too. As this is happening, skin becomes less supple and elastic.

Three out of four women in the menopause transition experience sudden reddening of the face and neck. This is called flushing, and it may worsen rosacea, a condition that causes redness and small bumps on the face. And some women in the menopause transition sweat more than usual for no clear reason.

By age 50, 2 in 5 women also show signs of hair loss. Stress, health problems, certain medications, and nutritional problems can also play a role in midlife hair loss. Losing hair around the center part and spreading out over the crown is called female pattern hair loss. This type of hair loss is partly genetic.

Many skin and hair issues of midlife can be treated. Some women taking hormone therapy for other menopause symptoms notice improvements in their skin and hair. For specialized skin and hair treatment, your ob-gyn can refer you to a dermatologist.

Talking With Your Ob-Gyn

Most menopausal symptoms can be managed. Some lifestyle tweaks and self-care remedies can make a big difference in your quality of life. More disruptive symptoms may need medication or other treatment approaches.

Learn about treatment options so you can discuss them with your ob-gyn. Track your symptoms so you can address each one at an office visit. You can use anything for tracking—a phone app or a notebook, or the Menopause Symptom Tracker listed in the Resources at the end of this chapter. Symptom tracking will make it easier for you and your ob-gyn to talk about your concerns and come up with a management plan together.

RESOURCES

Caring for Your Skin in Menopause
aad.org/public/everyday-care/skin-care-secrets/anti-aging/skin-care-during-menopause
Details on dry skin, bruising, hair loss, and more from the American Academy of Dermatology Association.

Hot Flashes: What Can I Do?
nia.nih.gov/health/menopause/hot-flashes-what-can-i-do
Webpage from the National Institute on Aging that focuses on proactive things you can do for hot flashes.

How to Find an Ob-Gyn
acog.org/FindAnObGyn

Webpage from ACOG with tips on finding generalist ob-gyns and those who specialize in areas like pelvic floor disorders and gynecologic cancer.

Menopause Symptom Tracker
acog.org/SymptomTracker

Online, printable tracker from ACOG that you can use to record symptoms and share with your ob-gyn.

Menopause Topics: Symptoms
menopause.org/patient-education/menopause-topics/symptoms

A review of common signs and symptoms of menopause from The Menopause Society.

My Menopause
acog.org/MyMenopause

Web resource from ACOG with information on the menopause transition, signs and symptoms, treatments, and self-care. Includes the latest information from the experts in ob-gyn care, menopause stories from real women, expert columns on how to manage symptoms, Q&A articles, videos, and more.

CHAPTER 5

Choosing Your Menopause Care Team

Sasha's journey with menopause care has included several doctors. At 46, she talked with a psychiatrist about sleep disturbances, a common early symptom of the menopause transition. Soon after, when she began having hot flashes, urinary tract infections, and what she calls "raging premenstrual syndrome," her family doctor recommended she see an ob-gyn. Her new ob-gyn offered hormone therapy for her hot flashes, but when she had side effects from the treatment, she talked with an ob-gyn who is a certified menopause specialist about other options. "It's important to advocate for yourself," Sasha says. "Find clinicians who know menopause care and listen to your concerns."

Choosing who will care for you during your *menopause transition* is important for your long-term health and well-being. It may be an *obstetrician–gynecologist (ob-gyn)*, a primary care doctor, or another health care professional. This chapter discusses the types of professionals who treat menopausal symptoms, how they are trained, and how they can work together.

In the past, many women suffered silently through their symptoms or delayed talking with a doctor. There's no reason to delay if you're bothered by *hot flashes*, night sweats, sleep problems, and other symptoms that seem to be related to your menopause transition. You can seek care when symptoms are bothersome, and you can be an active decision-maker in your medical care. And your care should be a partnership well beyond your last period.

Ob-Gyns Who Provide Menopause Care

There are different types of ob-gyns who treat menopausal symptoms and conditions that develop during midlife.

Obstetrician-Gynecologists

Ob-gyns are experts in obstetric and gynecologic care, including menopause care. After medical school, ob-gyns receive 4 years of residency training. To be board-certified, they must pass written and oral exams. They must also maintain their certification through continuing education and periodic exams. A certified ob-gyn can become a Fellow of the American College of Obstetricians

& Gynecologists (ACOG). Fellows of ACOG use "FACOG" after their names so you can identify them.

Ob-gyns can manage many treatments for women going through the menopause transition. They can prescribe *hormone therapy*, *antidepressants*, medications for vaginal dryness and low sex drive, and much more.

Urogynecologists

Urogynecologists are doctors who study obstetrics and gynecology or urology and then go on to do training in urogynecology and reconstructive pelvic surgery. In all, they have 7 years of obstetric, gynecologic, and surgical training after medical school. These doctors diagnose and treat conditions that may become more common during midlife, including

- *urinary incontinence* or leakage and *overactive bladder*
- sexual function disorders
- *pelvic organ prolapse*
- *accidental bowel leakage*, bowel pain, and related issues

Later in this book, we'll look at how a urogynecologist can work with you to diagnose, manage, and treat issues related to urinary health (Chapter 12, "Urinary Incontinence") and *pelvic floor disorders* (Chapter 13, "Pelvic Organ Prolapse").

Gynecologic Oncologists

Ob-gyns who go on to study female cancer and precancer are called gynecologic oncologists. They have 7 to 8 years of training in obstetrics, gynecology, cancer research, and treatments for gynecologic cancer. They perform surgery and manage *chemotherapy*, *radiation therapy*, and other therapies. Some of the conditions that gynecologic oncologists treat include

- breast cancer
- cancer of the *cervix*, *ovaries*, *fallopian tubes*, *vagina*, *vulva*, and *uterus*
- noncancerous conditions, such as pelvic masses
- precancerous changes in the uterus or on the cervix
- sexual function disorders related to cancer and its treatment

Reproductive Endocrinologists

Ob-gyns who go on to study disorders related to *hormones* and *fertility* treatment are called reproductive endocrinology and infertility (REI) specialists. In all, they have 7 years of ob-gyn and REI training after medical school, which includes more than a year of research training. In addition to *infertility*, REIs provide medical and surgical treatments for conditions such as

- *abnormal uterine bleeding*
- *endometriosis*
- fertility preservation
- *fibroids*
- *polycystic ovary syndrome (PCOS)*
- sexual function disorders

REI specialists are the go-to specialists when you have fertility issues during *perimenopause*.

> **How can I tell if a doctor will be right for me?**
>
> Some doctors make appointments for consultations. This means you can visit with the doctor and ask questions but not have a physical exam. The goal would be to learn if you feel comfortable with how they explain their approach to care. If you have a short list of doctors that you think seem promising, you can call their offices to see if they will make an appointment to learn more about them and discuss your specific health concerns. Check with your insurance to see if they will cover this kind of appointment. Most insurance plans do.
>
> –DR. GLORIA RÍCHARD-DAVIS

How to Find an Ob-Gyn

Whether you're just entering perimenopause or have been dealing with menopausal symptoms for a while on your own, talking with an ob-gyn is a good idea. If you don't already have one, there are several ways to find an ob-gyn:

- Ask your primary care doctor or other health care professional for recommendations.
- Ask your friends and family about their experiences with their ob-gyns.
- Look for the "find a doctor" tool at the website of your health insurance plan or call the number on the back of your insurance card.
- Look for a "find a doctor" tool on the website of your local hospital.
- Use an online directory to find and compare doctors near you.

When you have the names of some ob-gyns, use the internet to learn about their education and qualifications. You can also call their offices with questions. Always remember to ask whether they accept your health insurance.

If at any point you would like more support, look for a health care professional who has extra training in menopause care. This could include certification from The Menopause Society (previously known as the North American Menopause Society). Professionals with this certification use the letters MSCP after their names, which stands for The Menopause Society Certified Practitioner.

It may also be helpful to look for doctors who are familiar with your unique needs. People of color, those in the LGBTQ+ community, people with a history of traumatic experiences, and others may want to work with doctors who understand their communities and backgrounds. Read the box "Finding Care That's Right for You" for more information.

Finding Care That's Right for You

Sometimes finding a doctor who fits your needs is challenging. People of color, people of various religious faiths, or those with social concerns may want to find a doctor who understands the interaction of their medical and social needs. The same may be true for people with disabilities. Lesbian, gay, transgender, nonbinary, and queer people may want doctors who understand how the experience of menopause may be different for them. And survivors of sexual assault, abuse, discrimination, or other traumas may need doctors and medical facilities to be trauma-informed. This means that the medical space and interactions with doctors and staff are designed to help people feel welcome and safe.

These approaches can help you find doctors who meet your specific needs:

- Ask people in your community for recommendations.

- Ask patient advocacy groups for possible recommendations.

- Search online for directories of doctors who represent your community or are allies.

- Check hospital system websites for inclusive health care teams. Read doctor bios to see if any have a special interest in working with certain communities.

- Call medical offices and talk with the staff. Ask if their care teams are trauma-informed and what that means to them. Check their websites for inclusive images and language.

- Advocate for your needs to the extent that you feel able. You do not need to describe past struggles or traumas, though you can refer to these if you want to. It is fine to say, "I had a doctor who didn't seem to listen to me," or "I feel safer with doctors who understand my life experience."

Other Doctors and Health Care Professionals

There are other doctors who treat menopausal symptoms, including specialists who focus on one aspect like sleep problems or mood and memory challenges.

Primary Care Doctors

Primary care doctors manage and treat common health issues, including symptoms of menopause. After medical school, primary care doctors gain clinical experience through different areas of medicine so they can care for all types of conditions. For more complex issues, they may refer people to doctors with special medical training. Some primary care doctors specialize in women's health concerns.

Sometimes primary care doctors and ob-gyns work with nurse practitioners (NPs). NPs have master's or doctoral degrees in advanced practice nursing. State laws govern which health care services NPs can provide. These laws state whether they need to work with doctors or can practice independently. Some NPs use the credential APRN (advanced practice registered nurse) or FNP (family nurse practitioner). Some NPs are trained in treating menopause and have the MSCP certification from The Menopause Society.

> **I've heard about MDs and DOs. What's the difference?**
>
> An MD has a Doctor of Medicine degree. A DO has a Doctor of Osteopathic Medicine degree. Both degrees require medical school training and residencies. MDs and DOs can both prescribe medications and be licensed in all states. The main difference is that MDs practice what is called allopathic medicine. This means they use medication, surgery, and other treatments. DOs practice osteopathic medicine, which focuses on the ways the mind, body, and spirit work together. DOs also receive extra training in a hands-on technique for diagnosing and treating illnesses.
>
> –DR. CHERYL IGLESIA

Endocrinologists

Endocrinologists are doctors who study the body's hormones and treat conditions of the endocrine system. After medical school, these specialists complete 3 years of residency, often in internal medicine, and a 2- to 3-year fellowship in endocrinology, *diabetes*, or *metabolism*. They can treat a variety of conditions, including

- cancers of the endocrine glands
- diabetes
- infertility

- menopausal symptoms
- metabolic disorders
- *osteoporosis*
- thyroid problems

Endocrinologists can manage hormone therapy for menopausal symptoms.

Sleep Specialists

Sleep specialists are doctors, often neurologists, with expertise in sleep medicine. They can help you develop healthy sleep habits, provide treatments that improve sleep, and prescribe medication and devices. After medical school, these specialists complete 4 years of training in internal medicine, family medicine, neurology, psychiatry, or pediatrics followed by a 1-year fellowship in sleep medicine. Sleep specialists can treat

- *insomnia,* which includes trouble falling asleep, staying asleep, or getting quality sleep
- narcolepsy, a condition that causes daytime sleepiness
- *obstructive sleep apnea*
- restless leg syndrome

Other clinicians also work in sleep medicine. These include psychiatrists, psychologists, neurologists, nurses, and respiratory therapists. Chapter 9, "Sleep Problems," covers how sleep specialists work to diagnose and manage sleep issues.

Mental Health Specialists

Several types of health care professionals are licensed to diagnose mental health conditions and provide counseling. Some mental health specialists can also prescribe medications. For guidance on when to seek mental health treatment and what that might look like, read Chapter 8, "Mood and Memory."

Psychiatrists. These medical doctors provide counseling and prescribe medications. After medical school, they study psychiatry for 4 years. Some go on to extra fellowship training in a specialty such as sleep medicine, pain medicine, or addiction medicine.

Psychologists. These are doctors who provide counseling. In most states, they cannot prescribe medications. They have doctoral degrees in clinical psychology, counseling, or education.

Psychiatric or mental health nurses and nurse practitioners. These professionals provide counseling. Depending on the state in which they practice and their qualifications, they may prescribe medications, provide telehealth care, or work closely with psychologists. Advanced psychiatric or mental health nurses have master's or doctoral degrees in nursing with a focus on psychiatry.

Counselors, therapists, and social workers. These professionals also provide counseling. They cannot prescribe medications. Counselors and therapists have master's degrees in fields related to mental health, such as psychology or marriage and family therapy. Social workers have master's or doctoral degrees in social work.

Psychiatric pharmacists. These pharmacists specialize in mental health treatment. Some can prescribe medications. Psychiatric pharmacists have doctoral degrees. Many also have residency training in psychiatric pharmacy.

Registered Dietitians

Registered dietitians are experts in healthy eating. They apply the science of nutrition to support people who are coping with disease or weight management. Some dietitians have specialized training in *obesity*, diabetes, nutrition for cancer or *kidney disease*, sports nutrition, and other areas. These professionals have graduate degrees and have passed an exam in nutrition. You can read more about how dietitians can help during the menopause transition in Chapter 14, "Weight and Menopause."

Dermatologists

Dermatologists are doctors who specialize in skin, hair, and nail conditions. They provide medical and cosmetic consultation and treatments for many conditions, including

- acne, dermatitis, and eczema
- conditions that cause excess hair growth (on the face or abdomen, for example)
- dryness and thinning of the skin
- female pattern hair loss and receding hair

After medical school, dermatologists have 4 years of training in skin conditions and related issues. For more on skin and hair changes during the menopause transition, read Chapter 4, "Menopause Signs and Symptoms."

Physical Therapists

Physical therapists can help people improve their physical movement and bodily functions. They use a range of methods, including guided physical exercise, therapeutic ultrasound, heat and cold applications, electrical stimulation, and more.

Some physical therapists have extra training in pelvic floor therapy. This type of therapy is sometimes recommended for treatment of **urgency urinary incontinence**, accidental bowel leakage, pelvic organ prolapse, vaginal or pelvic pain, and sexual health issues.

Taking Charge of Your Care

Once you know who you want to manage your care, plan to partner with them. Remember that the care you receive during the menopause transition can help set you up for a healthy future. Voicing your goals, values, and preferences can help your ob-gyn and other health care professionals understand your treatment goals. There are steps you can take to make sure you and your health care professionals are on the same page:

- Keep track of your medical records and test results so you can discuss them with different professionals. You may have easy access to this information via an online patient portal.

- Check in regularly to make sure your care teams have the most up-to-date test results, medication lists, and treatment plans. If you see several health care professionals, they may not have access to each other's records. Talk with office staff about the best ways to share information so that everyone who cares for you is fully informed.

- Talk about your goals for treatment, including self-care. Keep notes of what you decide with your care team. Update these notes at each appointment. This way, you'll develop an ongoing record.

- Remember to track your symptoms, including hot flashes, mood shifts, and tiredness. Also track your response to any medical or self-care approaches you're trying. This way you can see how your body and mind adjust to them over time.

- Consider smartphone apps designed for health care planning. Some apps help you access your medical records, track your current health issues, schedule appointments, and request prescription refills. Apps are available to track your moods, sleep, physical activity, symptoms, and so on. Some can help you manage behaviors that you want to change. Some can track your medications and remind you to take them.

Before using an app, do your research. Read about privacy policies to be sure the app will not share your medical information with others.

RESOURCES

Find a Dermatologist
find-a-derm.aad.org

Searchable directory from the American Academy of Dermatology Association.

Find & Compare Providers Near You
medicare.gov/care-compare/?providerType=Physician

A directory of medical professionals and health care facilities, searchable by location, specialty, or name. This tool from the U.S. Centers for Medicare and Medicaid Services lists clinicians and facilities that accept Medicare and other types of insurance.

Find an Endocrinologist
endocrine.org/patient-engagement/find-an-endocrinologist-directory

Physician referral directory for the Endocrine Society, the largest organization of endocrinologists in the world.

Find a Health Professional
reproductivefacts.org/find-a-health-professional/

Directory from the American Society for Reproductive Medicine that includes ob-gyns and other specialists in reproductive medicine.

Find LGBTQ+ Friendly Healthcare Near You
lgbtqhealthcaredirectory.org/

Health care database from GLMA: Health Professionals Advancing LGBTQ+ Equality.

Find a Nutrition Expert
eatright.org/find-a-nutrition-expert

Searchable directory from the American Academy of Nutrition and Dietetics of credentialed nutrition and dietitian providers.

Find a Physical Therapist Near You
choosept.com/find-a-pt

Searchable directory from the American Physical Therapy Association.

Find a Provider
voicesforpfd.org/find-a-health-care-professional

Directory to use when looking for a specialist in pelvic health from the American Urogynecologic Society.

How to Find a Certified Menopause Practitioner
menopause.org/patient-education/choosing-a-healthcare-practitioner

Directory from The Menopause Society listing health care professionals who have the training to use the credential MSCP (The Menopause Society Certified Practitioner).

NAMI HelpLine
nami.org/help

Helpline and links from the National Alliance on Mental Illness that offers free information, resource referrals, and support for mental health.

Referral Directory
aasect.org/referral-directory

Searchable directory of sex therapists and educators from the American Association of Sexuality Educators, Counselors, and Therapists.

Seek a Specialist
foundationforwomenscancer.org/resources/seek-a-specialist/

Tool from the Society of Gynecologic Oncology's Foundation to help you find ob-gyns who treat cancer of the female reproductive organs.

Sleep Center Directory
sleepeducation.org/sleep-center

Searchable directory from the American Academy of Sleep Medicine.

My Menopause
acog.org/MyMenopause

Web resource from ACOG with information on the menopause transition, signs and symptoms, treatments, and self-care. Includes the latest information from the experts in ob-gyn care, menopause stories from real women, expert columns on how to manage symptoms, Q&A articles, videos, and more.

Part II

DETAILING SIGNS AND SYMPTOMS

CHAPTER 6

Hot Flashes and Night Sweats

Sandi's first experience with night sweats took her by surprise. She was 50 and woke up one night soaked. "I had to get out of bed and change my nightshirt. I threw the covers off and turned the fan on high," she says. Sandi's night sweats happened twice a week for about 3 years. She also had hot flashes every couple of hours during the day. "It's like someone flipped a switch. I felt intense heat spreading throughout my body, and my face got flushed, too." Ten years later she still gets mild hot flashes, but not as often. Patience helped her get through, Sandi says, and knowing that others were going through similar things.

As many as 8 in 10 women in the *menopause transition* get *hot flashes* and night sweats, otherwise known as vasomotor symptoms. The term "vasomotor" refers to the blood vessels getting wider or narrower in response to a change in the body. When your blood vessels widen, more blood flows through them, and this releases heat.

When hot flashes or night sweats strike, they cause a feeling of heat most often rising across the upper body, shoulders, neck, and head. In the first few seconds, skin temperature and blood flow increase in parts of the body. Some women sweat and their heartbeat quickens. Others feel a sense of anxiety. Each episode can last between 3 and 10 minutes.

In a large U.S. study, about half of women who experienced hot flashes and night sweats said they were only mildly bothersome. That said, vasomotor symptoms can be disruptive. They are the most common reason that women seek health care related to menopause. This is partly because hot flashes and night sweats are linked to other menopausal symptoms, such as sleep problems, tiredness, irritability, depressive symptoms, and lower quality of life.

A broad range of treatments gives us many options for improving quality of life for women with disruptive vasomotor symptoms. Later in this chapter, we'll cover effective treatments—with and without *hormones*—for hot flashes and night sweats. We'll also cover other things you can do for your symptoms.

Vasomotor Symptoms: The Basics

Let's start with the things that everyone who is approaching or in *perimenopause* should know. First, vasomotor symptoms vary, sometimes dramatically. How often you have hot flashes or night sweats is different from person to person and, in perimenopause, can differ month to month. Several hot flashes a day is typical, but they may range from mild to intense. Women tend to report more hot flashes during the day than night sweats at night, maybe because they are less alert to what's happening at night. But night sweats are often more bothersome.

Second, hot flashes usually begin at the start of perimenopause. Typically, perimenopause begins in the late 40s, though it's possible for symptoms to start earlier. You may notice hot flashes before you start skipping **menstrual periods** or around the same time. Hot flashes tend to become more frequent the closer you get to your final period. For most women, hot flashes peak in the year following your last period, then come less often before they stop altogether.

> **Am I guaranteed to get hot flashes?**
>
> Vasomotor symptoms are likely during perimenopause, but they aren't guaranteed. Some women never have hot flashes or night sweats, while others have them so often it disrupts their lives. And you could have hot flashes that are so mild you don't register them as a symptom of perimenopause. Remember that if you do develop hot flashes, or they get worse over time, talking with your ob-gyn can help you find solutions. Together you can discuss whether medical treatment could be right for you.
>
> –DR. NANETTE SANTORO

Third, as uncomfortable as night sweats can be, you may not be fully aware of how often they are happening. In some studies, women in the menopause transition wore devices on their skin that detected vasomotor symptoms at night. The devices detected more night sweats than the women did. Still, even if they aren't noticed as much as hot flashes, night sweats can be more disruptive because they interfere with good-quality sleep and daily functioning.

Fourth, hot flashes may go on after menopause. It's common to have hot flashes for up to 5 years after the last period. For some, hot flashes persist well beyond the menopause transition. In a U.S. study, hot flashes continued to affect 1 in 5 women in their late 50s, 1 in 10 women in their 60s, and 1 in 20 women in their 70s. Your likelihood of having hot flashes for a long time is higher if you started having them very early in your menopause transition.

Finally, scientists don't yet fully understand the cause of hot flashes and night sweats. Multiple bodily systems interact with the brain to cause them. These two systems are known to be involved:

- Reproductive hormones—Researchers know that women with lower levels of *estrogen* and higher levels of *follicle-stimulating hormone (FSH)* are more likely than others to report severe hot flashes and night sweats. There are specialized nerve cells in the brain that control the production of FSH. As FSH rises and estrogen declines through the menopause transition, these nerve cells become more active and send signals to the brain's thermostat. This is what kicks off hot flashes. But we also know that while everyone goes through hormonal changes during perimenopause, not everyone has severe or even any hot flashes or night sweats. This suggests that other systems in the body also play a role.

- Body temperature regulation—There is a separate set of nerve cells that pick up the initial signal for hot flashes and then transmit it to the rest of the body. The body is designed to be comfortable within a certain range of temperature. Perimenopause appears to narrow the core temperature range that your body tolerates comfortably. When your body temperature shifts outside this range, it triggers warming responses (such as shivering) or cooling responses (such as sweating). During the menopause transition, even small increases in body temperature are perceived as being outside the core range. This may cause the blood vessels to widen, triggering hot flashes and night sweats to release body heat.

Who Gets Hot Flashes and Night Sweats

Many studies have been done to understand why the experience of hot flashes and night sweats is so variable. We know that individual hormones and *genes* play a role. So do certain behaviors. Whether someone reports symptoms also relates to their sensitivity to symptoms and how comfortable they are talking about personal health issues. But some specific circumstances have been linked to frequent and bothersome hot flashes and night sweats.

Uterus or Ovary Removal

Women who have had their *uterus* removed *(hysterectomy)* are more likely to report hot flashes and night sweats, even in cases where the *ovaries* remain. Those who've had their ovaries and *fallopian tubes* removed, and who do not go on *hormone therapy*, report more frequent and severe symptoms.

Breast Cancer Treatment

Two in 3 women who are treated for breast cancer report hot flashes and night sweats, often severe. Symptoms are even more likely among women whose menopause was induced medically—for example, as a side effect of *chemotherapy*—and women treated with *tamoxifen* or *aromatase inhibitors*, medications that lower estrogen levels.

Race and Ethnicity

The experiences of menopause may vary depending on which racial or ethnic group a woman identifies with. For example, in the United States, Black women are most likely to report hot flashes and night sweats and describe them as bothersome. White and Hispanic women report symptoms at similar rates. Asian American women are the least likely to report hot flashes and night sweats. Studies around the world have also shown racial and ethnic variation based on how women self-identify, but this doesn't mean the differences are due to biology. One possibility is that women's varying descriptions of menopause reflect differences in language, education, and other social factors, even though their bodily changes are the same. Another possibility is that biology and culture interact in ways we don't yet understand.

Smoking and Certain Medications

Current smokers are more likely to report hot flashes and night sweats than nonsmokers. Those exposed to second-hand smoke are also at higher risk. Hot flashes are also linked to several medications, including some *antidepressants*, chemotherapy, and drugs that affect levels of reproductive hormones.

Body Weight

Women with *obesity* are more likely to report vasomotor symptoms than other women. Obesity has been linked to more frequent hot flashes and night sweats early in the menopause transition, and less frequent hot flashes later. Hot flashes and night sweats are also more commonly reported by those who gain weight during the menopause years. It's possible that body shape affects the body's temperature regulation or hormonal systems.

Mood Issues

Higher levels of anxiety, *depression*, and stress are linked to more frequent and bothersome hot flashes and night sweats. Studies show that vasomotor symptoms often continued for many years among women who were anxious or depressed going into perimenopause, who had more stress, or who were more sensitive to symptoms.

Childhood Neglect or Abuse

Hot flashes and night sweats are more likely to be reported by those who have a history of neglect or abuse in childhood. It's possible that abuse has long-term effects on the nervous system and hormone function, leading to increased risk of vasomotor symptoms in midlife. Also, adults who experienced abuse or neglect are more likely to have depression and anxiety, which are also known triggers of vasomotor symptoms.

Violence and Trauma at Home

Intimate partner violence is linked to worse menopausal symptoms generally. Women with a history of partner abuse are more likely to report night sweats. Women with current symptoms of *post-traumatic stress disorder (PTSD)* are also more likely than others to report hot flashes and night sweats.

Gender-Affirming Care

Transgender men and nonbinary people may experience menopausal symptoms as a result of gender-affirming health care. For example, if a transgender man or nonbinary person has their ovaries and uterus removed, they may experience vasomotor symptoms immediately. Those taking *testosterone* during their gender transition may also have vasomotor symptoms.

Hot Flash Triggers

Certain behaviors or situations may increase the chance of a hot flash. If you're seeking to manage your hot flashes, pay attention to your symptoms. Track when your hot flashes happen. This may help you see patterns and avoid possible triggers, plus it will give you a record to share with your *obstetrician–gynecologist (ob-gyn)*. Some of these things may trigger hot flashes.

Heated Spaces

During the menopause transition, the body seems to become less tolerant of heat. Relatively small increases in heat may trigger a hot flash. As you learn to manage hot flashes, one tool may be thermostat regulation in living and working spaces.

Spicy Foods

Spicy foods are often blamed for triggering hot flashes. Capsaicin—a natural substance in chili peppers—causes the body to generate additional heat.

Hot Drinks and Caffeine

Hot drinks and caffeine cause blood vessels to expand, increasing blood flow. Caffeine may also make the heart beat faster. One study found that hot flashes were more than twice as likely during or after caffeine use. This includes caffeine found in coffee, tea, soda, or chocolate.

Alcohol

You wouldn't be alone in blaming red wine. Some research suggests that alcohol can trigger hot flashes. This may be because, like caffeine, alcohol can cause blood vessels to expand.

Smoking

Cigarette smoking is both a risk factor for hot flashes and a trigger. Smoking affects how estrogen is processed in the body. It's also possible that **nicotine**, the addictive drug in tobacco, can generate heat.

Anxiety

Studies have compared women with differing levels of anxiety who report hot flashes. Those with moderate anxiety may be three times as likely to have hot flashes compared with women who do not have anxiety. And women with high anxiety may be five times as likely to report hot flashes. It's not clear how anxiety relates to vasomotor symptoms. If you have anxiety that doesn't go away or gets worse over time, talk with your ob-gyn. Read more in Chapter 8, "Mood and Memory."

Managing Hot Flashes and Night Sweats

Many women like to start with natural approaches to manage hot flashes. Ob-gyns have found that lifestyle changes can help some women immediately, including

- wearing layers of clothing, so you can easily take off layers to cool down
- avoiding spicy food, alcohol, caffeine, and hot drinks
- sitting still in a cold room when possible
- quitting smoking

Some women prefer to start with natural approaches to manage night sweats, too, including

- avoiding triggers like alcohol, spicy food, caffeine, and smoking before bedtime
- taking a warm bath or shower 1 to 2 hours before bed, which has been found in studies to produce a cooling effect
- keeping the bedroom at an ideal temperature for sleeping, which is 60 to 67 °F (15.5 to 19.5 °C)
- layering the bed with light blankets made of natural fibers
- chilling the bed with cooling gels or an ice pack under the pillow
- keeping iced water nearby in a flask designed to hold cold water for a long time
- changing night clothes if you wake up sweaty to avoid being chilled by wet clothes

These approaches have worked for many women going through the menopause transition. And now, more recent research points to the potential benefits of mind–body techniques in managing vasomotor symptoms. Mind–body techniques explore the interactions between the brain, body, and behaviors, and how these affect health. You may be able to change your hot flashes—or the way you experience them.

Cognitive Behavioral Therapy

Cognitive behavioral therapy (CBT) aims to change unhelpful ways of thinking and behaving. Some studies have found that CBT programs developed for menopausal symptoms are effective for women in the menopause transition, including breast cancer survivors. Women in these studies had fewer bothersome hot flashes and night sweats, more restful sleep, improved mood, and better emotional and physical functioning. Some of these benefits lasted at least 6 months.

> **How can I be positive about hot flashes when I'm so uncomfortable?**
>
> If your hot flashes are causing you enough discomfort that you can't enjoy your life, it may be time to talk with your ob-gyn. Perimenopause and menopause are times of life that coincide with other key life events: success in career, managing aging parents or maturing children, being in long-term romantic relationships or navigating this stage solo and independently, and sometimes the onset of new diseases. If menopausal symptoms and changes are making it difficult to do the things you want and need to do, then it may be right for you to start medical or hormonal therapy with the help of your ob-gyn.
>
> –DR. CARRIE ANN TERRELL

Hypnotherapy

In one recent study, hypnotherapy or hypnotic relaxation therapy greatly decreased the frequency of hot flashes. The treatment involved guided relaxation sessions that focused on cooling images for 15 minutes a day. The women in the studies also reported improved sleep and reduced anxiety.

Mindfulness-Based Stress Reduction

Mindfulness-based stress reduction is a form of meditation. It is taught by instructors in weekly classes over 8 weeks. In a study, women who took the program became less bothered by their hot flashes and night sweats, although the severity and frequency of these symptoms did not change. That benefit continued for at least 3 months. Participants also reported better sleep, decreased anxiety and stress, and improved quality of life.

Medical Treatment for Hot Flashes

If you've tried self-care and it's not helping your vasomotor symptoms, there are safe and effective medications you can discuss with your ob-gyn. The most effective medical treatment is hormone therapy. If you can't use hormone therapy for medical reasons, or if you prefer to avoid it, several nonhormonal medications are available. Note that researchers are learning that managing severe hot flashes now may be important for long-term heart and brain health. Read the box "Hot Flashes and Future Heart and Brain Health" for more details. For now, talk with your ob-gyn about treatments that can help disruptive vasomotor symptoms.

Hormonal Medications

In the past, hormone therapy was called hormone replacement therapy. In recent years, the word "replacement" has been dropped because the goal of therapy is not to replace the estrogen or progesterone to the higher levels seen before the menopause transition. Instead, the goal is to take just enough estrogen to curb symptoms and improve quality of life. Here, we'll cover key facts about hormone therapy. For more detail, read Chapter 17, "Hormone Therapies."

When taken for hot flashes and night sweats, hormones are taken as a pill or absorbed through the skin with a patch, gel, or spray. This is called systemic hormone therapy. The hormones enter the bloodstream and are distributed around the body. This means systemic hormone therapy may also help with other menopausal symptoms, like vaginal dryness.

Sometimes, systemic hormone therapy consists of estrogen only. Those who have a uterus also need to take another hormone, called *progestin*, to reduce the risk of cancer in the uterine lining. Ob-gyns typically advise women to take the lowest doses of hormones for the shortest period of time needed to manage their symptoms. Many women can eventually stop hormones and not have a recurrence of their hot flashes or night sweats.

Another medication combines estrogen and a drug called bazedoxifene, which enables estrogen to be active only in certain parts of the body. That means the estrogen does not raise the risk of cancer of the uterus. This medication can be used to relieve hot flashes plus vaginal dryness, pain during *sexual intercourse*, and sleep problems. It can also help prevent bone loss.

Hot Flashes and Future Heart and Brain Health

Women with frequent or persistent hot flashes may be at higher risk of heart disease or brain disease than those whose hot flashes are less bothersome. That's a key message of recent menopause research.

In the United States, heart disease is the leading cause of death for women—ahead of all forms of cancer combined. But many women don't have heart disease on their radar. That's why the menopause transition is a time to make lifestyle changes that protect your heart and brain.

When estrogen levels decline during perimenopause, there is also a decline in the function of blood vessels, and they begin to accumulate plaque. This is called hardening of the arteries. Some of these changes are known to be related to aging and some may be related to menopause itself. This helps explain why women who experience natural menopause at a younger age have a higher risk of heart disease and **stroke** than women whose menopause comes later. Now we know that hot flashes are a signal of future heart disease risk.

Much of the recent evidence about menopause and long-term health comes from a large U.S. study that followed 3,000 women over several decades. In that study, women who reported frequent hot flashes at clinic visits during their menopause transition—they had hot flashes on at least 6 of the last 14 days—were twice as likely to have a heart attack, stroke, or heart failure during the next 20 years, compared with women who did not experience hot flashes. Frequent hot flashes early in the menopause transition, or that persisted beyond menopause, were connected to higher-than-average risk. Hot flashes are also linked to **inflammation** and specific warning signs for heart disease, like thickening of the blood vessel walls.

Researchers are still learning what these results could mean. One possibility is that hot flashes are a marker of heart disease and could be seen as a warning sign to address heart health earlier rather than later. But another possibility is that the hot flashes themselves raise the risk of future heart disease, so treating hot flashes now may help with that risk moving forward. It's not currently known if either of these interpretations is true, and more research is needed. Still, we know that the risk of heart disease increases with age.

Cardiovascular health also affects brain health. The midlife risk factors for heart disease are also linked to declining cognitive function. Studies have linked hot flashes and night sweats to brain processes that may raise the risk for future dementia.

Researchers are still learning about the connection between hot flashes, heart disease, and brain disease. Regardless of your experience of hot flashes, talk with your ob-gyn about steps you can take to lower your risk for serious disease. You can also read Chapter 19, "Heart Disease and Diabetes," for more on heart health.

Estrogen-Free Medications

The U.S. Food and Drug Administration (FDA) has approved two estrogen-free medications to treat hot flashes and night flashes:

- Fezolinetant—This medication is approved to treat moderate to severe hot flashes and night sweats. It works in the part of the brain that helps control body temperature. Fezolinetant is taken as a pill at the same time every day. The most common side effect is headaches. Rarely, the medication can cause stomach pain, diarrhea, *insomnia*, and back pain. There's also a rare risk of liver injury with this medication. Your ob-gyn should check your liver function with a blood test before you start taking it. Blood tests should also be done at 1, 2, 3, 6, and 9 months of treatment.

- Paroxetine mesylate—This medication is the only antidepressant that is FDA-approved for the treatment of hot flashes. It should be taken at the same time every day, usually at bedtime. Other antidepressants have been used for hot flashes even though they are FDA-approved only for depression treatment. These include venlafaxine, desvenlafaxine, fluoxetine, and escitalopram.

Some medications used for other conditions may also be used to treat hot flashes:

- Gabapentin—This medication is used to treat seizures and nerve pain. It is not FDA-approved for vasomotor symptoms, but studies have shown that it reduces the frequency and severity of hot flashes. The starting dose usually is taken at night because gabapentin can cause sleepiness. Your ob-gyn may have you work your way up to three doses per day. You can take gabapentin with or without food. Gabapentin may be used when antidepressants and fezolinetant are not effective or when side effects of these medications are a problem.

- Oxybutynin—This medication for overactive bladder may also reduce the frequency and intensity of hot flashes. It is taken by mouth, usually on an empty stomach and at the same time every day. It also comes as a skin patch that is applied every 3 or 4 days. Oxybutynin may be used when another treatment for hot flashes hasn't worked or can't be taken. Research suggests that long-term use in those older than 55 may increase the risk of cognitive decline. Talk with your ob-gyn about this risk.

- Clonidine—This is a medication that lowers **blood pressure**. It has also been used to reduce the frequency of hot flashes. Clonidine is used as a pill or skin patch. When taken by mouth, it should be taken at the same time every day to have the best effect. Like oxybutynin, this medication may be prescribed when another treatment hasn't worked or can't be taken.

Read Chapter 18, "Estrogen-Free Medical Therapies," for more details.

Talking With Your Ob-Gyn

If hot flashes and night sweats are disrupting your quality of life, make an appointment to see your ob-gyn. Whether you choose lifestyle changes alone or decide to try medication, your ob-gyn can help support and guide your decisions. If one approach doesn't work or stops working, together you can talk about other options to relieve your symptoms.

RESOURCES

Hot Flashes: What Can I Do?
nia.nih.gov/health/menopause/hot-flashes-what-can-i-do
Website from the National Institute on Aging with lifestyle changes to improve hot flashes and sleep, and links to additional menopause resources.

Relaxation Techniques: What You Need to Know
nccih.nih.gov/health/relaxation-techniques-what-you-need-to-know
This website from the National Center for Complementary and Integrative Health describes various relaxation techniques and links to other mind–body approaches. It also outlines the benefits for health conditions including menopause, sleep problems, stress, anxiety, blood pressure, and more.

My Menopause
acog.org/MyMenopause
Web resource from ACOG with information on the menopause transition, signs and symptoms, treatments, and self-care. Includes the latest information from the experts in ob-gyn care, menopause stories from real women, expert columns on how to manage symptoms, Q&A articles, videos, and more.

CHAPTER 7

Abnormal Bleeding

Ro expected her periods to change as she got older. In her mid-40s, she would have one day of heavy bleeding and then a day of lighter flow, but there seemed to be a rhythm. Then things changed dramatically. "I started bleeding for up to 3 weeks," she says. "It got so heavy, clot after clot, some the size of a chicken egg." Ro had no pain and assumed her heavy bleeding was a normal part of perimenopause. Eventually, an ob-gyn diagnosed a polyp in her uterus. Ro had it removed with a brief procedure under anesthesia, and she hasn't bled since. "Looking back, I think the heavy bleeding was caused by the polyp, not my cycle," she says. "My final period may have been some time ago, though I haven't had other menopausal symptoms."

Changes in menstrual bleeding are one of the first signs that *perimenopause*, the transition between regular cycles and the last period, has begun. But there are certain conditions that can cause vaginal bleeding, too. This is why it's important to be aware of your bleeding patterns before perimenopause so you can identify differences.

In this chapter, we'll describe the menstrual changes that are typical during perimenopause. We'll also discuss the conditions that may cause abnormal bleeding. If you recognize the signs and symptoms of abnormal bleeding, make an appointment to see your *obstetrician–gynecologist (ob-gyn)*.

While this chapter talks about abnormal bleeding that happens before *menopause*—the final period—remember that bleeding or spotting after you have gone 12 months without a period is not normal. There could be many causes, including infection or a *benign* growth, but bleeding after menopause should always be checked out by your ob-gyn.

Why Bleeding Changes in Perimenopause

During your reproductive years, two *hormones* work together to regulate menstrual bleeding: *estrogen* and *progesterone*. Among women who *ovulate* regularly, the levels of these hormones rise and fall in a regular pattern throughout the *menstrual cycle*.

As you move through perimenopause, *ovulation* occurs less regularly, and the predictable rise and fall of hormones changes. Generally, the menstrual cycle shortens, or there may be fewer days of bleeding. As perimenopause goes on, the flow may be lighter or heavier, or there may be spotting instead of a period. Later in perimenopause, you may skip a period one month and have a normal or unusually heavy or long period the next month. This happens because ovulation during the *menopause transition* is unpredictable and less frequent.

Bleeding changes can create anxiety even when you know what's happening in your body. Talking with your ob-gyn can help you understand your individual experience and confirm that your changes are typical of perimenopause. Track the changes and bring details to your next ob-gyn visit. You can use a phone app, a notebook, or the Abnormal Bleeding Diary at the ACOG website (see the Resources section for the link).

When Bleeding Should Be Evaluated

You'll likely know what's normal for you when it comes to monthly bleeding. Any change from *your* normal is called **abnormal uterine bleeding**, even when these changes are an expected sign of perimenopause. Some changes in bleeding can be concerning, though, and affect your quality of life. If you experience any of these changes, call your ob-gyn:

- Bleeding that soaks through one or more tampons or pads every hour
- Bleeding that is so heavy you have to double up on pads
- Bleeding that lasts more than 7 days
- Flooding or gushing when you stand up
- Passing blood clots the size of a quarter or larger
- Irregular periods when the number of bleeding days varies by more than 7 to 9 days
- Bleeding or spotting after **sexual intercourse**
- Bleeding between cycles
- Menstrual cycles longer than 35 days or shorter than 21 days (measured from the first day of bleeding of one period to the first day of bleeding of the next period)

Sudden, unusual episodes of abnormal bleeding can also happen in perimenopause. This is called acute abnormal uterine bleeding. If you are changing pads or tampons every hour for more than 2 hours in a row, and you also have chest pain, have shortness of breath, and are lightheaded or dizzy, seek emergency medical care right away. You should be treated to control the bleeding. If you have lost a lot of blood, you may need **intravenous (IV) fluids** or a blood *transfusion*. When your condition is stable, your ob-gyn will look for the cause of your bleeding.

Conditions That Can Cause Abnormal Bleeding in Perimenopause

Several conditions of the *uterus* can cause abnormal vaginal bleeding. Some of these conditions are benign despite any discomfort or pain that comes with them. Other conditions can be cancer or precancer.

Fibroids

These common growths, also called *leiomyomas,* develop from the muscle tissue of the uterus. *Fibroids* can cause longer, more frequent, or heavy menstrual bleeding, more pain during periods, and bleeding between periods. The size, shape, and location of fibroids can vary. They may be inside the uterus, on its outer surface, within its wall, or attached by a stem. Fibroids are rarely cancerous, but they can grow very large.

Polyps

Polyps may develop in the lining of the uterus (the *endometrium*) and cause irregular or heavy bleeding. Although most uterine polyps are not cancer, some can have cancer cells. Uterine polyps should be removed with surgery and biopsied to be sure cancer is not present. Removing them also reduces the risk of polyps growing and leading to more abnormal bleeding.

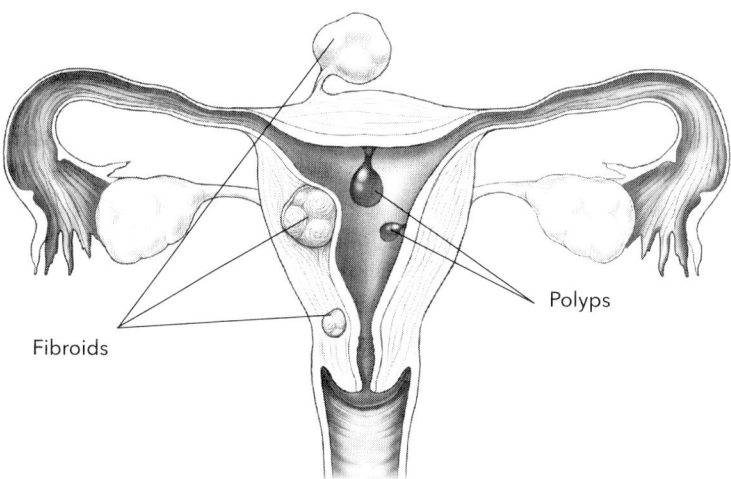

Fibroids and polyps. Fibroids are benign growths that may form inside or sometimes outside the uterus. Polyps, which are usually benign, attach to the inner wall of the uterus.

Adenomyosis

In this condition, the endometrium grows into the wall of the uterus. Signs and symptoms of *adenomyosis* may include heavy menstrual bleeding and menstrual pain that worsens with age. This condition does not lead to cancer.

Endometrial Hyperplasia

When the lining of the uterus grows too thick, it is called *endometrial hyperplasia*. This condition is not cancer, but in some cases, it can lead to cancer of the uterus. The most common sign of hyperplasia is abnormal uterine bleeding. Endometrial hyperplasia is most often caused when the *ovaries* make estrogen but not enough progesterone, which may happen during perimenopause.

Endometrial Cancer

This is cancer of the uterine lining. Common signs are irregular menstrual bleeding, spotting, and bleeding between periods. *Endometrial cancer* is caused by overgrowth of endometrial cells. The lining of the uterus may get thicker in places and form a mass of tissue called a tumor. The most common type of endometrial cancer, type 1, grows slowly. It is most often found only inside the uterus. Type 2 is less common. It grows more quickly and often spreads to other parts of the body.

Testing for Abnormal Bleeding in Perimenopause

You can talk with your ob-gyn about your bleeding changes during an office visit. Your ob-gyn should review your personal and family health history, including your current or past health conditions, surgical procedures, pregnancy history, medications, supplements, and the *birth control* method you may be using. A physical exam and *pelvic exam* will allow your ob-gyn to look for signs of diseases that can cause abnormal bleeding. A pelvic exam can also check for abnormalities, such as growths on the uterus or ovaries.

In some cases, your ob-gyn may order lab tests. A *complete blood count (CBC)* checks the blood for a range of conditions. These could include *anemia*, thyroid disease, infections, or bleeding disorders. A blood ferritin level checks iron stores—low iron levels can cause fatigue even if anemia is not found. Pregnancy and *sexually transmitted infection (STI)* testing may also be done, especially if there's a chance you could be pregnant or have been exposed to an STI. Some STIs can cause vaginal bleeding between periods and after sex.

Based on your symptoms, age, and weight, other tests may be needed. Some tests create images of your uterus and others are used to take a tissue sample for testing. Many of these procedures can be done in your ob-gyn's office.

Some tests require an empty *bladder*. Some require that you don't eat or drink for several hours beforehand. Ask your ob-gyn how to prepare and what to expect.

Transvaginal Ultrasound Exam

In an *ultrasound exam*, sound waves are used to create a picture of the inside of your *pelvis*. A *transvaginal ultrasound exam* uses a *transducer* that is shaped like a wand. It is covered with a latex sheath, like a *condom*, and lubricated before it is inserted into the *vagina*. You may be asked to empty your bladder before the test. You may feel some mild discomfort, but usually there is no pain with this procedure.

Hysteroscopy

Hysteroscopy uses a *hysteroscope*, a thin, lighted telescope that is inserted through the vagina and *cervix* and into the uterus. The hysteroscope sends an image of your uterus to a video screen. A fluid, such as saline (salt water), is put through the hysteroscope into the uterine cavity to expand it. This fluid helps your ob-gyn see the uterine lining and openings of the *fallopian tubes*. If you need a *biopsy* or other procedure, your ob-gyn can use small instruments passed through the hysteroscope to collect tissue samples.

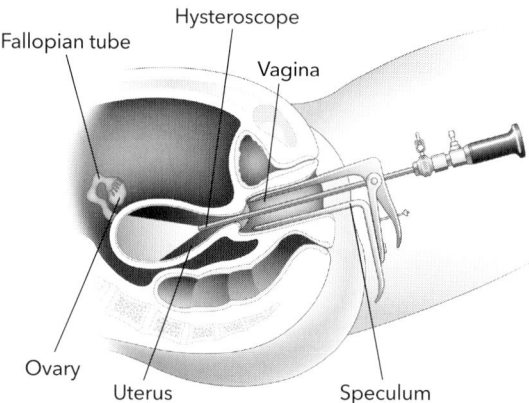

Hysteroscopy. During hysteroscopy, a thin, lighted tube is inserted into the uterus to view its lining. Some conditions can be treated with instruments passed through the hysteroscope.

Before hysteroscopy begins, you may be given a medication to help you relax, or a local *anesthetic* may be used to block the pain. If you have *general anesthesia*, you are not awake during the procedure.

Sonohysterography

Sonohysterography is a special kind of ultrasound exam. It is also called saline infusion sonography, or SIS. Fluid is put into the uterus through the cervix using a thin plastic tube. Sound waves are then used to create images of the lining of the uterus. The fluid helps show more detail than when ultrasound is used alone.

Sonohysterography is done when your bladder is empty. You may want to take an over-the-counter (OTC) pain medication, such as ibuprofen or acetaminophen, beforehand. Ask your ob-gyn what would be best.

Endometrial Biopsy

Endometrial biopsy uses suction to remove a small sample of tissue from the endometrium. A thin tube is passed through the cervix and into the uterus to take a sample. The sample is then sent to a lab where it is looked at under a microscope.

Endometrial biopsy is uncomfortable and can cause painful cramping. Taking ibuprofen or acetaminophen before the procedure may help with pain. Your ob-gyn may also use a numbing medication on your cervix to reduce pain.

Medications for Abnormal Bleeding in Perimenopause

Together you and your ob-gyn will discuss test results, diagnoses, and possible treatments. Depending on the cause of bleeding during perimenopause, medications are often tried first to treat irregular or heavy menstrual bleeding.

Combined Hormonal Birth Control

This is birth control that combines estrogen and *progestin* in a pill, patch, or vaginal ring. One effect is to thin the endometrium, which lightens menstrual flow and makes bleeding more regular. Combined hormonal birth control can be used to treat problems with ovulation, *polycystic ovary syndrome (PCOS)*, and fibroids.

When taken or used daily without a break, these methods can reduce the number of periods or stop them completely. Estrogen and progestin medications should not be used if you have a history of blood clots in the leg or lungs.

Progestin-Only Hormonal Methods

Progestin-containing methods of birth control, which include the hormonal *intrauterine device (IUD)*, progestin-only pills, and the birth control injection, keep the endometrium from growing too thick before a *menstrual period*. The hormonal IUD and injections may stop bleeding completely after 1 year of use.

Hormone Therapy

Treatment with estrogen and progestin can thin the endometrium and stop heavy bleeding caused by hormonal shifts during perimenopause. In addition, *hormone therapy* can treat other perimenopausal symptoms, such as *hot flashes*, night sweats, and vaginal dryness.

Irregular bleeding can continue after starting hormone therapy, but over time it may diminish or go away completely. Before deciding to use this therapy, weigh the benefits and risks based on your symptoms and your personal and family medical history. Read Chapter 17, "Hormone Therapies," for more details.

GnRH Medications to Treat Fibroids

These medications, also called *gonadotropin-releasing hormone agonists* or antagonists, directly or indirectly stop the ovaries from making estrogen and progesterone. This then stops the menstrual cycle and reduces the size of fibroids. These medications are used only for short periods, usually 6 months or less, so their effect on fibroids is temporary. Once you stop taking medication, fibroids may return to their original size.

> **Can fibroids go away by themselves?**
>
> Estrogen levels in the body have long been thought to cause fibroid growth. In women who take medication to reduce estrogen production, fibroids can decrease in size. Fibroids may also get smaller as the body makes less estrogen during perimenopause. But this is not the case for everyone. Talk with your ob-gyn about your symptoms and the best treatment for you if you have fibroids.
>
> —DR. CHARLES KILPATRICK

Tranexamic Acid

This prescription medication helps the blood to clot, which in turn reduces bleeding. *Tranexamic acid* comes in a tablet, is taken three times a day at the start of period bleeding, and should not be taken for more than 5 days at a time. It should not be used if you have a history of blood clots in the legs or lungs.

NSAID Medications

These OTC medications, also called *nonsteroidal anti-inflammatory drugs*, reduce *prostaglandins*, chemicals made by the body that cause the muscles of the uterus to contract. Reducing prostaglandins can lessen their effect on the uterus and reduce bleeding during periods. NSAIDs include ibuprofen and naproxen.

Antibiotic Medication

These medications kill or slow the growth of *bacteria*. Some bacterial infections can cause abnormal bleeding. If you have an infection, including an STI, you may be given an *antibiotic*.

Medication for Bleeding Disorders

If you have a bleeding disorder, your treatment may include medications so that your blood clots more readily, which can help reduce abnormal uterine bleeding. Your ob-gyn may refer you to a hematologist, a doctor who specializes in blood disorders.

Procedures to Treat Abnormal Bleeding in Perimenopause

If medication does not reduce your bleeding, your ob-gyn may recommend a surgical procedure.

Uterine Artery Embolization

Uterine artery embolization is used to treat fibroids without removing the uterus. Tiny particles (about the size of grains of sand) are injected into the blood vessels that lead to the uterus. The particles cut off the blood flow to a fibroid and cause it to shrink. You may have cramping and fever soon after the procedure, as well as vaginal discharge for up to a month. You may pass fibroid tissue through your vagina. It may take 2 to 3 months before you see a change in your heavy bleeding. Your fibroids may continue to shrink for a year or more after the procedure.

Hysteroscopic Polypectomy or Myomectomy

These procedures can be used to remove fibroids or polyps without removing the uterus. Using hysteroscopy means the procedures can be done through the vagina and no cutting into the abdomen is needed. This makes recovery much quicker than procedures that use incisions. You may have light vaginal bleeding or spotting and cramping for a few days to a few weeks after a procedure. There's a possibility that fibroids may return after a *myomectomy*.

Endometrial Ablation

Endometrial ablation destroys most of the lining of the uterus to stop or reduce menstrual bleeding. Endometrial ablation should be considered only after medication or other therapies have not worked. Endometrial ablation is not appropriate for those who are pregnant or may be planning for a future pregnancy.

There are several different methods of doing ablation. The type of pain medication and your recovery will depend on the method your ob-gyn has experience with. After the procedure, you may have nausea, frequent urination for a day, cramping for 1 or 2 days, or watery discharge mixed with blood for a few weeks. Ask your ob-gyn when you can go back to exercising, having sex, or using tampons. It may take several months before you see the full effects of ablation.

After ablation, the uterine lining can no longer be evaluated with imaging or biopsy. So if you have *postmenopausal* bleeding, a surgical procedure may be recommended to find the cause.

Hysterectomy

This is surgical removal of the uterus. *Hysterectomy* is used to treat fibroids and adenomyosis when other types of treatment have failed or are not an option. It is also used to treat endometrial cancer. Depending on the reason for having the surgery and your age, the ovaries and fallopian tubes may also be removed.

Hysterectomy is usually done with a laparoscopic, robotic-assisted, or vaginal procedure. Laparoscopic and robotic-assisted procedures use small cuts on your abdomen. Vaginal procedures are done through the vagina, without cutting your skin. Less commonly, an open procedure (with a larger incision in the lower abdomen) may be done. The choice will depend on why you are having the surgery and other factors, including your ob-gyn's experience.

Depending on the procedure, some people can go home the same day as their surgery or the next day. Afterward, you may feel discomfort or soreness around any incisions. Talk with your ob-gyn about pain relief. You should also ask when you can get back to normal activities.

For those in perimenopause, periods stop after a hysterectomy. If your ovaries are removed at the time of hysterectomy, you may have menopausal symptoms right away. Even if you still have your ovaries after hysterectomy, you may experience menopausal symptoms earlier than you would have otherwise.

> **If I have a hysterectomy, do I still need to see my ob-gyn?**
>
> You should continue to see your ob-gyn after you have a hysterectomy. Depending on the reason for your hysterectomy, you still may need pelvic exams and cervical cancer screening. At each annual wellness visit, you and your ob-gyn should talk about your medical history, any new symptoms, and whether you need a pelvic exam, Pap test, or HPV screening at that visit. Your ob-gyn can help with other concerns, too, such as urinary incontinence, pelvic pain, and problems with sex. They can also track your vaccine history and health screenings.
>
> –DR. ANDREW KAUNITZ

MRI-Guided Ultrasound Surgery

This is a form of "knifeless surgery" for fibroids that does not remove the uterus. It requires lying on your stomach in a *magnetic resonance imaging (MRI)* machine. This gives your doctor a detailed picture of the inside of your uterus. Focused ultrasound waves are then used to heat and destroy fibroids.

You can usually get back to your normal activities within a day of having MRI-guided ultrasound surgery. Improvements in bleeding happen within a few months. This procedure is done at specialized clinics and is not widely available.

There are other surgical options, too, including radiofrequency ablation. This procedure can be performed with the aid of a *laparoscope* or hysteroscope to identify and then heat the fibroid with radiofrequency waves. The heat causes the fibroid to shrink and die. Radiofrequency ablation is a newer procedure, but so far it has been shown to improve uterine bleeding, reduce fibroid size, and improve quality of life.

Before and After Your Procedure

Once you know which procedure you will have, you and your ob-gyn should discuss how to prepare for it. Keep these things in mind:

- If there's a chance you could be pregnant, you may be given a pregnancy test. These procedures should not be done during pregnancy.

- If you have off-and-on abnormal bleeding, or bleeding that will not go away, you may be given a medication to stop the bleeding before the procedure.

You and your ob-gyn should also talk about what to expect in recovery. Most people go home the day of their surgery, but if your pain is not well controlled, you may spend a night in the hospital.

If you have general anesthesia, you will be in the recovery room for a few hours. You may feel sleepy and nauseated. If you have outpatient surgery, you will stay in the recovery room until your pain is well controlled, you can stand up without help, you can tolerate liquids, and you can completely empty your bladder. You must have someone drive you home.

You may feel tired for a few days. Your ob-gyn will let you know when you can get back to your normal activities. For minor procedures, this is often 1 to 2 days afterward. For more extensive or complex procedures, like a hysterectomy, it can be longer, perhaps as long as 4 to 6 weeks.

At home, your pain can be managed with ibuprofen or acetaminophen. In some cases, you may go home with a prescription for pain medication. If you develop a temperature of 101 °F (38.3 °C) or higher, contact your ob-gyn right away. Also watch for pain that is severe or gets worse, heavy vaginal bleeding, foul-smelling vaginal discharge, worsening redness, pain or pus around incisions, flu-like symptoms, nausea or vomiting, or difficulty urinating. Call your ob-gyn if you have any of these symptoms.

Your ob-gyn should follow up with you soon after your procedure to discuss biopsy or other results. More treatment may be needed in some cases.

Bleeding After Menopause

Changes in vaginal bleeding are common during perimenopause, but any bleeding after the final period is not normal. If you have gone 12 months without a period, you should not have bleeding or spotting. Postmenopausal bleeding can range from light spotting all the way to heavy flow, often without pain.

Some causes of postmenopausal bleeding are benign. For example, after menopause the endometrium may become too thin from lack of estrogen. This condition, called endometrial atrophy, can cause bleeding. But postmenopausal bleeding can also be a sign of serious conditions like uterine cancer.

You should not self-diagnose the cause of your postmenopausal bleeding, and it should never be ignored. This is especially important for Black women, who have historically been twice as likely as White women to die of uterine cancer—read more about this in the box "Health Disparities and Uterine Cancer." Make an appointment with your ob-gyn right away if you have bleeding or spotting after menopause.

Health Disparities and Uterine Cancer

Postmenopausal bleeding is an early symptom of uterine cancer. For Black women, who have higher rates of fibroids and irregular menstrual cycles, heavy or unpredictable bleeding is often interpreted as normal. This means that Black women have historically not received the same testing for abnormal bleeding that other groups have received. This also means Black women often have advanced disease when it is finally diagnosed. Black women are twice as likely as White women to die from uterine cancer.

There is no evidence that genetic causes are at work in the higher rates of uterine cancer among Black women. But there is strong evidence that racial bias may play a role in the treatment of Black women and other women of color. Doctors may not be aware of their own bias. Unequal treatment in medicine also stems from racism in the health care system and other parts of society. Racism shapes the policies, funding, and systems that have served–or not served–communities throughout history. This means that women of color may encounter barriers to resources that help ensure good health outcomes.

In recent years, ob-gyns and other doctors have become more aware of the needs of Black women and testing for abnormal bleeding. This is an important step in providing health care that meets all peoples' needs, regardless of race and ethnicity. Any time you have concerns about the quality of your care, tell your doctor. If you are not happy with the response, talk with the director of the clinic or hospital department where your doctor works.

It's also OK to think about switching doctors. Patient advocates, friends, and family may be able to help you find a different doctor. If you have health insurance, your insurance company may be able to help you find a new doctor, too. Any bleeding after menopause should be checked, so you should ensure you are receiving the care you need.

RESOURCES

Abnormal Bleeding Diary
acog.org/AbnormalBleeding
Online, printable form from ACOG that you can use to record bleeding changes and share with your ob-gyn.

ACOG Explains: Hysterectomy
acog.org/HysterectomyVideo
Watch this video to learn about the common reasons for a hysterectomy, different types of hysterectomy, and what side effects to expect in the recovery period.

Educational Materials
foundationforwomenscancer.org/resources/educational-materials/
This website from the Foundation for Women's Cancer offers a range of resources. These include a guide to endometrial cancer, guides and factsheets on other cancers affecting women, and free courses for people with cancer and their caregivers. Also in Spanish and Mandarin Chinese.

Uterine Fibroids Toolkit: A Patient Empowerment Guide
swhr.org/resources/uterine-fibroids-toolkit-a-patient-empowerment-guide/
The Society for Women's Health Research offers a range of toolkits, including one on uterine fibroids. The toolkits cover diagnosis, treatments, and tips for talking with your ob-gyn and other clinicians.

Uterine/Endometrial Cancer/GTD
foundationforwomenscancer.org/gynecologic-cancers/gynecologic-cancer-types/uterine-endometrial-cancer-gtd/
This webpage from the foundation of the Society of Gynecologic Oncology covers risk factors, symptoms, your first medical appointment, diagnosis, treatment, and more. Their Survivorship Toolkit helps you create a personalized health plan and record.

My Menopause
acog.org/MyMenopause
Web resource from ACOG with information on the menopause transition, signs and symptoms, treatments, and self-care. Includes the latest information from the experts in ob-gyn care, menopause stories from real women, expert columns on how to manage symptoms, Q&A articles, videos, and more.

CHAPTER 8

Mood and Memory

For Miranda, perimenopause was a tearful transition that started at 47. "I couldn't control my emotions," she says. "I cried on the train and was worried that I'd start crying at work." She struggled with appearing "weak" among her colleagues and losing her professional confidence. Miranda's doctor recognized that she had started her menopause transition and recommended a low-dose antidepressant. "She said she'd had a lot of success with it among women in menopause to control anxiety-related symptoms, and it helped me." A workplace menopause group also restored Miranda's confidence. "Being with people I'd seen doing great, hearing them say, 'I can't work, I can't even remember my dog's name'—I wouldn't have thought I was a support group person, but for me it was very positive."

Sadness, anxiety, and forgetfulness are part of life. For some women, they become more frequent and problematic during the *menopause transition*. Thanks to hormonal changes and midlife stress, the years around *menopause* are known for mood shifts and "brain fog." Some women even develop anxiety and *depression* for the first time during these years. Talking with your *obstetrician–gynecologist (ob-gyn)* can help you understand the reasons for these changes. Together you can discuss self-care and medical treatment, if needed, to improve your quality of life.

Menopause affects the brain for a few reasons. *Estrogen* helps regulate mood and cognitive function during the reproductive years. When estrogen declines during *perimenopause*, the result for many is forgetfulness, confusion, and lack of focus. Decreasing estrogen disrupts sleep, which itself can result in problems with brain function. And estrogen decline plays a role in existing anxiety and depression. Having more severe menopausal symptoms, like *hot flashes* or night sweats, may increase the risk of these symptoms.

In this chapter, we'll talk about the difference between feeling low or on edge and having a depressive disorder or anxiety disorder. We'll look at brain fog symptoms, especially memory problems, and discuss what's typical at this stage of life versus what's concerning. We'll talk about when to seek professional help for changes in mental health and brain health. And we'll address science-based ways to take care of your brain.

Am I Just Feeling Down or Is It Depression?

There's a lot going on in midlife, and you may feel sad, angry, or apathetic about things happening in your life and in the world around you. When you go through periods of sadness, you may lose interest in your usual activities for a few days. You may want to spend more time alone or cry about things that are bothering you. These symptoms are common during perimenopause. Studies have shown that women are three times more likely to have bouts of sadness in late perimenopause than they did before.

When a sad mood lasts for 2 weeks or more and interferes with everyday life, it may be depression. People with depression may have some or most of these symptoms:

- Crying often
- Feeling anxious, restless, or cranky
- Feeling empty, hopeless, guilty, or worthless
- Avoiding things that used to give them pleasure
- Feeling tired and lacking energy
- Having trouble concentrating, remembering, or making decisions
- Having less or no interest in sex
- Having trouble falling or staying asleep, waking early, or sleeping too much
- Eating too much or too little, maybe with weight changes
- Having physical aches or pains that don't seem to have a cause, including stomach problems
- Thinking about death or about taking their own life

Some women are at higher-than-average risk of depression during the menopause transition. If you have a history of depression, trauma, or *premenstrual syndrome (PMS)*, be alert to changes in your mood. Other risk factors for depression include smoking, financial stress, and limited social support. Women with hot flashes and sleep problems are also more likely to become depressed. Physical conditions that increase the risk of depression include heart disease, *stroke*, chronic pain, and *chronic fatigue syndrome*.

Depression is a mood disorder. It's not the result of something you've done or haven't done, and it's not something that will just go away by itself. You may need treatment to feel better. This is why it's important to understand how you're feeling so you can get the help you need. And remember that you are not alone.

One in 4 women with no history of depression have enough symptoms during the menopause transition to be diagnosed with a depressive disorder.

When you talk about your symptoms at an office visit, your ob-gyn may ask you to take a depression *screening test*. This is a set of questions about your symptoms. It asks about changes in your mood, sleep, appetite, energy, concentration, and more.

> **My friend uses melatonin to fall asleep. Is this safe?**
>
> Melatonin is a hormone produced by a gland in the brain. It helps maintain the cycles of sleeping and being awake. Melatonin supplements are made in a lab and marketed for insomnia because they cause drowsiness. For most people, melatonin is safe to take for short periods of time. Talk with your ob-gyn before starting melatonin so you know what dose to use. Let your ob-gyn know if you're taking an antidepressant, as melatonin may reduce the effectiveness of antidepressants, and may also worsen depression.
>
> –DR. ANDREW KAUNITZ

Is This Nervous Energy or Is It an Anxiety Disorder?

Occasional anxiety is a normal part of life, and it becomes more common during perimenopause. In a U.S. study, half of women between 40 and 55 had experienced tension, nervousness, or irritability in the previous 2 weeks. If you were anxious before perimenopause, it may continue. But some women with no history of this condition find that their anxiety rises in the years leading up to their last period. Worries related to family, health, and finances are common triggers of anxiety.

Anxiety disorders are different. They bring anxiety that doesn't go away and sometimes gets worse over time. They can cause many of these symptoms:

- Feelings of worry that are hard to control
- Feeling restless, irritable, or on edge
- Having a sense of impending danger
- Becoming easily tired
- Having a hard time concentrating, remembering, or making decisions
- Getting headaches, stomach aches, or other aches and pains that don't seem to have a cause
- Having trouble falling or staying asleep

- Avoiding things, people, or situations that seem threatening
- Having intrusive or compulsive thoughts and behaviors that disrupt daily life

Some women are at higher risk of anxiety disorder during perimenopause. If you have a history of anxiety, stressful life events, or PMS, be watchful. Hot flashes and night sweats are also linked to high anxiety. Other risk factors include having certain health conditions, such as thyroid problems, irregular heartbeat, Lyme disease, and vitamin B_{12} deficiency. There's also a higher risk of anxiety disorder for women who are worried about finances.

As with depression, there is a screening test for anxiety disorders. It may include questions about persistent worrying, restlessness, and irritability.

Treatment for Depression and Anxiety

If your emotional health issues are mild, you may be able to manage them yourself using lifestyle approaches (read the box, "Self-Care for Your Mood, Anxiety, and Brain"). If your symptoms are more severe, you and your ob-gyn should talk about them and plan for you to see a mental health specialist or neurologist.

Self-Care for Your Mood, Anxiety, and Brain

Healthy behaviors can support sleep, brain health, and mental health during the menopause transition and beyond. The behaviors that ease depression and anxiety are also important for maintaining long-term brain health. It is estimated that 2 in 5 cases of dementia could be prevented or delayed by lifestyle changes.

Remember that while small changes add up, these suggestions are not meant to pile on to your to-do list. Ob-gyns often hear women talk about being overwhelmed. Work, home, family, pets, and other responsibilities can add up, and doing more isn't always the right answer. Still, there are things you can try, including the following.

Get regular exercise. Exercise releases endorphins, natural chemicals in the body that improve mood. Physical activity is one of the best treatments for depression, anxiety, and stress. Symptoms may improve within a few weeks of starting a regular exercise routine. Higher-intensity aerobic workouts are especially helpful, but all types of physical activity have benefits. Exercise has other benefits as well. Being active throughout life

- strengthens muscles and increases flexibility
- helps build and maintain strong bones
- relieves stress and increases energy
- improves sleep quality

(continued)

Self-Care for Your Mood, Anxiety, and Brain (continued)

The Centers for Disease Control and Prevention (CDC) recommend 150 minutes of moderate-intensity aerobic activity a week, along with muscle-strengthening activities on 2 days or more a week. Another option is to do 75 minutes of vigorous-intensity aerobic activity and 2 days of muscle-strengthening activity a week. Exercising more—a total of 300 minutes (5 hours) of moderate-intensity activity a week—can help with weight loss and bring more health benefits.

Eat nutritious foods. Research has shown that diets high in fruits and vegetables may reduce some mental health symptoms. A Mediterranean diet, which includes vegetables, fruits, nuts, seeds, legumes, whole grains, fish, and extra virgin olive oil, may help keep the brain healthy. Although the American diet is high in processed foods—foods changed from their natural state and typically containing little fiber and plenty of added sugar, salt, and fat—it's best to minimize their intake. There's some evidence that highly processed foods can negatively affect brain health.

Limit substance use. Quitting smoking, reducing or stopping drinking, and avoiding illegal drugs protect your brain health. Smoking raises the risk of dementia, while quitting can lead to reduced anxiety and depression. Alcohol is linked to anxiety, depression, suicidal feelings, and psychosis. Even moderate alcohol use shrinks parts of the brain linked to memory and judgment. Chronic substance use impairs multiple brain functions and can lead to mental health disorders. If you are looking for support with substance use, review the Resources section in this chapter.

Practice mind-body techniques. Mindfulness therapies can relieve mood issues and improve quality of life. Meditation, yoga, and relaxation can support anxiety treatment. Meditation, mindfulness-based stress reduction, hypnosis, and yoga programs may also improve brain health during the menopause transition.

Spend time in nature. Spending time outdoors has benefits for mood, self-esteem, and energy. It can reduce stress and worry and may help with attention and memory. For this reason, outdoor exercise has more brain benefits than indoor exercise.

Antidepressants are medications that work to balance the chemicals in the brain that affect your moods. There are many types of antidepressants for anxiety and depression. If one type does not work for you, another may be better. Your ob-gyn may prescribe antidepressant medication, or they may refer you to an expert in mental health care. Antidepressants are often most effective when they are combined with counseling.

It often takes at least 3 to 4 weeks of taking the medication before you start to feel better. Everyone is different, so what works for one person may not work for you. Be easy on yourself while finding the medication that's right for your symptoms.

Antidepressants can cause side effects. They may include loss of sexual desire, difficulty reaching *orgasm*, headaches, nausea, diarrhea, sleepiness, *insomnia*, and feeling jittery. Side effects often are temporary. If they bother you, communicate with your doctor.

Psychotherapy or "talk therapy" is especially helpful when you're dealing with current or past life stressors. You may have one-on-one therapy (with just you and the therapist) or group therapy, where you meet with a therapist and other people with problems similar to yours. Another option is family or couples therapy, in which you and family members or your partner may work with a therapist.

Be wary of over-the-counter products that claim to heal your mood, ease your anxiety, or maintain your brain health. They may be unsafe or a waste of your money (read the box "Supplements for Mood and Memory: Are They Safe?").

Supplements for Mood and Memory: Are They Safe?

Brain supplements. Skip these. No dietary supplement has been shown to preserve thinking skills, improve brain function, or delay or prevent dementia in adults 50 and over. There's no scientific evidence for brain health supplements. Experts say the best nutrients for brain health come from a healthy diet.

Depression and anxiety supplements. Proceed cautiously. For most supplements that claim to support mental health, there is little or no evidence that they help. Vitamin D supplements have been shown to have no effect on depression, but they are recommended for other reasons, including helping the body absorb calcium. So keep taking vitamin D if your ob-gyn has recommended it.

Talk with your doctor before taking any dietary supplement marketed for anxiety or depression. Dietary supplements do not have to be reviewed by the U.S. Food and Drug Administration for safety or effectiveness, and many of the claims made for these products are unproven. Read Chapter 16, "Lifestyle Changes and Alternative Approaches," for more on nonprescription approaches to treating menopausal symptoms.

Is This Brain Fog or Am I Just Tired?

When people talk about brain fog during the menopause transition, they often mean they have a lack of focus, slow thinking, and forgetfulness. Studies show that about 3 in 5 women in midlife have difficulty recalling words and numbers, need to make lists and reminders, and forget why they're doing something.

Declining estrogen is often the culprit. Estrogen affects the levels of serotonin and dopamine, the natural chemicals in the brain that regulate mood and certain cognitive functions, including memory and focus. Brain fog is typical during perimenopause, even when a woman is getting enough good-quality sleep. Although they can be distressing, these changes are usually temporary and improve after a woman has her final *menstrual period*.

Minor issues can become much more challenging when a woman isn't sleeping well and is having symptoms of confusion or forgetfulness. Women in the menopause transition often struggle to fall asleep. If this is your experience, you may also wake often and find your nights are less restful. Insomnia is linked to poorer cognitive function, and it tends to endure beyond menopause itself. Women who've been through menopause have much higher rates of insomnia compared to men or to women who are not yet menopausal.

The risk to brain health seems to be about the quality of sleep—how fragmented it is—rather than the total number of hours. This may be why night sweats are linked to worse cognitive performance. The good news is that treating night sweats with *hormone therapy* or effective alternatives may lead to better sleep quality and improved brain health and function. There's also some evidence that hormone therapy may help protect against dementia later in life if it is started early in perimenopause and continued long-term. More studies are needed. You can read more about hormone therapy in Chapter 17, "Hormone Therapies."

Is This Brain Fog or ADHD?

Distraction, disorganization, and struggling to focus can be symptoms of attention-deficit/hyperactivity disorder (ADHD). There is little research on menopause and ADHD, though ob-gyns hear about it from patients. It's common for women in the menopause transition to find their ADHD symptoms are getting worse, or to be diagnosed with ADHD for the first time.

Here again, changing estrogen levels, and the resulting change in levels of other brain chemicals, could explain ADHD symptoms that get worse in midlife. It's possible that women with ADHD are more vulnerable to mood disorders during the menopause transition. If you're struggling with ADHD or related symptoms, talk with your ob-gyn.

> **How does cognitive behavioral therapy help with anxiety and depression?**
>
> Cognitive behavioral therapy or CBT is a short-term, goal-oriented therapy. With CBT, you can learn specific skills that help you change the way you think about and cope with problems. Goals can include helping you feel calmer and more accepting of situations and then responding in better ways. CBT may also be used to reduce insomnia and improve sleep quality.
>
> —DR. CARRIE ANN TERRELL

Is This Brain Fog or Early Dementia?

During perimenopause, 7 in 10 women report problems with their memory. Memory problems can be upsetting if you have relatives with early dementia, or if you've read headlines linking menopausal symptoms to the risk of developing dementia. You may wonder which you're dealing with—menopause and natural aging, or early dementia?

If you or a family member is concerned about your cognitive function, talk with your ob-gyn. Table 8-1, "Normal Aging vs. Early Dementia," lists signs and symptoms to think about. Before your appointment, track any changes related to memory and thinking so you're ready to share details with your doctor. You and your ob-gyn may talk about other possible causes, such as untreated anxiety or depression, stress, sleep deprivation, and some physical illnesses, such as thyroid disorders or vitamin B_{12} deficiency.

Table 8-1   Normal Aging vs. Early Dementia

Sign or Symptom	Normal Aging	Possible Dementia
Memory changes	Sometimes forgetting a name or appointment, and remembering later Forgetting a conversation you had a year ago Writing reminders and lists	Forgetting information you just learned or forgetting recent events Asking the same questions multiple times
Struggling with familiar tasks	Occasionally needing help to figure out the audio system	Difficulties getting dressed, following a recipe, paying bills, or doing household chores Taking much longer to do things

(continued)

Table 8-1 Normal Aging vs. Early Dementia (continued)

Sign or Symptom	Normal Aging	Possible Dementia
Visual and spatial challenges	Needing a new prescription for eyeglasses	Difficulty with balance, reading, or placing objects on a table Difficulty judging distance and contrast, causing unsafe driving
Communication challenges	Sometimes having trouble recalling the right word	Forgetting simple words Struggling to join in or follow conversations Substituting words—like "the thing you sleep on" for "bed"
Confusion about time and place	Not remembering which day of the week it is or why you went into that room	Feeling lost in familiar places and not knowing how you got there Losing track of dates and seasons
Misplacing things	Forgetting where you put your wallet or keys Retracing your steps to find them	Putting things in unusual places, like the remote control in the freezer Not being able to retrace your steps to find them again

To maintain your brain health long-term, it's important to manage any chronic diseases, including **diabetes** and **high blood pressure**. Persistently high blood pressure, high **cholesterol** levels, excess belly fat, and poorer cardiovascular health in midlife are all linked to increased risk of dementia later. And get your hearing checked. Poor hearing is a risk factor for cognitive problems, perhaps because the brain does not get enough stimulation.

If your doctor rules out physical health causes for your cognitive symptoms, ask if you should see a specialist. If needed, your ob-gyn can refer you to a mental health professional or a neurologist.

RESOURCES

Get Help Right Now
cdc.gov/howrightnow/get-help/index.html
Webpage from the CDC that lists hotlines for people dealing with suicidal feelings, disasters, sexual assault and domestic abuse, and mental health conditions. It also has a hotline for veterans in crisis.

How to Boost Mental Health Through Better Nutrition
nutrition.org/how-to-boost-mental-health-through-better-nutrition/

Article from the American Society for Nutrition and the American Psychiatric Association on eating better for your mental health. Includes links to articles on the Mediterranean diet.

Menopause Topics: Mental Health
menopause.org/patient-education/menopause-topics/mental-health

Information on mental health and menopause from The Menopause Society.

SAMHSA's National Helpline
samhsa.gov/find-help/national-helpline
800-662-HELP (4357)
800-487-4889 (TTY)

Free, confidential help for substance use from the Substance Abuse and Mental Health Services Administration. Available 24 hours a day, 7 days a week, in English and Spanish.

Tips and Strategies to Manage Anxiety and Stress
adaa.org/tips

Resources from the Anxiety & Depression Association of America, including blogs, videos, and webinars.

My Menopause
acog.org/MyMenopause

Web resource from ACOG with information on the menopause transition, signs and symptoms, treatments, and self-care. Includes the latest information from the experts in ob-gyn care, menopause stories from real women, expert columns on how to manage symptoms, Q&A articles, videos, and more.

CHAPTER 9

Sleep Problems

Caroline, whose periods stopped at 48, says the most bothersome part of perimenopause was its effect on her mental health and her sleep. "The sleep part really surprised me," she says. "With menopause you always hear about the night sweats and hot flashes. Those symptoms were annoying, but not as bad as the anxiety and insomnia." Caroline still has postmenopausal challenges but says talk therapy helps with her anxiety, and she combines this with an antidepressant and another prescription to help her sleep. She's also thinking about ways to improve her exercise routine. Her network of friends has helped, too. "It's so important that we talk about menopause and share our stories," she says.

How did you sleep last night? It's a common question, but during the *menopause transition*, the answer can be far from easy. Changes during *perimenopause* can rob you of sleep even if you don't have a history of sleep problems. The risk of *insomnia*, the most common sleep disorder, is high during midlife—and higher still if you have **hot flashes** or **depression**. Modern life doesn't help, with its longer work hours, increasing family responsibilities, and more time spent on phones and other devices.

Many people are not aware of how damaging lost sleep is for their health and well-being. Disrupted or insufficient sleep can affect health both now and in the future. Women are more prone to sleep problems in general, and these problems tend to get worse during the menopause transition.

In this chapter, we'll cover why sleep problems become so common during this time in life and how they make it harder to function in your daily life. We'll explore self-help strategies for sleeping better as well as medical treatments that may improve your sleep. And we'll cover the difference between sleep problems and sleep disorders and how you can get help.

What Happens to Sleep in Perimenopause

Adults typically need 7 to 9 hours of sleep every night. Routinely getting less than 7 hours leads to fatigue, low energy, agitation, daytime sleepiness, poor memory, lack of concentration, and impaired work performance. Short term, not getting enough sleep increases the risk of

- mood shifts, irritability, and anger
- accidents at home, at work, or on the road
- unwanted weight gain
- depression and substance use

Long term, the effects of inadequate sleep become more concerning, increasing the risk of

- earlier onset of diseases associated with aging, including **high blood pressure**, **diabetes**, and heart disease
- mild cognitive decline and dementia
- earlier death

Among women in the menopause transition, as many as 6 in 10 report sleep problems. These problems may be related to the transition, aging, or may signal the onset of a sleep disorder. When sleep changes stem from the transition, declining reproductive *hormones* play a role.

In younger women, **progesterone** helps with sleepiness and sleep cycles. Meanwhile, *estrogen* interacts with chemical messengers in the body that are involved in sleep. It also helps regulate body temperature and serves as a natural antidepressant. As the levels of these hormones fluctuate in perimenopause, sleep problems may come and go. Common perimenopausal changes that disrupt sleep include

- hot flashes and night sweats
- anxiety and depression
- frequent nighttime urination

Some other causes of sleep problems are not unique to perimenopause but may be more common in midlife, including

- stress related to health, work, finances, relationships, or family concerns
- use of certain medications, such as **antidepressants** for depression and anxiety, beta-blockers and diuretics for high blood pressure, **corticosteroids** for *autoimmune disorders*, bronchodilators for asthma, and medications for *seizure disorders* and thyroid diseases
- some health conditions, including **obstructive sleep apnea (OSA)**, sleep-disordered breathing, heart disease, lung disease, nerve disorders, pain, and restless leg syndrome

- use of some over-the-counter products, including decongestants, ginseng, and vitamin B_1 at high doses

Research also shows that sleep problems in the menopause transition differ based on racial and ethnic backgrounds. For example, Black, Asian, and Hispanic women report shorter sleep times, poorer sleep quality, and more interrupted sleep than White women. Some of these differences may be related to chronic stress and things that lead to stress, like discrimination.

Key Steps for Improving Your Sleep

Sleep hygiene is the term for behaviors and environmental changes that can help you sleep better. For people who don't have sleep disorders, improvements in sleep hygiene can be very effective. The focus should be on changing any habits that don't help and then developing bedtime routines and preparing your bedroom to promote good sleep.

Prioritize Sleep

When life's pressures close in, it's easy to think you can sleep less tonight to get a jump on tomorrow's tasks or responsibilities. Over time, this pattern of shorting yourself on sleep can become a habit. One way to break this cycle is to resolve to make sleep a top priority, just as you would prioritize eating better or exercising more.

> **What's the connection between sleep and mental health disorders?**
>
> A mental health disorder is a pattern of thoughts, feelings, or behaviors that interferes with your normal routine. Some common disorders include anxiety disorders and mood disorders. They both can lead to restlessness and sleep problems, but conditions like depression can sometimes make you sleep more. If your sleep troubles come with anxiety, worry, mood swings, or feeling irritable or hopeless, talk with your ob-gyn. Together you can discuss the signs of mental health conditions and who you can see for evaluation and treatment.
>
> –DR. NANETTE SANTORO

Set Your Sleep Hours

Go to bed and wake up at the same time each day, even on weekends. Use alerts to remind you to start getting ready for bed and keep your wake-up alarm time consistent. And stop using the snooze button. This can lead to patterns of fragmented sleep. It's best to get up when the alarm goes off and start your day.

Avoid Caffeine, Nicotine, and Alcohol Close to Bedtime

Substance use close to or just before going to bed can have a significant impact on sleep quality and, in some cases, whether you can even fall asleep.

- Caffeine—Consuming caffeine in the evening can throw off your internal clock. Drinking fully caffeinated coffee even 6 hours before bedtime can disrupt sleep. If you have sleep problems, limit yourself to one caffeinated drink in the morning, or switch to decaf. Also think about how much caffeinated soda and chocolate you have later in the day.

- *Nicotine*—The nicotine in cigarettes and vape pens promotes wakefulness. It's best to not smoke or vape close to bedtime and even better to quit completely. If you're planning to quit and thinking about nicotine patches, pills, or lozenges to help with withdrawal, talk with your ob-gyn about their effects on sleep.

- Alcohol—A drink before bed may seem to help you fall asleep, but alcohol can affect sleep quality and cause you to wake during the night. Over time, habitual drinking, especially before bed, continues to disturb sleep. It's not something the body gets used to. Occasional light drinking may be less problematic for sleep, but the closer to bedtime you drink, the worse it is for sleep quality.

Get Regular Exercise

Daily physical activity helps promote better sleep. It's also a key to managing stress, depression, and anxiety, all of which can affect sleep quality. When you exercise outdoors, the benefits are even greater. During the day, especially the morning, exposure to natural light is a key influence on your internal body clock. Even gray skies are much brighter than indoor lighting.

Manage Stress

Stress is strongly linked to worse sleep. Pondering unresolved issues, lying in bed worrying about sleep, and checking the time are likely to make your night worse. Relaxation and mindfulness practices have been shown to reduce stress and improve sleep. Take a half hour before bed to try something you find calming. You can read about relaxation practices in the box "The Mind–Body Connection and Better Sleep."

The Mind-Body Connection and Better Sleep

Mind-body practices are low-risk, and most can be done at home. They are best used in combination with other approaches, such as sleep hygiene improvements and medications. You may need to practice any technique regularly for weeks or months to see if it works for you.

(continued)

The Mind-Body Connection and Better Sleep (continued)

- Relaxation techniques—Guided relaxation exercises are available online. Some use imagery and mindfulness techniques to relax the mind and body. Relaxation practices may help with chronic insomnia, but more research is needed.
- Meditation and mindfulness practices—These approaches relax the mind, potentially soothing the thought processes that disrupt sleep. Some studies have found sleep benefits for women with breast cancer and older adults.
- Yoga—The practice of yoga has appeared helpful for sleep in studies involving perimenopausal and **postmenopausal** women.
- Tai chi—Some studies suggest that tai chi may be helpful for sleep problems in older adults. There is not enough evidence on whether it can treat insomnia.
- Acupuncture—Some evidence suggests that auricular acupuncture (on the outer ear) may improve insomnia.
- Music-based approaches—In a few studies, people with insomnia report some benefits from listening to music.
- **Biofeedback**—This therapy uses sensors to measure heart rate, breathing, and muscle tension. It aims to help you take control of these bodily functions, which may be helpful as you wind down before bedtime. But biofeedback has not been shown to specifically improve sleep quality.

Reduce Night Noise and Light

Even if you're used to it, noise at night (like traffic, music, and clunky plumbing) disrupts your brain activity. Ear plugs may help. So might "white noise," a steady background sound like a humming air conditioner or humidifier. White noise can also include the sounds of gentle rain coming from a device that's timed to turn itself off.

Small amounts of light can also disrupt sleep, partly because light suppresses melatonin, a hormone that helps promote sleep. Sleeping with a light on leads to less restorative sleep and more brain fog in the morning. Light exposure during sleep is also linked to health problems, including diabetes, high blood pressure, and *obesity*. Solutions include blackout shades to keep the room dark or a well-fitted sleep mask. You can also turn off devices and cover indicator lights with black tape. If you get up at night, keep the lighting low.

Unplug From Electronics

Shut off your cell phones, tablets, and laptops an hour before bedtime. Using these devices increases mental arousal. The short-wavelength blue light from screens may also disrupt your internal clock. If you must use a device before bed, dim the screen.

Experiment With Other Strategies

Researchers are still learning which behaviors and aspects of the environment make the biggest difference for improving sleep. Sleep strategies vary in their effects from person to person. Feel free to try the following and see what might work for you.

- Reconsider napping—Some sleep advice online says to avoid daytime naps, but most studies find that they don't disrupt nighttime sleep. There are exceptions, though, so find what works for you.
- Make it comfortable—Ventilate your bedroom and reduce the temperature. Ideally, the room you sleep in should be 60 to 67 °F (15.5 to 19.5 °C) overnight. Replace worn pillows and consider a new mattress if needed.
- Avoid going to bed hungry—Hunger can wake you up. But avoid eating dinner too close to bedtime. Eating just before bed can impair digestion and cause heartburn.
- Warm up—Try taking a warm shower or bath an hour or two before bedtime. Some studies have found that this can improve sleep quality and reduce the time it takes to fall asleep.
- Consider dietary changes—Some researchers have found a postmenopausal link between insomnia and a diet high in refined carbohydrates, such as white rice, pasta, and baked goods. Alternatives include whole grains, oats, and beans.
- Dedicate your bed to sleep and sex—Some people find that not using their bed for eating, reading, watching TV, or phone calls helps establish a mental connection between bed and sleep, and this makes falling asleep easier.
- If you can't sleep, get up—If you're still awake 20 minutes after going to bed, get up and do a calming activity, like relaxation, journaling, stretching, or reading. Avoid turning on overhead lights.
- Talk about sleep with your bed partner—If a partner disrupts your sleep due to different schedules, snoring, or other sleep habits, talk about options for sleeping separately for a while and see if it improves your sleep quality.
- Rethink sharing your bed with a pet—If a restless pet disrupts your sleep, try taking a break and note whether your sleep improves without them in bed.

- Talk with your ob-gyn about over-the-counter (OTC) products—You've likely seen whole shelves at the pharmacy devoted to OTC sleep aids. Some might help you, but it's best to ask your ob-gyn before spending your money on OTC remedies. Read the box "Over-the-Counter Sleep Aids: Are They Safe?" for details.

Over-the-Counter Sleep Aids: Are They Safe?

Many products are marketed as sleep aids and sold without a prescription. Check with your doctor before using any OTC products. Some can have side effects and interact with other drugs. The American Academy of Sleep Medicine does not recommend OTC sleep aids for chronic insomnia, because of limited data about safety and effectiveness.

- Antihistamines—Most OTC sleep aids contain diphenhydramine, which is used to treat allergies. This medication is not addictive but can quickly become less effective. Side effects can include daytime grogginess, a dry mouth, and constipation. In older people, they may cause dizziness or falls. Check to see if the product contains other active ingredients, such as a pain reliever.

- Melatonin—Used correctly, lab-made melatonin supplements may help people fall asleep a little more quickly and sleep a little longer. Melatonin is not habit-forming. Studies have shown that the amount of melatonin in supplements is often very different from the amount stated on the label. Look for the "USP Verified" mark for more accurate labeling.

- Cannabinoids—Products made from the cannabis plant may contain THC (which can get you high), CBD (which does not get you high), or both. They may be edible, smoked, or vaped. The effects on sleep vary and the evidence is mixed. Products may not contain the dose indicated on the label. THC can disrupt sleep cycles. Your sleep may get worse when you stop using them.

- Magnesium—This mineral may help soothe brain activity and affect levels of natural melatonin, but studies on sleep have had mixed results. Magnesium supplements are safe in low doses. They may cause drowsiness, muscle weakness, nausea, and (in high doses) heart rhythm problems. You can get magnesium safely from eating fish, soy milk, beans, green leafy vegetables, and some nuts and seeds.

- Herbal products—Chamomile or valerian products may bring on drowsiness. Kava is sometimes used for anxiety, stress, or restlessness, but it carries a risk of liver damage.

What Happens With Sleep Disorders

There are more than 80 types of sleep disorders, and some are more common than others. This chapter will discuss insomnia, OSA, and restless leg syndrome, as they are among the most common.

Insomnia

If you've made changes to help with better sleep and still can't get the quality sleep you need, you may have insomnia, the most common sleep disorder. Insomnia is sometimes its own diagnosis and sometimes a symptom of an underlying health condition. You may have insomnia if you

- have a hard time falling asleep or staying asleep
- are a light sleeper when you do sleep
- feel fatigued during the day
- find your daily functioning or mood worsening
- worry about sleep and what will happen if you do not sleep
- feel like you need to sleep at times that are out of sync with your work or social schedules

In the U.S., 3 in 10 adults have symptoms of insomnia. This includes 1 in 10 whose insomnia is bad enough to affect their daytime functioning. Many of these people are women in the menopause transition. Insomnia increases the risk of high blood pressure, heart disease, and diabetes.

> **What type of doctor treats sleep problems?**
>
> Sleep specialists are medical doctors who are usually neurologists, pulmonologists, or psychiatrists with training in sleep medicine. They can diagnose sleep disorders, often with a sleep study, and advise on the best treatment options. If you think you need to see a sleep specialist, talk with your ob-gyn or primary doctor. Based on your symptoms, they should be able to refer you to a specialist who can help.
>
> –DR. CARRIE ANN TERRELL

Obstructive Sleep Apnea

If you seem to be sleeping through the night yet wake up feeling tired, you may have OSA. This disorder causes breathing to stop and restart many times during the night. Sleep is interrupted when you wake up just enough to restart breathing, but you're often not aware this cycle is happening. The next day, you may feel sleepy, moody, and forgetful. OSA is important to recognize and to treat because it raises the risk of depression, diabetes, high blood pressure, heart disease, and stroke. Often a person learns they have a problem when a bed partner notices snoring or pauses in breathing overnight.

OSA is generally more common in men—until the menopause transition, when the gender gap narrows. After menopause, as many as 2 in 3 women develop this disorder but many are not diagnosed or treated. While men with this disorder tend to snore heavily, women's symptoms may be more subtle.

Obesity is a major risk factor for obstructive sleep apnea. Diabetes and other metabolic diseases also increase the risk. OSA is diagnosed with an overnight sleep test.

Restless Leg Syndrome

With this condition, sleep is disrupted due to irresistible urges to move the legs. Sometimes this comes with burning, tingling, or other uncomfortable sensations in the legs. It can be due to an underlying medical condition, so your ob-gyn may recommend additional testing or refer you to sleep specialist if this is the reason for your poor sleep.

Treatments for Sleep Disorders

Depending on the disorder, treatments may include medication in combination with mind–body approaches (for insomnia) and breathing machines (for obstructive sleep apnea).

Cognitive Behavioral Therapy

Cognitive behavioral therapy (CBT) for insomnia, also called CBT-I, combines talk therapy with behavioral approaches that change your sleep habits. For example, you might limit the time you spend in bed, training yourself to associate bed with sleep only. CBT-I usually involves 4 to 8 sessions with a clinician over several weeks. The American Academy of Sleep Medicine highly recommends CBT-I for insomnia, and the U.S. Department of Veterans Affairs offers a free CBT-I app. See the Resources section at the end of this chapter for information.

Devices to Treat Sleep Apnea

If you have OSA, a CPAP machine may be recommended. CPAP stands for "continuous positive airway pressure." At night, you breathe through a mask over your nose and mouth, and a pump keeps your airway open. This can feel awkward at first, though most people get used to it. Various surgeries can also treat this condition. Mild to moderate cases can be treated with mouthguards.

Medications

Sleep medications have become safer than in previous decades. Still, they are usually prescribed for short-term use, and not every night. This is because some sleep medications can disrupt your sleep cycle or lead to dependence. Your doctor will likely expect you to work on sleep hygiene, too. Medications may include the following:

- Antidepressants—At lower doses, some sedating antidepressants, like trazodone and mirtazapine, can help with insomnia. Doxepin can help some people stay asleep.

- Orexin receptor antagonists—These medications block the action of a brain chemical that helps you stay alert. Suvorexant can help people fall asleep and stay asleep.

- "Z" drugs—Zolpidem and zaleplon can help people fall asleep. Eszopiclone can help people fall asleep and stay asleep. These work similarly to an older type of sleep medication but are less habit forming. A downside is that they can increase the risk of car accidents and falls.

- Melatonin agonists—Ramelteon can help people fall asleep. It is a prescription medication, not the supplement that is sold in pharmacies and online.

- *Hormone therapy*—Combined hormone therapy—using estrogen and progesterone—is not prescribed for sleep problems, but those using it for hot flashes and night sweats may find that they fall asleep more easily, stay asleep longer, and sleep more soundly. Research suggests that women using the estrogen patch with oral progesterone have the most sleep benefits.

- Gabapentin—This medication, also sometimes used for night sweats, can be used for restless leg syndrome.

When to Talk With Your Doctor

By itself, sleep hygiene is unlikely to "cure" significant insomnia or other sleep disorders. If you are consistently sleeping poorly, you'll notice the effects. If you rely on caffeine to get through the day or count on weekends for "catching up on sleep," review your sleep situation. It's time to talk with a doctor if

- you routinely have trouble falling asleep, staying asleep, or both

- you go to bed at a reasonable time and feel like you're sleeping OK, but are often tired or exhausted during the day

- your insomnia causes significant stress or anxiety
- a bed partner has noticed that you snore or your breathing often pauses while you're asleep

You can talk with your *obstetrician–gynecologist (ob-gyn)* or primary doctor about your sleep symptoms, the possible causes, and what you've tried to do about it. Keeping a sleep diary can be very helpful for this discussion. Your doctor may refer you to a mental health specialist or sleep specialist for a treatment plan that may include a sleep study. This involves staying overnight in a specialized sleep center where your sleep stages are monitored as you sleep. Sleep studies can help diagnose OSA, restless leg syndrome, and other disorders.

RESOURCES

CBT-i Coach
mobile.va.gov/app/cbt-i-coach

Free app from the U.S. Department of Veterans Affairs that can guide you through creating good sleep routines, improving your sleep environment, and addressing insomnia.

Sleep Disorders
sleepeducation.org/sleep-disorders/

Guide from the American Academy of Sleep Medicine that describes a wide range of sleep disorders, their symptoms, and treatments.

NSF Sleep Diary
thensf.org/nsf-sleep-diary/

Resource from the National Sleep Foundation that includes a sleep diary and tips for using it.

What Is Obstructive Sleep Apnea in Adults?
site.thoracic.org/advocacy-patients/patient-resources/what-is-obstructive-sleep-apnea-in-adults

Detailed FAQ on sleep apnea symptoms and treatments from the American Thoracic Society.

Women & Sleep Apnea
swhr.org/swhr_resource/women-sleep-apnea/

Sleep apnea guide from the Society for Women's Health Research with daytime and nighttime clues, who's at risk, and why it matters.

My Menopause
acog.org/MyMenopause

Web resource from ACOG with information on the menopause transition, signs and symptoms, treatments, and self-care. Includes the latest information from the experts in ob-gyn care, menopause stories from real women, expert columns on how to manage symptoms, Q&A articles, videos, and more.

CHAPTER 10

Sexual Health

Kari started missing periods in her late 40s. A year later, her periods stopped. Her perimenopause was short, but it had a big impact on her sex life. "My sex drive started to wane, and I had vaginal dryness," she says. Kari spoke with her ob-gyn, who recommended some treatments that didn't work for her. Meanwhile, Kari and her partner found a lubricant that worked and felt natural. Then she tried vaginal estrogen prescribed in tablet form. "This has been magic," Kari says. "It's a little pill you insert twice a week, and it's been a miracle drug for me. With all the trial and error, this is the thing that has worked the best."

It can be challenging to find positive messages about sex and aging. Movies and television readily focus on the sex lives of young people. But aging doesn't spell the end of sexual activity. People over 50 may engage in everything from masturbation, kissing, and fondling to oral sex and vaginal *penetration*. Even among those who aren't sexually active now, interest in sexual expression can remain high, regardless of age.

In the most recent National Poll on Healthy Aging, more than half of women aged 50 to 64 reported being sexually active in some way in the last year. Among those 65 to 80, the number was 3 in 10. Overall, women 50 to 80 reported being satisfied with their sexual activity. But 1 in 4 said menopausal symptoms interfered in some way with their ability to have or enjoy sexual activity.

This is where *obstetrician–gynecologists (ob-gyns)* come in. They understand that sex activity, including solo sex, can improve well-being, increase vitality, relieve stress and anxiety, and increase the joy of living. And they know from many years of clinical experience that the right health care can help preserve sexual fulfillment. If loss of desire, reduced arousal, vaginal dryness, vulvar irritation, pain, or other menopausal symptoms have affected your interest in or ability to be comfortable with sex, you and your ob-gyn can work together to find solutions.

In this chapter, we'll talk about how changes in sexual health, interest, and response may be related to the *menopause transition*. We'll discuss the treatments and self-care that may help. And we'll look at how to talk with your ob-gyn, how to talk with a partner, and how to protect your sexual health if you start a new relationship.

Sexual Health in Midlife

If you're wondering why **sexual intercourse** or other activity doesn't feel the same anymore, physically or emotionally, you're not alone. While some people maintain sexual desire and functioning as they age, many others struggle. The sections below outline some changes that are common. If you read something that sounds familiar, make an appointment to see your ob-gyn.

Problems With Desire, Arousal, and Orgasm

People with low desire for sex typically do not have sexual fantasies and are not motivated to be sexually active. Low desire can be caused by age-related health problems, side effects of medication, anxiety, **depression**, relationship issues, or low levels of sex **hormones**. People with low arousal find it hard to become physically excited during sexual activity, even if they feel desire. Low arousal can be caused by some of the same things as low desire.

For some women, low desire or arousal may be caused by **sexual interest/arousal disorder**. This disorder is more than loss of sexual interest. It may be diagnosed when a lack of interest in sexual activity comes with no fantasies and no response to sexual stimulation, goes on at least 6 months, and causes significant worry.

Some women report a reduction or loss of sensation in the **vulva**, **vagina**, or **clitoris**. And others may report an inability to achieve **orgasm**. Not being able to have an orgasm can be caused by anxiety, depression, stress, medication, and health problems. But it can also be caused by an orgasm disorder, which may be diagnosed if the inability to reach orgasm goes on for at least 6 months and causes persistent worry. Fortunately, there are treatments for these conditions.

Discomfort During Sex

This is a major complaint during the menopause transition. Declining **estrogen** causes vaginal dryness and irritation, and many women also report genital itching, burning sensations, and vaginal discharge. Some women even report vaginal discomfort doing nonsexual activities, including exercise, or just sitting for too long. Left untreated, all of these can lead to an avoidance of intercourse and the discomfort that may come with it.

Pain During Sex

Painful sex affects 3 in 4 women in their lifetimes, and it is more common during **perimenopause** and after the last period. Pain may be located around the vulva, in the area surrounding the opening of the vagina, within the vagina, or in the **perineum** (the area between the vagina and **anus**). It's also common to feel pain in the lower back, pelvic region, **uterus**, or **bladder** when having sex. Genital and pelvic pain can be caused by the following:

- *Genitourinary syndrome of menopause (GSM)*—This is a collection of symptoms that are caused by declining estrogen. Symptoms may include vaginal and vulvar dryness; a narrower, shorter, and less elastic vagina; and tissue that easily tears and bleeds.

- *Dyspareunia*—This is pain with penetration. If your vaginal muscles clench when you attempt intercourse or try to use sex toys, or if you have burning or pain with penetration, you may have *genito-pelvic pain and penetration disorder*. The causes may be physical, emotional, or both. For example, tight *pelvic floor* muscles can sometimes be related to past trauma. Treatment involves addressing the underlying causes.

- *Pelvic organ prolapse*—Prolapse happens when one or more organs in the *pelvis*—the vagina, uterus, bladder, *urethra*, small intestine, or *rectum*—drop from their normal position. It's caused by a weak pelvic floor, the collection of muscles, *ligaments*, and connective tissues that hold these organs in place. When a pelvic organ drops, it may bulge into another organ. In some cases, the organ may bulge into or out of the vagina. This can lead to pain during intercourse or an inability to have sex with penetration.

- Other medical conditions—Vaginal infections, *sexually transmitted infections (STIs)*, *pelvic inflammatory disease*, bladder or bowel syndromes, mood disorders, and tenderness in the pelvic floor or abdominal wall can all cause pain during sex. Pain can also result from past trauma, including sexual or physical abuse.

Midlife Health Problems

Overall health plays a big role in whether someone continues to see sex as important. Typically, people in midlife and beyond who have had recent sexual declines also report health problems like *diabetes* or heart disease. Conditions such as **high blood pressure**, **urinary incontinence**, cancer, or **stroke** can affect interest in sexual activity. And certain prescription medications, especially for anxiety and depression, can cause sexual problems. Also, adults with health problems may believe they should not have sex, or they may find sex tiring or uncomfortable. They may also assume sexual problems are just part of aging and not talk with a doctor or seek treatment.

Mental Health Challenges

Mental health is key, as well. Anxiety and depression become more common during the menopause transition, and those with these conditions have a higher risk of sexual problems. In particular, anxiety about the changes in your body can interfere with enjoyment of sex, but worries about anything going on in your life can affect your desire for sexual activity. Sexual issues can also be caused by past trauma, substance use disorders, sleep problems, and relationship struggles. Depression and depressive symptoms are also strongly associated with a lack of interest in sex.

Changes in Sexual Relationships

As partners move through midlife together, sexual problems can affect communication between them. Male partners can develop sexual side effects of medication, such as erectile dysfunction, or orgasmic dysfunction. Female partners can have sexual side effects from health conditions or medication. Changes can be so significant that partners avoid talking about them. Licensed sex therapists or couples counselors can help you talk about what you're going through and any relationship issues that interfere with your ability to have a satisfying sexual life. For discussion of how to talk with a partner on your own, read the section "When to Talk With a Partner."

Treatments for Sexual Problems

Talking with your ob-gyn is the first step toward finding answers. Bring a list of symptoms to your office visit so you can discuss specific issues, like vaginal dryness or pain, and how they feel. Being able to explain which aspects of sexuality and sexual response—interest, arousal, orgasm, or sexual pain—are bothering you will help direct the conversation.

Your ob-gyn may review your health history and ask about your partners, relationships, life stressors, sleep, body changes, and substance use. Your ob-gyn may also do a *pelvic exam*. This might include using a cotton swab to gently touch different areas so you can identify where you have the most pain or discomfort. It may also include taking small skin samples for a *biopsy* to rule out infections or skin issues.

If needed, your ob-gyn may refer you to a urogynecologist or a clinician with expertise in sexual dysfunction. This could be a sex therapist, psychologist, psychiatrist, relationship counselor, pelvic floor physical therapist, or pain specialist. Depending on the problem and any underlying issue, treatments may start with psychological or sex therapy. Other options may include topical *hormone therapy* or oral medications.

> **It's hard for me to talk about sex. How can I start the conversation with my ob-gyn?**
>
> You can open the door to discussion with a simple statement like "I have some concerns about my sex life," or "I've been having trouble with physical intimacy." Your ob-gyn should pick up on your comment and ask questions about what's going on. Your care should be a partnership with your ob-gyn, and your sexual health is as important as any other aspect of your health. So speak up and let your ob-gyn know what's going on.
>
> –DR. CHERYL IGLESIA

Cognitive Behavioral Therapy

Cognitive behavioral therapy, also known as CBT, addresses beliefs, thoughts, and behaviors that may be contributing to a sexual problem. It involves improving communication skills, and it may include sensory touch exercises without sexual pressure. CBT may be helpful for improving low sexual interest.

Mindfulness-Based Therapy

This therapy helps people be in the moment during sexual activity and be more aware of pleasurable sensations. It has been shown to improve sexual interest and arousal and help with difficulty reaching orgasm. Depending on the problem, self-care can also play a role in sexual comfort. Read the box "Self-Care for More Comfortable Sex" for some things to try.

Self-Care for More Comfortable Sex

When physical changes affect sexual comfort, it may be helpful to consider self-care measures. The following tips can help with some issues, but if pain is the biggest problem, see your ob-gyn.

- Use a lubricant—Water-soluble lubricants are a good choice if you experience vaginal irritation or sensitivity. Silicone-based lubricants last longer and tend to be more slippery than water-soluble lubricants. Do not use petroleum jelly, baby oil, or mineral oil with latex **condoms**. They can dissolve the latex and cause the condom to break.

- Try sexual activities that do not cause discomfort—For example, if penetration is difficult right now, you and your partner may want to focus on oral sex or mutual masturbation. You can also incorporate massage to maintain physical connection.

- Add steps to relieve discomfort before and after sex—These can include taking an over-the-counter pain reliever before intercourse and using cold to relieve burning after intercourse. You can wrap a frozen gel pack in a small towel and apply to the vulva for a few minutes.

- Make time for solo sex—Masturbation and tuning in to your body can help you learn what feels good in this stage of life. This can be satisfying on its own and can also help you talk with your partner about what you need.

- Make time for partner sex—Set aside a time when neither you nor your partner is tired or anxious. Tell your partner where and when you feel discomfort, as well as what activities you find pleasurable. It's also good to check in and ask if your partner's needs and desires have changed as well. If they feel something might be off with their sexual health, encourage them to see their doctor.

Sexual Skills Training

This addresses difficulty reaching orgasm. It may involve instruction in masturbation and using erotic stimuli, vibrators, or sex toys. Treatment may aim to improve communication with partners about sexual needs and preferences, increase comfort with your bodies, and challenge beliefs linked to sexual guilt and shame. Training may also be able to address a partner's health issues, including erectile dysfunction, and the impact on a relationship.

Pelvic Floor Physical Therapy

Pelvic floor weakness or tightness can result in pain during sex, trouble with penetration, and vulvar pain. Pelvic floor physical therapy helps restore muscle function and relieve pain. Physical therapists may use a range of techniques, including exercises, manual therapy, electric stimulation, *biofeedback*, and ultrasound. They may also recommend you work with vaginal dilators at home. These are tube-shaped devices in different sizes that you insert in your vagina and leave in place for short periods of time. When used correctly, dilators can help overcome vaginal muscle spasms and make penetration easier. And depending on the cause of your pain, *Kegel exercises* may also be recommended. Read more in the box "How Kegel Exercises Can Help With Sexual Function" for details on how these exercises are done.

Trigger-Point Injections

This approach can also decrease vaginal pain and sex-related pain. It is used to relieve chronic pain and spasms in the muscles and connective tissues. Trigger points in those tissues are sensitive to pressure. Injections of saline, *anesthetic*, or other drugs have been shown to reduce pain and improve sexual function.

Medications

Some medications can help treat sexual issues, such as low desire or pain during sex. Others can directly address uncomfortable changes in the vagina. Talk with your ob-gyn about the benefits, risks, and potential side effects. Medications include:

- Bremelanotide—This medication is used to treat low sexual desire. It's in a class of medications called *melanocortin receptor agonists*. Bremelanotide is usually prescribed for women who are still having periods and is given as an injection. It should be avoided if you have uncontrolled blood pressure. It is not approved by the U.S. Food and Drug Administration (FDA) for *postmenopausal* use.

How Kegel Exercises Can Help With Sexual Function

Kegel exercises can help strengthen your pelvic floor. That's the set of muscles and tissues that support your reproductive organs, bladder, and bowel. The pelvic floor can be weakened by pregnancy, vaginal childbirth, aging, repeated heavy lifting, overweight and **obesity**, and conditions that cause chronic coughing.

A stronger pelvic floor may improve your sexual health, reduce pelvic pain, and help you reach orgasm. Kegels can also reduce accidental leakage of urine, gas, or stool. And doing them may help guard against pelvic floor prolapse or prevent it from getting worse.

For some women, tightness of the pelvic floor is the cause of their sexual pain. If you have pelvic muscle tightness, avoid Kegels unless you know they won't make your problem worse. For others, it's important to do Kegels correctly. These are the steps:

- Squeeze the muscles that you use to stop the flow of urine. This contraction pulls the vagina and rectum up and back.
- Hold for 3 seconds, then relax for 3 seconds.
- Do 10 contractions three times a day.
- Increase your hold by 1 second each week. Work your way up to 10-second holds.

Make sure you are not squeezing your stomach, thigh, or buttock muscles. You also should breathe normally. Do not hold your breath as you do these exercises. If you're unsure about whether Kegels are right for you, talk with your ob-gyn.

- Estrogen—Topical estrogen is very effective at treating vaginal changes, vulvar dryness, and painful sex that stems from them. It can be used as a cream, ring, or tablet that's inserted into the vagina. Low-dose vaginal estrogen does not appear to raise the risk of *endometrial cancer*. It may also be safe to use after breast cancer, but you should check with your oncologist.

- Flibanserin—This medication also treats low sexual desire in women who are still having periods and don't have depression. It's in a class of medications called *serotonin receptor agonist/antagonists.* Flibanserin is taken by mouth. Side effects may include dizziness, sleepiness, nausea, and fatigue. You should avoid alcohol while taking this medication. It is also not FDA approved for postmenopausal use.

- Ospemifene—This oral medication is FDA approved for painful sex and moderate to severe postmenopausal vaginal dryness. It's in a class of medications called **selective estrogen receptor modulators (SERMs)**. These medications stimulate certain bodily tissues that respond to estrogen, but not others. Before taking ospemifene, tell your ob-gyn if you have a history of stroke, blood clots, high blood pressure, high **cholesterol**, diabetes, heart disease, or **lupus**. Studies show that ospemifene is not linked to an increased risk of breast cancer or endometrial cancer.

- Prasterone—This FDA-approved medication is inserted into the vagina for the treatment of moderate to severe pain during sex. It's made of a synthetic form of DHEA, a steroid naturally found in the body. When prasterone is placed in the vagina, the tissues convert it into **androgens** and estrogen, which restore lubrication. DHEA has been studied as an effective treatment for women with a history of breast cancer, who are at higher risk of severe vaginal dryness. Still, more studies are needed to learn if DHEA is safe for use after breast cancer recovery. This medication is not linked to endometrial cancer.

- *Testosterone*—If you follow social media, you may have heard that testosterone can help with low libido. Testosterone is not FDA approved to treat low sexual interest in women, in part because of the risks. These include cholesterol problems, excess hair growth, and acne. And there are no long-term studies that look at the effects of testosterone use on future breast cancer or cardiovascular disease.

  But there is some evidence that testosterone can help those with sexual interest or arousal disorders. For postmenopausal women with a disorder, testosterone can be considered. If this describes you, you and your ob-gyn can work together to determine if a trial of testosterone is a reasonable option despite the possible risks and unknowns. But avoid using testosterone pellets. There's not enough safety data on pellets, and there's a risk of getting too much of the hormone.

When to Talk With Your Ob-Gyn

The best time to talk with your ob-gyn is when you first notice discomfort, pain, or other symptoms that negatively affect your sex life. It's best not to delay. The sooner you seek help, the better.

There are good reasons to address sexual problems. Sexual activity benefits your health. It improves blood circulation, supports muscles and joints, and may help maintain brain health. And research suggests that among older adults, the quality of sex, frequency of sex, or both are linked to reduced risk of heart disease, prostate cancer, and breast cancer.

Midlife women and people of all sexual and gender identities, partnered or single, can talk with their ob-gyn about sexual intimacy and satisfaction in all its forms. Remember that your ob-gyn hears questions about sexual health every day. No questions or concerns are off limits.

> **How do I know if I'm having the right kind of sex at my age?**
>
> Fortunately, there is no "right kind of sex" at any time in life. Some midlife adults have penetrative sex less often and enjoy using vibrators and dildos, kissing and fondling, oral sex, and mutual masturbation instead. For others, romantic dates and cuddling are a means of expressing their sexuality and connection. But many midlife adults continue to enjoy the same types of foreplay and sex play they liked when they were younger. The question is what kind of intimacy is important to you now (and your partner, if you have one) and how you can get there.
>
> –DR. CARRIE ANN TERRELL

When to Talk With a Partner

If you have a partner, the best time to talk is when you first experience something that doesn't feel right. If pain or discomfort are your main concerns, it's likely your partner will want to know if there's treatment that can help. It is the same with low desire or trouble with arousal. If the problem is something that could benefit from therapy, your partner may be eager to know more.

Sex therapy is an effective way to explore the challenges in your relationship that are related to sex itself or the desire to be sexual with a partner. Sex therapy is a form of talk therapy and does not involve any physical contact with a therapist. Instead, a licensed sex therapist with specialized training in sexual health and sexual problems talks with you or you and your partner together, working to create a safe environment to work out issues and concerns.

Sex therapy can help you address any sexual problem that has an emotional or relationship component. Ideally, you would see a sex therapist with your partner. A sex therapist can help you adjust your thoughts, behaviors, and environments in ways that establish trust and relieve pressure. A sex therapist can help you address these issues and more:

- You and your partner have stopped having sex or are in conflict over sex.
- One of you is avoiding sex.

- Your low sexual desire is mostly about emotional or relationship challenges.
- Your sex-related problems are affecting your self-confidence.
- You're having difficulty with penetration or reaching orgasm.
- You or your partner has a history of *sexual abuse* or assault or *intimate partner violence*.
- You're in individual or couples therapy, and it's not helping address your sex issues.

If you think sex therapy could be helpful for you or your relationship, ask your ob-gyn to recommend a therapist or work with your insurance company to find one.

When You Have a New Partner

Rates of sexually transmitted infection have risen dramatically among older adults. Between 2012 and 2022, diagnosed cases of *syphilis*, *gonorrhea*, and *chlamydia* spiked in people over 55. In addition, more than half of diagnosed cases of *human immunodeficiency virus (HIV)* are in people 50 and older. In 2021, 1 in 6 new HIV diagnoses were in this age group.

Much of the educational messaging around sexual health is aimed at younger people. Some clinicians hesitate to talk about sexual health with older adults. As a result, these adults may lack up-to-date knowledge about sexual health, setting up a "senior epidemic" of STIs. If you start a new relationship in midlife, it's important to prioritize your health and your partner's. Here's how:

- Assume that a new partner could have an STI—Some STIs do not cause symptoms, or they can look like other conditions. Do not make assumptions about sexual health risk based on age, appearance, personality, relationship history, financial circumstances, sexual preferences, or your past relationship experiences.
- Get tested for STIs—Do this before having sex with a new partner. Your ob-gyn can do the testing. Let potential partners know that you do not have sex with anyone who has not been recently tested. Share your STI results with each other.
- Prioritize protection—Use a new condom for every act of vaginal, oral, or anal sex with a male partner. Use a *dental dam* for oral sex with a female partner.
- Talk about safer sex—Discussing dating and sexual experiences with friends can help empower you and them for safer sex conversations. Talk with your ob-gyn about how you can stay safe when starting a new relationship. And perhaps most importantly, talk with your new partner. Starting the

conversation shows you care about your health and theirs, and it can promote emotional connection.

RESOURCES

Find a Local Sex Therapist
aasect.org/referral-directory

Interactive directory from the American Association of Sexuality Educators, Counselors, and Therapists. Search by country and state.

PT Locator
aptapelvichealth.org/ptlocator

A resource from the American Physical Therapy Association for finding a licensed physical therapist or physical therapist assistant specializing in pelvic health.

In the Mood
aarp.org/membership/members-edition/in-the-mood

Website from AARP with resources on how to have great sex and improve relationships as you age. Includes tips for rekindling the spark, strengthening your sex life, healthy sex for people with diabetes, sex and dating trends, and more.

Sexual Health
healthinaging.org/a-z-topic/sexual-health

Website from the Health in Aging Foundation covering sexual problems, treatments, and lifestyle, with tips on safer sex and what to ask your doctor.

Sexual Health
ncoa.org/older-adults/health/physical-health/sexual-health

Website from the National Council on Aging with information on changing sex drive, changing bodies, the importance of intimacy, and more.

My Menopause
acog.org/MyMenopause

Web resource from ACOG with information on the menopause transition, signs and symptoms, treatments, and self-care. Includes the latest information from the experts in ob-gyn care, menopause stories from real women, expert columns on how to manage symptoms, Q&A articles, videos, and more.

CHAPTER 11

Vaginal and Vulvar Conditions

Sara's perimenopause started with vaginal changes. At 45, she needed lubricant to make sex comfortable, something she hadn't needed in the past. And despite having no history of urinary tract infections, she had two close together. After reading that the hormonal changes during perimenopause can lead to vaginal symptoms, Sara began looking for medical help. Through telemedicine she found a doctor who prescribed a vaginal estrogen cream, which Sara applies internally and externally. "After a couple of weeks, I had more natural lubrication and elasticity," she says. "A few months in, my vagina feels back to normal."

Changes in vaginal and vulvar tissues come as a surprise to many women in the *menopause transition*. It can feel hard to talk about what's happening, and it's important to know you're not alone. In surveys, up to 3 in 5 women report problems such as vaginal burning and irritation or pain during sex in the years after their last period. For some, these symptoms start in *perimenopause*. Symptoms can be uncomfortable, interfere with sleep and enjoyment of life, and change how women feel about themselves. They can also have a negative impact on intimate relationships.

Without treatment, the vaginal and vulvar symptoms of menopause are unlikely to get better and may even get worse. But many conditions are not properly diagnosed or treated. This may be because some women assume that vaginal and vulvar issues are unavoidable. They may not know they can talk about their symptoms. Or they may try to treat the problem themselves, perhaps believing the symptoms are caused by something familiar, like a *yeast infection*.

Understanding the *genital* and urinary changes that come with menopause can mean the difference between seeking treatment or suffering alone. Effective treatments are available that can ease you through midlife and beyond.

Changing Hormone Levels

Declining *estrogen* levels are the primary cause of discomfort and other symptoms of the *genitals* and *urinary tract*. Over time, the vaginal lining becomes thinner, dryer, and less elastic. The decrease in estrogen and other sex *hormones* may also thin the lining of the urinary tract.

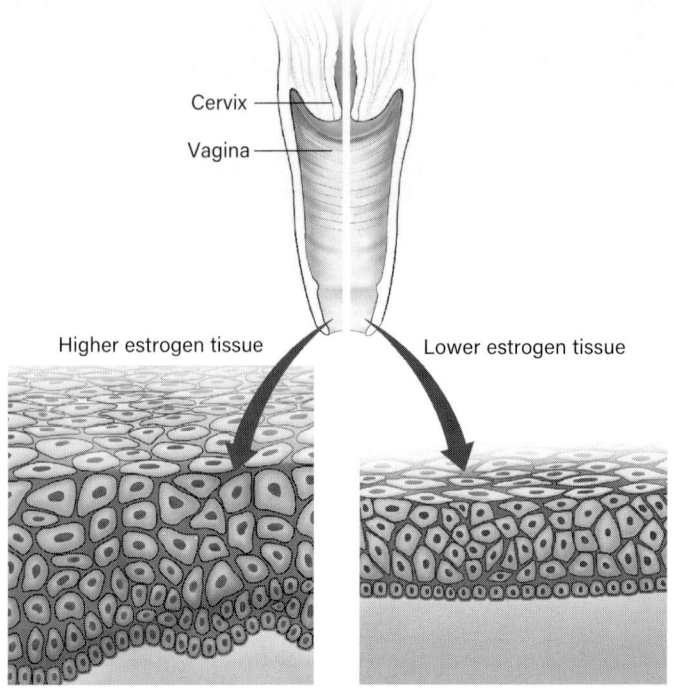

Changes in vaginal lining. During the reproductive years, when estrogen is relatively high (l.), the lining of the vagina receives more blood flow and is thicker and well lubricated. When estrogen is relatively lower, as happens after menopause (r.), the vaginal lining receives less blood flow and becomes thinner, dryer, and less lubricated. Women may feel the effects of lower estrogen in the lower vagina and around the urethra.

But there is another aspect that adds to vaginal discomfort: bacterial changes. Before menopause, the *vagina* is naturally acidic. Healthy *bacteria* in the vagina help protect it from infection. With menopausal changes, the vagina becomes less acidic. This can reduce the levels of healthy bacteria, which can lead to more frequent infections.

When women have increased urinary frequency or repeated ***urinary tract infections (UTIs)*** along with vaginal dryness, they may be diagnosed with ***genitourinary syndrome of menopause*** or GSM. Women with GSM can have most or all of these symptoms:

- Dryness—This may affect 9 in 10 women with vaginal symptoms. Most report that dryness is moderate to severe.

- Burning, irritation, and itching—This has been reported by 6 in 10 women with vaginal symptoms. Many also have irritation, soreness, and chafing of the *vulva*.

- Less lubrication during sex—This often leads to painful intercourse.

- Damage to genital tissues during sex—This may cause bleeding or spotting.

- Vaginal infections—Common infections include yeast infection and *bacterial vaginosis*.

- Other vaginal and vulvar changes—The vagina may become shorter and narrower as tissue changes. The vagina may lose the internal tissue folds that provided elasticity. Pubic hair may start thinning.

In a long-term study of vaginal changes related to menopause, 6 in 10 women reported symptoms of GSM 1 year after their final *menstrual periods*. Five years later, 8 in 10 had GSM. The takeaway? Moderate to severe vaginal, vulvar, and urinary symptoms do not get better on their own. If you have any of these symptoms, talk with your *obstetrician–gynecologist (ob-gyn)*, especially if they affect your quality of life.

Talking About Discomfort

Talking with your ob-gyn early on can help lead you to effective treatments that will improve your comfort. At an office visit, you and your ob-gyn can discuss what you're feeling and identify or rule out anything other than menopausal changes. You may also talk about factors that increase the risk of GSM, which include

- past removal of *ovaries* or cancer treatment that stopped menstrual periods

- lifestyle factors, such as smoking, heavy drinking, and not being active

- disorders of the urinary or reproductive systems

Your ob-gyn may recommend an exam to check the vulva and vagina for changes in skin color or texture as well as lesions or cracks in the skin. Sometimes a cotton swab is used to gently touch areas and identify where you have the most discomfort. If needed, your ob-gyn may recommend testing for *sexually transmitted infections (STIs)* or doing a *biopsy*, which means sending a small skin sample to a lab to help diagnose a skin condition or infection.

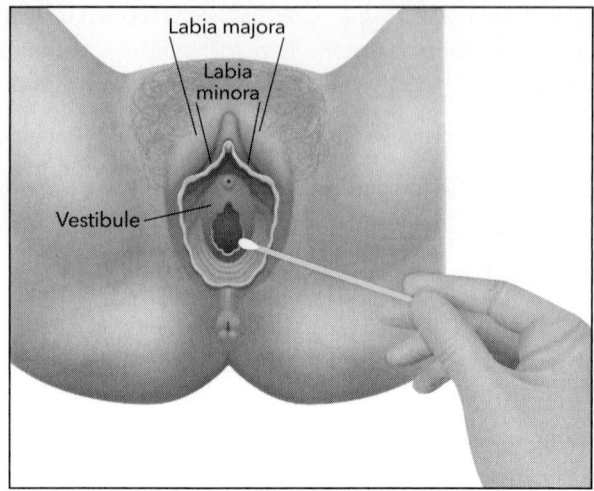

Cotton swab testing. Cotton swab testing starts with gentle touches to the thighs followed by the labia majora, labia minora, and entrance to the vagina, called the vestibule. The vestibule is tested at different positions. If you feel pain, you may be asked to describe it as mild, moderate, or severe.

Treatments for Vaginal Dryness

Once you and your ob-gyn know that your vaginal changes are related to menopause, you can start talking about treatments. Some are available over the counter. Others need a prescription. Estrogen-free treatments may be effective early on for mild-to-moderate symptoms. But it's possible that as time goes by, you may want to talk about hormonal medications, too, some of which are used on the skin.

Nonhormonal Treatments

Vaginal moisturizers are often a first-line treatment. They are designed to ease vaginal dryness with regular use and are available without a prescription. They work by trapping moisture in and around the vagina. Moisturizers may reduce itching, irritation, and pain, and help restore healthy acidity to the vagina.

In research trials, vaginal moisturizers containing polycarbophil or hyaluronic acid were effective. (Hyaluronic acid is a substance made in the body that helps tissues stay hydrated.) Food-grade oils (coconut, olive, and vegetable) can also work, but they can break down latex **condoms**. Oils can also cause allergic reactions, and they may upset the pH balance of the vagina. Talk with your ob-gyn before using one.

Vaginal lubricants ease vaginal dryness and friction and are used mostly for sexual activity. They are available over the counter. In a U.S. study, five water-based lubricants relieved dryness and pain during sex with no serious side effects. In another study, a vaginal lubricant containing hyaluronic acid improved vaginal dryness and lubrication during intercourse. For more information about sex during the menopause transition, read Chapter 10, "Sexual Health."

Hyaluronic acid for vaginal use is also sold over-the-counter as inserts, tablets, or gels. You place it in the vagina to help moisturize and protect tissues. Studies involving women in the menopause transition found that hyaluronic acid was effective at improving vaginal tissue and acidity and relieving pain during sex.

Local Hormone Treatments

Low-dose estrogen cream is very effective for vaginal and vulvar symptoms of menopause. Estrogen cream is applied directly to the vulva and in the vagina (that's why it's called "local"). The estrogen helps restore the natural thickness and elasticity of the vaginal lining and relieves dryness and irritation. Low-dose local therapy may also improve some urinary symptoms of menopause. Low-dose local estrogen does not appear to raise the risk of *endometrial cancer*. It may also be safe to use after breast cancer, but you should check with your oncologist.

Most vaginal estrogen medications are used daily for 1 to 2 weeks, then twice weekly or as needed. This treatment is available by prescription as vaginal creams or tablets. The vaginal ring releases estrogen over 3 months. Women often appreciate its ease of use and comfort. For more information, read Chapter 17, "Hormone Therapies."

> **Can I use topical estrogen long-term for GSM?**
>
> Topical estrogen for vaginal or vulvar dryness, or pain with intercourse, usually improves symptoms in a few weeks. The medication can be applied to the affected area with your finger. The time to improvement varies from person to person. The estrogen acts locally on tissues and does not go throughout the body, so you may continue to use it for as long as you like. Check with your ob-gyn if your symptoms return or do not get better with treatment.
>
> –DR. CHARLES KILPATRICK

Systemic Hormone Therapy

With this type of *hormone therapy*, estrogen is released into the bloodstream and travels to the organs and tissues where it is needed. Systemic hormone treatment is often prescribed for *hot flashes* and night sweats, but it can help relieve vaginal and urinary symptoms, too. Estrogen is available as pills, skin patches, gels or sprays applied to the skin, and a vaginal ring.

Those who still have a uterus also need to take *progestin*. This medication helps reduce the risk of endometrial cancer, which can develop over time when estrogen is used alone. Those without a uterus do not need to add progestin. Chapter 17, "Hormone Therapies," has more details on systemic hormone therapy.

Other Medications

Ospemifene is an oral medication approved by the U.S. Food and Drug Administration (FDA) for painful sex and moderate to severe *postmenopausal* vaginal dryness. It's in a class of medications called *selective estrogen receptor modulators (SERMs)*. These medications stimulate certain bodily tissues that respond to estrogen, but not others.

Before taking ospemifene, tell your ob-gyn if you have a history of *stroke*, blood clots, *high blood pressure*, high *cholesterol*, *diabetes*, heart disease, or *lupus*. Studies show that ospemifene is not linked to an increased risk of breast cancer or endometrial cancer.

Prasterone is an FDA-approved medication that's inserted into the vagina for the treatment of moderate to severe pain during sex. It's made of a form of DHEA, a steroid naturally found in the body. When prasterone is placed in the vagina, the tissues convert it into *androgens* and estrogen, which restore lubrication.

DHEA has been studied as an effective treatment for vaginal dryness in women with a history of breast cancer, who are at higher risk of severe vaginal dryness. Still, more studies are needed to learn if DHEA is safe for use after breast cancer recovery. This medication is not linked to endometrial cancer.

Other Disorders of the Vulva

In midlife, some vulvar symptoms that seem like GSM may actually have other causes, including skin conditions and *cysts*. Many vulvar conditions are uncomfortable, painful, or distressing, and some get worse over time. Some occasionally lead to cancer. It's important to talk with your ob-gyn and get the right diagnosis and treatment.

Itching and pain are two of the most common vulvar symptoms. If you have symptoms that do not go away, or that do not respond to treatment or local hormone therapy, your ob-gyn may recommend you see a doctor who specializes in vulvar skin disorders. Some disorders of the vulva include the following.

Vulvodynia

If vulvar pain lasts 3 months or longer and is not caused by an infection, skin disorder, or other condition, it may be caused by *vulvodynia*. During or after the menopause transition, the symptoms of vulvodynia may be mistaken for GSM. Vulvodynia is not caused by declining estrogen, but it may involve burning, stinging, irritation, and rawness. The entire vulva may be painful, or pain may be centered in a specific area. The pain may be constant, come and go, or happen only when the area is touched. Treatment for vulvodynia may include physical therapy for the *pelvic floor*, trigger point therapy, and *cognitive behavioral therapy (CBT)*. These may be used in addition to hormone cream, local pain relievers, or *antidepressants*.

> **I've heard about vaginal laser therapy for vaginal problems. What is it?**
>
> You may see energy-based treatments marketed as nonsurgical options for "vaginal rejuvenation." The FDA has not approved any laser or other energy-based treatment for vaginal cosmetic surgery. These treatments also have not been approved for treating menopausal symptoms, urinary incontinence, or other sexual problems. The FDA has warned that laser and other energy-based treatments can cause serious problems, including vaginal burns, scarring, pain with sex, and long-lasting pain. Your first resource for vaginal symptoms should always be your ob-gyn.
>
> –DR. CHERYL IGLESIA

Lichen Sclerosus

This skin disorder causes scarring and tightening around the genitals and *anus*. The scarring creates a pale, wrinkled look in a keyhole pattern around the opening of the vagina and anus. There may be white bumps and discolored spots. Lichen sclerosus can lead to itching, burning, tearing of the skin, or pain during sex. The condition can also shrink the *labia minora* and bury the glans of the *clitoris*. The condition may be linked to problems with the *immune system* and certain *genes*, and it carries a small risk of skin cancer. This is a chronic condition that can usually be managed with a steroid ointment.

Folliculitis

When bacteria infect hair *follicles*, it causes small, red, sometimes painful bumps. This can happen because of shaving, waxing, or even friction. Folliculitis can occur on the *labia majora*. It often goes away by itself. You can speed up the healing process by keeping the area clean, wearing loose clothing, and applying warm compresses. If the bumps do not go away or they get bigger, see your ob-gyn. You may need additional treatment.

Contact Dermatitis

Half of women with chronic vulvar itching or burning have contact dermatitis. It can be caused when the vulva is in contact with moisture, including sweat and urine. Other irritants may include cleansers, fragrances, lubricants, laundry detergents, hygiene products, medical products, and many more. Self-care includes avoiding products that irritate the vulva. Antihistamine medications can relieve itching and scratching. In some cases, a steroid ointment may be recommended for a limited time.

Bartholin Gland Cysts

The *Bartholin glands* are located under the skin on either side of the vaginal opening. They release a fluid that helps with lubrication during *sexual intercourse*. If the Bartholin glands become blocked, a cyst can form, causing a swollen bump near the opening of the vagina. If a cyst becomes infected, an *abscess* (containing pus) can form. If your cyst is not causing pain, you can treat it at home. Sit in a warm, shallow bath or apply a warm compress. But if it quickly gets larger, see your ob-gyn. The cyst may need to be drained, using a needle or other instrument, or even removed if it keeps coming back.

Lichen Planus

This condition causes scarring around the vulva and often inside the mouth. Symptoms include pain during sex, burning, soreness, itching, and increased vaginal discharge. Its effect on the skin can vary. Lichen planus can cause whiteness, pale or red streaks, or warty lesions. This condition may be linked to problems with the immune system. A full cure is unlikely, though it can be managed with steroid ointment, vaginal tablets, prescription pills, or injections. Dilators can be used to prevent scarring and structural changes in the vagina.

Lichen Simplex Chronicus

This condition causes thick, scaly patches on the vulva and intense itching. If you have this condition, you may struggle to resist scratching and rubbing. Lichen simplex chronicus can be related to excessive sweating or irritation from clothing or products. It may be linked to a yeast infection or another skin condition, like contact dermatitis or lichen sclerosus. Most women with this condition have a family history of seasonal allergies, asthma, or childhood eczema. Self-care is important to control scratching and manage new outbreaks. Treatment includes steroid ointment and anti-itch medication. Antihistamines or a type of *antidepressant* medication can also help relieve itching.

Squamous Intraepithelial Lesion

This is the presence of abnormal vulvar cells that have not yet become cancer. Squamous intraepithelial lesion (SIL) is common and often caused by *human papillomavirus (HPV)* infection. Signs include itching, burning, or abnormal skin. The skin may be bumpy or smooth, or a different color, like white, brown, or red. SIL can also affect the *cervix*, vagina, anus, and throat. It is usually found during a *pelvic exam* or skin biopsy.

SIL should be treated to prevent the development of cancer. It can be treated with laser therapy or surgery. Another option may be a cream that activates the immune system to fight abnormal skin cells.

Self-Care for Vulvar Conditions

It may seem easier to try treating a problem at home, but you should talk with your ob-gyn first to make sure you know what's causing your symptoms. Otherwise, you may mask the signs of a condition, such as itching, without treating the condition itself. You could even make it worse. Your ob-gyn can help you figure out which products you can buy for home care or recommend that you use a prescription treatment. Options may include the following.

Hydrocortisone Cream

This mild steroid cream is available at low strengths over the counter and at higher strengths by prescription. It is meant for short-term use and can reduce itching, redness, and swelling of the genital area. Do not put it in your vagina. Do not use if you have vaginal discharge that isn't normal for you, which could be a sign of infection.

Steroid Cream or Ointment

These products can be stronger than hydrocortisone. They should be used cautiously, as the long-term effects are not fully known. Long-term or improper use can cause bothersome side effects. Limit the amount used and do not apply it to normal skin. Use of steroids can raise your risk of yeast infections or outbreaks of genital herpes (if you have a history of this).

Antifungal Medications

These treat itching, burning, and rashes in the vagina or vulva caused by yeast infections. They are available as pills, creams, ointments, tablets, and sometimes vaginal inserts.

Antibiotics

Prescription antibiotic creams or pills treat vaginal and vulvar conditions caused by unhealthy bacteria and parasites. These include bacterial vaginosis and some STIs (*trichomoniasis*, *chlamydia*, and *gonorrhea*).

Other Products

Various over-the-counter products may relieve itching or irritation but will not cure the condition. Heavy-duty moisturizers help keep the skin hydrated. Local *anesthetic* gels may help reduce discomfort. Antihistamine ointments or pills may relieve discomfort linked to allergies, as in contact dermatitis. Antihistamines and anti-itch tablets can cause drowsiness and may be helpful if your symptoms interfere with sleep. Read the box "Caring for Vulvar Skin" for more on vulvar care.

> **Caring for Vulvar Skin**
>
> Taking care of vulvar skin mainly revolves around avoiding anything that could cause irritation. Follow these tips:
>
> - Do not douche or use feminine sprays or talcum powders.
> - Clean the vulva with water only.
> - Gently pat the vulva dry after bathing.
> - Apply an unscented cream without preservatives to retain moisture in the skin.
> - Rinse and dry after urinating to prevent skin irritation.
> - Avoid scented toilet paper and lotions and other products with multiple ingredients.
> - Buy unscented panty liners if you use them.
> - Use unscented lubrication for sexual intercourse.
> - Apply cool gel packs if your vulva is irritated or sore.
> - Wear 100 percent cotton underwear during the day and no underwear at night.
> - Avoid tight pants, tight underwear, or pantyhose (unless they have a cotton crotch).
> - Check your vulva every month for thickened skin patches, color changes, or sores. Use a mirror and your fingertips to check the inner and outer labia, around your vaginal and urinary openings, and between your vagina and anus. Talk with your ob-gyn about any changes.

What Menopause May Mean for Chronic Pelvic Pain

Chronic pelvic pain is pain that lasts for more than 6 months and goes beyond the genital area. In some cases, menopause can trigger a chronic pain disorder or make it worse. Some women develop *genito-pelvic pain and penetration disorder (GPPPD)*, a condition that causes difficulty or pain with vaginal *penetration*, or fear of penetration. Women with GPPPD may not be able to stop their pelvic floor muscles from clenching when they try to have sex. They often have burning around the entrance to the vagina during sexual activity.

The causes of GPPPD may be physical, emotional, or both. Typically, multiple factors contribute. These could include

- GSM

- skin disorders of the vulva, such as lichen sclerosus or a Bartholin gland abscess

- an inflammation or nerve issue

- pelvic floor muscle weakness, tightness, or dysfunction

- fibromyalgia or other full-body pain syndromes

- problems with the digestive system, such as *irritable bowel syndrome* or *Crohn's disease*

- problems with the bladder and urinary tract, such as UTIs or *cystitis*

- disorders of the uterus or ovaries, such as *fibroids* or *endometriosis*

- a history of sexual trauma or *intimate partner violence*

- anxiety, *depression*, or substance use disorder

Treatment for Pelvic Pain

If your chronic pelvic pain lasts 6 months or longer and causes you significant distress, see your ob-gyn. Treatment involves identifying and addressing the underlying causes. You may be referred to a sex counselor, psychologist, physical therapist, or pain specialist. Treatment options may include the following:

- Medication—GSM can be treated with local or systemic hormone therapy, ospemifene, or prasterone. Certain antidepressants and drugs for nerve pain might be an option. Medications are also used to treat vaginal infections, vulvar skin disorders, endometriosis, or other physical conditions that may be contributing.

- Pelvic floor physical therapy—This helps restore muscle function and relieve pain. Physical therapists may use a range of techniques, including exercises, manual therapy, electric stimulation, *biofeedback*, and ultrasound.

- Talk therapy—When sexual pain is accompanied by depression, anxiety, or social isolation, CBT can be useful. CBT helps you manage your thoughts and environment to lessen your pain perception and improve your coping skills. Mindfulness-based cognitive therapy can also be helpful.

- Sex therapy or counseling—Individual or couples counseling or sex therapy can help with emotional or relationship issues. Sex therapy may also include education. Learning about your body and the pelvic floor can be helpful.

- Trigger-point injections—These can relieve chronic pain and spasms in the muscles and connective tissues. "Trigger points" in those tissues are sensitive to pressure. Injections of saline, anesthetics, or other drugs can improve pain and function.

- Desensitizing and relaxing the genital area—Fingers or vaginal cones can help you gradually get used to touch and penetration. Dilators may ease tight pelvic muscles.

- Surgery—Rarely, pelvic pain that does not respond to other treatments can be relieved by surgery. Cutting or destroying nerves can block pain signals from reaching tissues and organs.

If you've had pelvic pain for more than 6 months, talk with your ob-gyn soon. It can take time to learn the cause of pelvic pain and more time to effectively treat it. It's a frustrating condition, but treatment is available. If needed, your ob-gyn can refer you to a specialist who may be able to help, such as a urogynecologist, gastroenterologist, or dermatologist.

RESOURCES

Improving Sexual Health: Vaginal Lubricants, Moisturizers, Dilators, & Counseling
rogelcancercenter.org/files/lubricants-moisturizers-counseling-guide.pdf
This PDF from the University of Michigan Health Center provides a detailed guide to helpful vaginal products.

Vulvar Self-Examination
vulvalpainsociety.org/about-vulval-pain/vulval-self-examination/
Web page from the Vulval Pain Society with guidance on how to check your vulva for signs of infection or disease.

My Menopause
acog.org/MyMenopause
Web resource from ACOG with information on the menopause transition, signs and symptoms, treatments, and self-care. Includes the latest information from the experts in ob-gyn care, menopause stories from real women, expert columns on how to manage symptoms, Q&A articles, videos, and more.

CHAPTER 12

Urinary Incontinence

Kristine had urinary incontinence on and off for years. At 54, her symptoms worsened and her ob-gyn recommended a physical therapist who specializes in pelvic floor issues. The therapy involves coaching for home exercises—Kegels, for example—and breathing exercises to help relieve abdominal pressure that can make incontinence worse. The therapist also manipulates the tissue that supports Kristine's pelvic organs. Scar tissue from cesarean births affects Kristine's muscle function and contributes to the incontinence, so her therapist works on breaking down that scar tissue. Several months in, the urge incontinence lessened, and Kristine is hopeful about further relief. "I'm so grateful I found this specialist," she says. "She'll continue to guide me well, I'm sure."

During the *menopause transition* and beyond, *urinary incontinence* becomes far more common. It may be a few drops of urine here and there, or a complete emptying of the *bladder*. Urinary leakage can affect your physical activity, everyday functioning, self-confidence, relationships, and quality of life.

This is not a condition that gets better on its own. One in 4 premenopausal women experiences involuntary urine loss, rising to more than half of women in midlife. Among women over 65, 3 in 4 are affected. And these numbers may not reflect how widespread the problem is because many women hesitate to talk with their doctors about it. But the truth is that most cases of urinary incontinence can be greatly improved or even cured with treatment.

In this chapter, we'll look at the different types of incontinence and other bladder conditions, what causes them in midlife, how they are diagnosed, and how treatment decisions are made. We'll also look at *accidental bowel leakage*, a condition that can create even more concern than urinary incontinence but also has effective treatments.

Types of Urine Leakage

Stress urinary incontinence is the most common type of incontinence. This is the involuntary loss of urine with physical effort or exertion, such as running, jumping, or rearranging planters on the patio. You may also leak urine when sneezing or coughing. In a U.S. study, 3 in 4 women with stress incontinence said their symptoms were bothersome—and of them, more than a quarter said they were "moderately to extremely" bothersome.

Urgency urinary incontinence is the involuntary loss of urine that comes with a sudden, strong urge to urinate. You may struggle to hold it in while rushing for the bathroom. This type tends to have a worse impact on quality of life than stress incontinence. In *postmenopausal* women—those who are 12 months or more past their final *menstrual period*—urgency incontinence becomes more common over time.

Mixed urinary incontinence is the involuntary loss of urine when there is urgency *and* when there is physical exertion, sneezing, or coughing.

Any type of incontinence can also involve pain while urinating or leaking urine while sleeping.

Overactive bladder (OAB) is the sudden urge to urinate, usually with frequent visits to the bathroom, including at night. OAB is about feeling an urgent need to urinate, while incontinence involves the loss of urine.

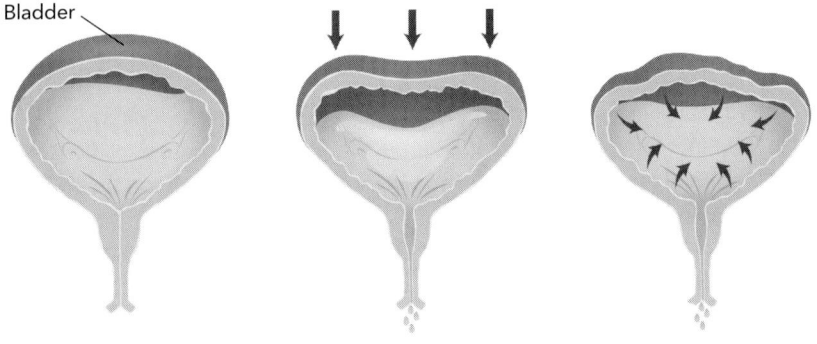

Urinary incontinence. When there is normal bladder function, the bladder is relaxed and the urethra stays closed until a person is ready to urinate. With stress urinary incontinence, the urethra is weak and does not stay closed when there is pressure in or around the abdomen, which might be caused by bending or lifting. With urgency urinary incontinence, the bladder muscles contract before a person is ready to release urine.

Urinary tract infections (UTIs) can sometimes cause urine leakage in addition to a sudden urge to visit the bathroom. In *postmenopause*, it's common to have recurrent UTIs. This is defined as at least two UTIs in 6 months, or three UTIs in a year. Studies suggest that up to 1 in 5 women between 65 and 70, and half of women 80 and older, have *bacteria* in their urine that can lead to UTIs. In older women, UTIs that aren't treated can worsen dementia and lead to a serious condition called *sepsis*.

Why Urinary Problems Are Happening Now

Urinary symptoms are caused by a combination of menopausal changes, aging, and other factors.

Declining Estrogen

Before *perimenopause*, the reproductive *hormones*, especially *estrogen*, helped support the urinary tract (the system that makes urine and removes it from your body). As estrogen levels decline, this tract weakens. The *sphincter muscles* in the bladder that control the release of urine also become less efficient.

Weakening Pelvic Floor

The *pelvic floor* is the term for the muscles and tissues that support the bladder, *uterus*, *vagina*, and *bowels*. Over time, the pelvic floor tends to lose strength and function. A weaker pelvic floor can also contribute to *pelvic organ prolapse*, a condition that causes one or more pelvic organs (often the uterus and vagina) to drop down. Prolapsed organs can press on the *urethra* and contribute to urine leakage. (Learn more in Chapter 13, "Pelvic Organ Prolapse.")

Number of Pregnancies and Births

Giving birth can weaken or damage the pelvic floor muscles. Your chance of stress or mixed urinary incontinence rises if you've ever given birth. Those who have had more than one baby are at higher risk.

Changing Vaginal Bacteria

Before menopause, the vagina supported more healthy bacteria that resist infection. During the menopause transition, changes in the vagina make it less able to fight off harmful bacteria or fungi. This, along with a weaker pelvic floor, allows harmful bacteria to enter the urethra and move up to the bladder. These bacteria can then cause UTIs.

Problems With Nerves and Muscles

People with *diabetes*, *multiple sclerosis*, Parkinson's disease, spinal cord damage, or past *stroke* can have problems with nerves and muscles. The nerve signals from the brain to the bladder and urethra may be disrupted. The muscles that control those organs can lose function and allow urine to leak.

Other Pelvic Problems

The outlet of the bladder into the urethra can become blocked by bladder stones or other growths. The urethra may develop an abnormal pouch called a *diverticulum* that causes urine leakage or dribbling. A *fistula* is an abnormal connection from the urinary tract into the vagina, which allows urine to leak out. A fistula can also develop between the large and small bowel and the bladder. Pelvic surgery, *radiation therapy*, pelvic cancer, and childbirth are other common causes of a fistula.

Other Health Issues

Chronic respiratory diseases, especially with coughing, contribute to urinary incontinence. Certain medical procedures raise the risk, too, like surgery to remove the *ovaries* and some cancer treatments. Medications that may contribute to urinary symptoms include *diuretics*, mental health medications, certain pain relievers, allergy treatments, and more.

Weight Gain

Weight gain is common during the menopause transition. Any excess weight can increase the risk of incontinence. Women with *obesity* are more than four times as likely to develop incontinence as women of average body type. We'll talk about midlife weight concerns in Chapter 14, "Weight and Menopause."

Lifestyle Factors

Your risk of urinary leakage increases with smoking, heavy drinking, caffeine use, and not being physically active. Smoking and caffeine can irritate the bladder and increase the need to urinate. Alcohol is a diuretic, which means it causes the body to increase urine production and in turn the need to urinate. And sitting for long periods of time can make incontinence worse.

Interpersonal Violence

In an international study, women who had been targets of emotional, physical, or sexual violence reported more urinary symptoms during the menopause transition. They also reported declining physical and mental health.

What You and Your Ob-Gyn Can Do

When you talk with your *obstetrician–gynecologist (ob-gyn)* about urinary problems, you'll be one of many patients who have shown up with this problem this week. Among women who are past their final menstrual period, urinary incontinence is more common than diabetes, **high blood pressure**, and *depression*.

A correct diagnosis is important for effective treatment. Your ob-gyn should ask about your symptoms, their impact on your quality of life, and your goals for treatment. They may ask you to keep a bladder diary for several days or fill out a questionnaire about your symptoms. (See the box "How to Keep a Bladder Diary.") You may need a physical exam to check for pelvic organ prolapse and pelvic muscle strength. Your ob-gyn may recommend a urine test to screen for UTIs.

> **How to Keep a Bladder Diary**
>
> Tracking your symptoms is a great way to help you and your doctor figure out what's going on and how to treat it. Symptom diaries are also effective tools for helping you change your own behaviors and form healthier habits. To keep a diary, you record the following over 24 hours:
>
> - How much fluid you drink and when (include all fluids)
> - When you went to the bathroom to void
> - How much urine you passed (use a "toilet hat" that fits under the seat and catches urine)
> - Any leakage episodes and what you were doing at the time
>
> Repeat these steps for 3 to 5 days. If you have accidental bowel leakage, you can also record your bowel movements and episodes of diarrhea, constipation, and **fecal incontinence**.

Other tests may be done as well, including a "cough stress test" while standing or lying down on an exam table to see if urine leaks when you cough. In some cases, your ob-gyn may order tests to assess how your urinary system is functioning, including whether your bladder is completely emptying when you urinate.

There are several effective treatments for urinary incontinence. Depending on test results and how much your symptoms bother you, you may choose from lifestyle and behavioral approaches, devices, pelvic floor physical therapy, medications, and surgical solutions. Often, several treatments are used together for the best results. Your ob-gyn may also recommend you see a pelvic floor physical therapist or a urogynecologist, a doctor who specializes in pelvic floor conditions.

Approaches to Try First

A good starting point for incontinence treatment is behavioral changes, which vary based on your situation. Steps could include:

- Manage weight—Losing even a small amount of weight can help decrease urine leakage.
- Manage fluid intake—If you have leakage in the early morning or urgency at night, you can try limiting how much you drink several hours before bedtime. Limiting yourself to 8 cups of fluids throughout the day may also help. (If your urine has no color, you may be drinking too much.)
- Train your bladder (timed voiding)—With bladder training, you time your urination according to a schedule. This gradually increases the amount of

urine your bladder can hold and helps you go longer between bathroom visits. Bladder training takes several months.

- Change your diet—Some common drinks and food are bladder irritants, including coffee, cola with caffeine, chocolate, alcohol, and spicy foods. Try skipping these foods and drinks for a week or two and see if it makes a difference in urgency or frequency.

- Do pelvic floor exercises—*Kegel exercises* help tone the muscles of the pelvic floor, which may help improve bladder control. Many women benefit from doing Kegels, but you should not do them if you've been diagnosed with tight or overactive pelvic floor muscles. Here's how they're done:

    1. Squeeze the muscles that you use to stop the flow of urine. This pulls the vagina and *rectum* up and back.
    2. Hold for 3 seconds, then relax for 3 seconds.
    3. Do 10 contractions three times a day.
    4. Increase your hold by 1 second each week. Work your way up to 10-second holds.

As you do these exercises, breathe normally. Make sure you are not squeezing your stomach, thigh, or buttock muscles. You can do Kegel exercises while working, driving in your car, or watching television, but don't do them while urinating. Before you start, talk with your ob-gyn or pelvic floor specialist to be sure you're doing them correctly.

Devices and Physical Therapy

If behavioral changes aren't effective enough at managing symptoms, you and your ob-gyn may talk about bladder support devices or pelvic floor physical therapy.

Bladder Support Devices

A *pessary* is a small silicone device that's inserted into the vagina to lift the bladder and urethra. Pessaries can help with stress or mixed urinary incontinence and provide immediate control of symptoms. They come in several shapes and sizes. Your ob-gyn can fit you for the right pessary, then you can insert, remove, and clean it yourself. Pessaries are also used for some types of pelvic organ prolapse.

Pelvic Floor Physical Therapy

This type of therapy helps up to 8 in 10 people with stress incontinence that happens with major physical exertion. It helps half of people whose stress incontinence happens during moderate exercise, too. Your physical therapy and exercises will be tailored to you and will include techniques to practice at home. Your physical therapist might use manual therapy to release tight muscles or internal vaginal pressure probes to help restore pelvic floor strength. They may also use *biofeedback*, electrical stimulation, or ultrasound to help you do the exercises effectively.

Medications

Medications can reduce the symptoms of urgency urinary incontinence and overactive bladder. They are less effective for stress urinary incontinence. Other medications can help prevent recurrent UTIs.

Medications That Control Muscles

Certain drugs help control muscle spasms and bladder contractions that contribute to urgency incontinence. These medications are available as pills or patches. These medications can help but are unlikely to cure the problem. Possible side effects include dry mouth, dry eyes, and constipation.

Medications That Help the Bladder Store Urine

There are medications that help the bladder to store more urine and stop leakage. Talk with your ob-gyn if you have high blood pressure. Some of these medications are not recommended for people with poorly controlled high blood pressure or certain liver or kidney conditions.

Botox Injections

Botox can be injected into the muscle of the bladder to relax it. This can be done in a doctor's office with numbing medication. Botox helps relieve the symptoms of overactive bladder, and the benefits typically last 3 to 9 months. In a 6-month trial, a single injection of Botox was twice as likely to completely resolve urgency urinary incontinence, compared to other medications that controlled bladder contractions. But Botox had a higher risk of side effects, including UTIs and issues with emptying the bladder.

Local Hormone Therapy

Using *hormone therapy*, specifically an estrogen cream, tablet, or ring in the vagina, may help with urinary incontinence. Vaginal estrogen therapy also increases the presence of "good" bacteria in the vagina and is a good preventive for recurrent UTIs. Vaginal estrogen does not raise the risk of blood clots or stroke. Systemic estrogen therapy, with or without *progestin*, does not appear to prevent or treat urinary incontinence or UTIs. If you have a history of hormone-sensitive cancer, discuss vaginal estrogen with your oncologist. For more information, read Chapter 17, "Hormone Therapies."

Low-Dose Antibiotics

Your ob-gyn may prescribe preventive *antibiotics* for 6 months or more. If your UTIs occur only after sex, you may take a single dose of antibiotics right after having sex. This can be a highly effective strategy, but there is a small risk of creating bacteria that are resistant to antibiotics. You and your ob-gyn should talk about this and the possible side effects of using antibiotics, including nausea, diarrhea, or skin rashes.

Nerve Stimulation Treatments

Nerve stimulation may be a useful approach for people whose incontinence has not responded to other treatments. There are two options:

- Sacral neuromodulation—A thin wire is placed under the skin of the low back and close to the nerve that controls the bladder. The wire is attached to a battery device placed under the skin nearby. The device sends a mild electrical signal along the wire to improve bladder function. This is thought to influence reflexes related to urination. Trials have shown that it can reduce or cure urgency incontinence.

- Percutaneous tibial nerve stimulation (PTNS)—A thin needle is inserted near a nerve in the ankle and connected to a machine. A signal is sent through the needle to the nerve, which sends the signal to the pelvic floor. PTNS usually involves weekly 30-minute office sessions for a few months. In a study, women who received PTNS once a week for 12 weeks saw improvements in urinary frequency, urgency, incontinence, and needing to urinate at night.

Surgical Treatments

Several surgeries and other procedures may help with certain types of incontinence.

Using Slings to Support the Urethra

Different types of slings can be used to lift or provide support for the urethra, which in turn prevents or reduces urine leakage. These slings include:

- Synthetic midurethral sling—This is a mesh "hammock" for the urethra. It is the most common surgical treatment for stress incontinence. In studies, the midurethral sling is more effective than pelvic floor physical therapy 1 year after treatment. This is a quick procedure, and most people go home the same day. Risks include possible injury to pelvic organs during surgery and *complications* from mesh. Complications include vaginal bleeding, pelvic pain, or pain during sex. Synthetic mesh also carries a small risk of eroding through the vaginal tissue, which may require additional surgery to correct the problem.

- Traditional sling—Also called an autologous sling, a traditional sling is made from a strip of your own tissue taken from your lower abdomen or thigh, threaded under your urethra. Traditional sling surgery is used if your body can't tolerate mesh or if you are having surgery for urethra repair at the same time. After traditional sling surgery, you will likely have to stay in the hospital for several days. This surgery has a risk of subsequent UTIs, difficulty urinating, and new or continued incontinence. If these problems occur, the sling may need to be adjusted.

Using Stitches to Lift the Urethra

Also called *colposuspension*, this procedure uses stitches placed on either side of the *bladder neck*. This lifts the urethra back into its normal position. This procedure is highly effective, but slings have been shown to be as effective with fewer complications. Colposuspension involves either an abdominal incision or smaller cuts done with *laparoscopy*. After an abdominal incision, you may need to spend several days in the hospital. After laparoscopy, you may be able to go home the same day. If you have problems emptying your bladder after surgery, the stitches may need to be loosened or removed.

> **What should I expect during recovery from incontinence surgery?**
>
> The time needed to recover varies depending on how the surgery was done. Discomfort may last for a few days or weeks. Some women may find it hard to urinate for a while or notice that they urinate more slowly than they did before surgery. They may need to use a catheter to empty their bladders a few times each day, even when back at home. Talk with your surgeon about things to avoid during recovery, including heavy lifting. You should also talk about when it's okay to resume driving, exercise, and sexual intercourse.
>
> –DR. CHARLES KILPATRICK

Using Bulking Agents

If your urinary sphincter muscle is not working well, urethral bulking may help. A safe synthetic substance is injected into the tissues around the urethra and the neck of the bladder. This can narrow the opening of the urethra, which may reduce leakage. It is usually done in your doctor's office with local *anesthesia*. Bulking agents are less effective than surgical procedures. Repeated injections are sometimes needed. Bulking agents do not usually cure the incontinence but can reduce symptoms. This procedure is usually done if symptoms recur after surgery or if surgery isn't appropriate for you.

Using Dual Procedures

Among women with pelvic floor disorders, as many as 4 in 5 have both stress incontinence and pelvic organ prolapse. During surgery for the prolapse, it might make sense to address the incontinence, too. Some women who are at risk of stress incontinence but don't yet have symptoms may also benefit from this approach.

Managing Accidental Bowel Leakage

Some people also experience accidental bowel leakage, also known as fecal incontinence. This may be loose or solid stool or mucus leaking from the rectum. Accidental bowel leakage is not directly connected to menopause. It becomes more likely, though, with age and when urinary incontinence has developed. Sedentary lifestyles, obesity, certain medications, and smoking also raise the risk. Accidental bowel leakage is linked to depression, social isolation, shame, and sexual difficulties.

> **What is biofeedback training for accidental bowel leakage?**
>
> Biofeedback is a training technique that helps you improve the function of the anal sphincter muscles. In biofeedback, sensors are placed inside or outside the anus. These sensors provide visual feedback on a monitor so you can see if you are contracting and relaxing muscles correctly. Like exercising any other type of muscle, you can strengthen the anal sphincter muscles over time. By helping you identify your anal muscles, biofeedback can improve your ability to sense stool or gas in the rectum.
>
> –DR. CHERYL IGLESIA

Finding the cause of accidental bowel leakage is an important step in finding the right treatment. Talking honestly with your ob-gyn offers the best chance of finding the best treatment for you. At an office visit, your ob-gyn should ask about your medical history and symptoms. You may be asked to keep a record each time you pass stool. Write down whether you had regular bowel movement or leakage of stool or gas. Also, write down any other symptoms and what you were doing at the time. This symptom record will help your ob-gyn diagnose why you are having problems.

You should also tell your ob-gyn about any prescription or over-the-counter products or herbal remedies you may be taking. Some medications and supplements can cause constipation or diarrhea and may add to your symptoms. You and your ob-gyn should review the results of your physical exam and any tests that might have been ordered. There are also some self-care strategies for accidental bowel leakage you may want to try:

- Managing anal pain—Care for the skin around the *anus*, which can become irritated. Try using zinc oxide ointment around the anus and wearing disposable underwear or using underwear pads.

- Dietary changes—Certain foods may make your leakage worse. Use a food diary to figure this out. Some people have problems with dairy products, foods that contain gluten, fatty foods, spicy foods, alcohol, or caffeine. If you have constipation, aim for 25 grams of fiber daily and drink plenty of water.

- Medications—Over-the-counter products help treat diarrhea and gas leakage and prevent constipation. If you need stronger medications, your doctor can prescribe them.

If these approaches are not effective enough, talk with your doctor about other treatments, including the following:

- Bowel training can help you have bowel movements at the same time each day.

- Biofeedback during pelvic floor muscle training or injections of bulking agents can help improve the function of your anal sphincter muscle.

- Electrical stimulation therapy can improve the function of nerves that control the bowel.

- Anal plugs and vaginal balloon devices can be used to control bowel movements.

- Surgery can repair a torn anal sphincter muscle.

Sacral neuromodulation, used for urgency urinary incontinence, may also be effective for fecal incontinence.

Talking With Your Ob-Gyn

Incontinence can be embarrassing, annoying, and costly. But you don't have to suffer in silence. If you've started using pads to soak up urine every day, or your urine leakage is interfering with work or intimate relationships, it's time to talk with your ob-gyn. Together you can discuss your symptoms and the best treatment for you. And follow-up will be important. Studies continue to look for ways to better treat incontinence and other urinary problems in postmenopausal women.

RESOURCES

Bladder Diary
niddk.nih.gov/health-information/urologic-diseases/bladder-control-problems/diagnosis
This tool from the National Institute of Diabetes and Digestive and Kidney Diseases helps you track your urinary symptoms.

Incontinence Education and Support for Patients, Caregivers, and Professionals
nafc.org
Website from the National Association for Continence with an A–Z guide to conditions and tips for talking with your doctor.

Patient Guides to Incontinence
urologyhealth.org/educational-resources
Website from the American Urological Association including a patient guide to incontinence, and additional guides addressing overactive bladders, stress urinary incontinence, women's health and menopause, topical estrogen treatment, and more.

PT Locator
aptapelvichealth.org/ptlocator
A directory that helps patients find licensed physical therapists and physiotherapists who specialize in pelvic floor health and physical therapy.

Voices for Pelvic Floor Disorders
voicesforpfd.org
Website from the American Urogynecologic Society covering pelvic floor disorders, with information on incontinence and related conditions, UTIs, bladder control, bowel control, painful bladder syndrome, various medical and surgical treatments, videos, and more.

My Menopause
acog.org/MyMenopause
Web resource from ACOG with information on the menopause transition, signs and symptoms, treatments, and self-care. Includes the latest information from the experts in ob-gyn care, menopause stories from real women, expert columns on how to manage symptoms, Q&A articles, videos, and more.

CHAPTER 13

Pelvic Organ Prolapse

At 54, Elaina didn't feel anything unusual when standing or walking, but when she felt her vagina with her fingers, she knew something wasn't right. "There was a bulge in my vagina that shouldn't be there, and I wondered if it was a cyst," she says. Her ob-gyn diagnosed a uterine prolapse and cystocele (when the bladder drops into the vaginal wall) but noted her symptoms were mild. The prolapse was not affecting Elaina's sex life and not causing urinary retention. She and her ob-gyn agreed that no treatment was needed unless her symptoms got worse. If that happens, Elaina plans to try a pessary, a device placed in the vagina that supports organs that have dropped.

elvic organ prolapse is a disorder in which one or more of the pelvic organs drop from their normal position. It can happen at any age, but most women who develop symptoms do so in the years after their final period, when they are *postmenopausal*.

The pelvic organs include the ***vagina***, ***uterus***, ***bladder***, ***urethra***, and ***rectum***. These organs are held in place by ***pelvic floor*** muscles, ***ligaments***, and layers of connective tissue. Prolapse happens when these tissues and muscles can no longer support the pelvic organs, and they slump low in the pelvis.

A key prolapse symptom is feeling a bulge and pressure in the vagina. Prolapse can also cause problems with intercourse, urinating, or passing bowel movements. Some types of prolapse are mild and don't need treatment. Other types that affect your normal activities or lower your quality of life may need treatment. And despite how it might feel, prolapse is not a tumor or cancer.

In this chapter, we'll look at different types of prolapse, their symptoms, and what causes them. We'll cover how you can relieve discomfort related to a prolapse, and the ways that your ***obstetrician–gynecologist (ob-gyn)*** can help. Treatment focuses on improving your symptoms and quality of life. Not all types of prolapse need intervention. Options can include waiting and watching to see if the prolapse gets worse, using nonsurgical approaches, or having surgery. If nonsurgical treatments aren't effective enough, you may want to see a urogynecologist, an ob-gyn who specializes in treating pelvic support and urinary problems.

Symptoms of Pelvic Organ Prolapse

Symptoms of prolapse can come on gradually and may not be noticed at first. Many women have no symptoms. Sometimes an ob-gyn finds the prolapse during a physical exam. And sometimes a sexual partner may notice something is different.

In mild cases, an organ may drop only a short distance and cause few, if any, problems. Mild prolapse may not need to be treated. When the prolapse is severe, an organ may push out of the vaginal opening. Other symptoms of more severe prolapse may include

- feeling of pelvic fullness or pressure
- leakage of urine
- difficulty emptying the bladder
- problems having a bowel movement
- lower back pressure or pain
- discomfort or pain with intercourse
- problems inserting tampons or applicators

Causes of Prolapse

The most common cause of organ prolapse is pregnancy and vaginal childbirth, but these often do not cause prolapse right away. Most women who develop a prolapse do so near the end of their *menopause transition*. Other causes can include

- aging and loss of tissue and muscle strength
- repeated heavy lifting
- constipation and straining to have bowel movements
- chronic coughing caused by smoking or medical conditions like asthma
- overweight and *obesity*
- disorders affecting the connective tissues, such as *rheumatoid arthritis* or *lupus*, and conditions affecting joints and ligaments

Prolapse may run in families. Some women may be born with weaker pelvic floor muscles. Prolapse can also happen in certain professions. For example, female paratroopers experience a lot of stress on the pelvic floor as part of their job. Prolapse can also happen after a *hysterectomy*.

> **Does prolapse always get worse over time?**
>
> This is a great question and one that has not been studied well. We used to think that the prolapse would only worsen over time. We have noticed that this is not always true, and for some women prolapse stays the same or even improves with time. In general, more severe prolapse is not likely to improve with time, and those with overweight or obesity may see their prolapse progress. If symptoms get worse, you and your ob-gyn can talk about the first steps in treatments.
>
> —DR. CHARLES KILPATRICK

Types of Prolapse

The types of prolapse have different names depending on which parts of the body are affected. Mild prolapse is common, and the degree of the prolapse and symptoms help guide treatment.

Anterior Vaginal Wall Prolapse

Anterior vaginal wall prolapse happens when the tissue between the bladder and vagina (the anterior, or front, vaginal wall) weakens and stretches. This allows the bladder to drop down from its normal place and into the vagina. It's also referred to as a cystocele or herniation of the bladder into the vagina. Sometimes an anterior vaginal wall prolapse can create a kink in the urethra and make it difficult to empty the bladder. When this happens, a woman may need to reach into the vagina and push up the bladder to pass urine.

Posterior Vaginal Wall Prolapse

A *posterior vaginal wall prolapse* happens when the tissue between the rectum and the vagina (the posterior, or rear, vaginal wall) weakens and stretches. This allows the rectum to bulge into the vagina. This is also referred to as a rectocele. A large prolapse may make it hard to have a bowel movement. Some women need to insert a finger into the vagina to push the bulge out of the way in order to pass stools.

Uterine Prolapse

A *uterine prolapse* happens when the uterus drops into the vagina. The distance it drops may vary. Mild degrees of prolapse are common. Mild uterine prolapse often does not cause symptoms and usually doesn't need surgery. Women with more severe uterine prolapse often have a feeling of pelvic pressure or a pulling feeling in the vagina or lower back. The *cervix* may stick out from the vagina. This can lead to cervical sores and bleeding caused by rubbing on underwear.

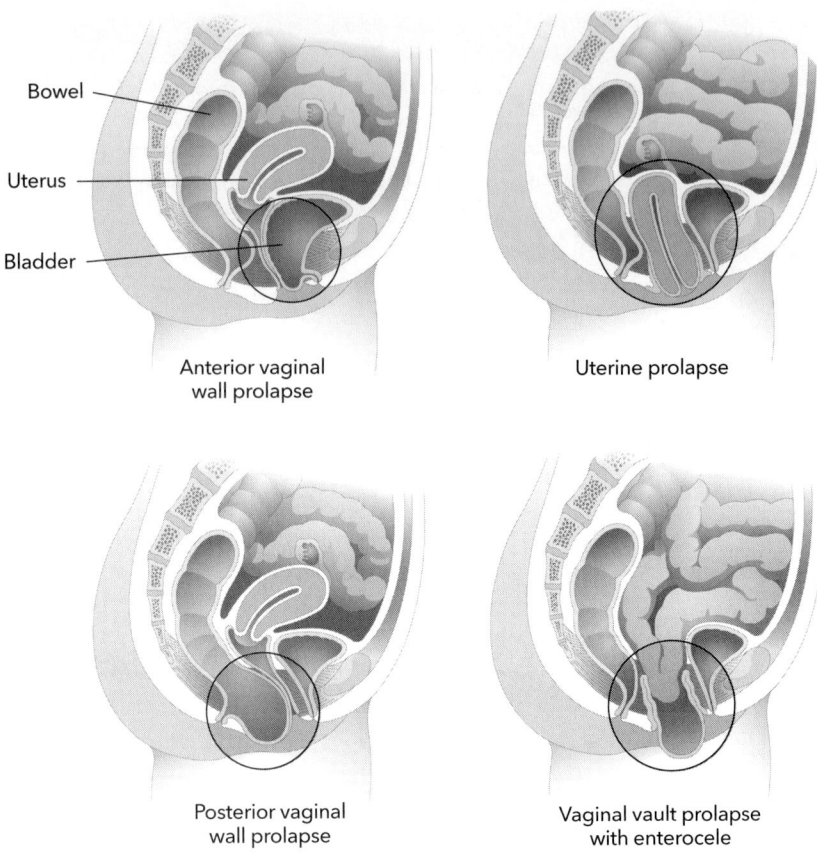

Types of pelvic organ prolapse. There are several types of prolapse that have different names depending on the part of the body that has dropped. Anterior vaginal wall prolapse involves the bladder, uterine prolapse involves the uterus, posterior vaginal wall prolapse involves the rectum, and vaginal vault prolapse involves the top of the vagina. Women who have vaginal vault prolapse may also have an enterocele. This forms when the small intestine bulges into the vagina.

Vaginal Vault Prolapse

Vaginal vault prolapse happens when the vagina loses its support and drops. This can happen in women who have had their uterus removed. The degree of prolapse varies. Symptoms can include changes in bladder, bowel, and sexual function. It's also possible for the small intestines to bulge into the vagina. This is referred to as an enterocele.

In some cases, more than one type of prolapse can happen at the same time. For example, both the uterus and bladder might shift down, or the uterus, bladder, and rectum. You can find short videos on the different types of prolapse at ACOG's page on Understanding Pelvic Organ Prolapse (find link in the Resources section).

Talking With Your Ob-Gyn

Diagnosing the type of prolapse is key to the right treatment plan. To figure this out, your ob-gyn may recommend vaginal and rectal exams while you are lying down on an exam table or standing. You may be asked to strain or cough during the exam to see if you leak urine. Your ob-gyn may ask about bowel function and may recommend a test to see how well your bladder empties.

You should also talk about how much your symptoms bother you and your goals for treatment. Your ob-gyn has heard many stories of prolapse symptoms and their effects on quality of life. This is your time to share how your symptoms may be affecting or limiting your physical activity or sex life, or if symptoms seem to be getting worse.

> **Will prolapse treatment improve my sex life?**
>
> Good sex starts with feeling good in body and mind. Any pain or discomfort of the pelvis can lead to distress, lack of confidence, and a desire to avoid sex or the pain that may come with it. The good news is that prolapse treatment can help your sex life as much as your overall health. By treating symptoms, resolving pelvic discomfort, and stopping leakage of urine or stool, many women feel better about themselves and sexual activity. Talk with your ob-gyn or a urogynecologist if one of your treatment goals is to improve your sex life.
>
> –DR. CHERYL IGLESIA

Many women with prolapse do not need treatment. At regular checkups, your ob-gyn should keep track of your concerns. If symptoms start to bother you, it may be time to talk about treatment. Bothersome symptoms can include more severe bulging and pelvic pressure, sexual problems, or worsening issues with urinary function or bowel movements. There is no guarantee that any treatment—including surgery—will relieve all symptoms. Even so, treatment is likely to lead to significant relief. After talking together, your ob-gyn may recommend that you see a urogynecologist. For more on urogynecologists, read Chapter 5, "Choosing Your Menopause Care Team."

The best treatment for you depends on your age, your sexual activity, how much the symptoms bother you, and how advanced the prolapse is. Other health problems may also play a role in treatment decisions. Surgery may carry risks if you have *diabetes*, heart disease, or breathing problems, or if you smoke. If you are still in *perimenopause* and hope to have more children, this will also affect your treatment choices.

Nonsurgical Treatments for Prolapse

The first option for mild prolapse may be waiting and watching to see if symptoms change. Sometimes the degree of prolapse gets worse, but other times it can improve. Mild cases of prolapse may never progress. Some health conditions can affect whether prolapse gets worse over time, including obesity. If symptoms warrant treatment, these are the options that ob-gyns and urogynecologists usually recommend.

Pelvic Floor Exercises

Kegel exercises help tone the muscles of the pelvic floor and the muscles that surround the openings of the urethra, vagina, and rectum. Doing Kegels regularly may strengthen the support muscles and slow the progression of some types of prolapse. They may also help with *urinary incontinence* caused by a prolapse. Your ob-gyn or a pelvic floor physical therapist can help you be sure you're doing these exercises the right way, and there are apps to provide daily reminders of when to exercise. For a guide to doing Kegels, read Chapter 12, "Urinary Incontinence."

Pessaries

A *pessary* is a device inserted into the vagina to support the pelvic organs. As many as 9 in 10 women can be fitted with a pessary and experience immediate relief, so it's a good first step in treatment. Pessaries are usually made of soft silicone and are available in several shapes and sizes. Your ob-gyn can help find the pessary that fits you comfortably, depending on your symptoms and type of prolapse. Common pessary types include

- ring pessary with support for bladder prolapse

- ring pessary with knob for prolapse and urinary incontinence

- Gellhorn pessary for advanced pelvic organ prolapse

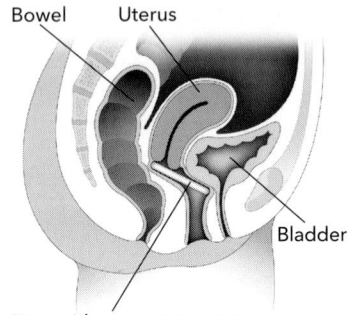
Ring with support pessary

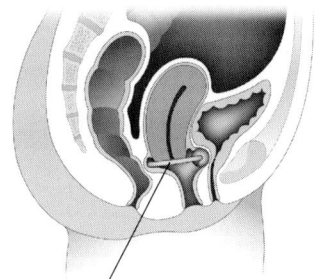
Ring with support and knob pessary

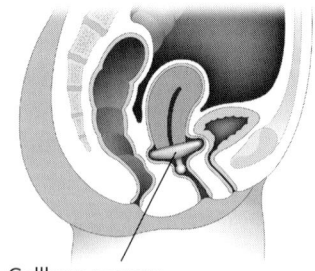
Gellhorn pessary

Pessaries. Pessaries are inserted into the vagina to support the pelvic organs. They are available in several shapes and sizes and can be used short-term or long-term.

Many women become comfortable removing, cleaning, and replacing their own pessary. They see their ob-gyn once a year to discuss how the pessary is working. Women who aren't able to manage the pessary themselves need appointments every 3 to 4 months.

A small number of women may find that the pessary irritates the vaginal wall. If this happens, the pessary can be removed for 2 to 4 weeks, and a vaginal *estrogen* cream may be used to help with healing. More frequent pessary changes or a different pessary style may be needed after the irritation has healed.

Lifestyle Changes

Sometimes changes in lifestyle or diet may be enough to bring symptom relief. For example, if urinary incontinence at night or early in the morning is your main prolapse symptom, it can help to limit how much you drink several hours before bedtime. Limiting yourself to 8 cups of fluids throughout the day may also help. (If your urine has no color, you may be drinking too much.)

Bladder training may be useful. With this training, you time your urination according to a schedule. This gradually increases the amount of urine your bladder can hold and helps you go longer between bathroom visits.

For women with bowel problems, increasing the amount of dietary fiber can stop constipation and straining during bowel movements. Sitting with your feet slightly raised may help with the sensation of bulging in the vagina. Also, sometimes losing a small amount of weight can help improve prolapse symptoms.

Surgery for Prolapse

If other options do not work and if your symptoms are severe, you may want to consider surgery. In the U.S., about 1 in 10 women who have given birth have prolapse surgery at some point in their lives. Prolapse surgery is the most common surgery among women in their 60s.

Surgery may relieve some, but not all, prolapse symptoms. Generally there are two approaches: 1) repairing the pelvic floor and 2) shortening, narrowing, or closing off the vagina to create support for the organs above. It's important to talk with your surgeon about which option is best for your situation. You and your surgeon will consider

- the type of prolapse and how much it is affecting you
- your overall health and history of other surgeries
- your family goals and plans for pregnancy
- possible recovery time and risks related to surgery

Surgery to repair the pelvic floor is called *reconstructive surgery*. This approach restores pelvic organs as close as possible to their original position. Surgery may be done through an incision in the vagina, an incision in the abdomen, or with *laparoscopy*, and sometimes with robotic surgery assistance.

Surgery to shorten or close off the vagina is called *obliterative surgery*. Vaginal intercourse is not possible after this is done. Women who choose this type of surgery have decided that vaginal intercourse is less important than relief of their symptoms.

More than one type of surgery may be done at the same time. This is called a dual procedure or a combined procedure. For example, in women who have uterine prolapse, a hysterectomy may be combined with supporting the vagina. Or a slumping vagina may be supported and the front vaginal wall repaired at the same time. Combined procedures may reduce the risk of the prolapse happening again.

Sometimes a procedure is added that may prevent worsening urinary incontinence after surgery. Combined procedures may be recommended when a person has both prolapse and bothersome *stress urinary incontinence*. Some surgeons prefer to do prolapse surgery first, and if stress urinary incontinence develops, address that later. To find out more about treatments for urine leakage, read Chapter 12, "Urinary Incontinence."

How Prolapse Surgery Is Done

If you're thinking about surgery, consider your options. Talk with your surgeon about which procedures may be best for your type of prolapse. You should also discuss risks and possible *complications*.

Using Your Own Tissues

When a surgeon uses your own tissues to fix uterine or vaginal vault prolapse, it's called "native tissue repair." This surgery is done through an incision in the vagina. The prolapsed organ is attached with stitches to a muscle or ligament in the pelvis. Recovery time is shorter compared to procedures done with an abdominal incision. Postsurgical complications may include pain during sex and urinary incontinence. Rarely, there may be injury to the bladder, *urinary tract*, or *bowels*. Injury can lead to constant leaking of urine or leaking stool or gas through the vagina. But again, this is rare.

Colporrhaphy

Colporrhaphy treats prolapse of the front or back wall of the vagina. The surgeon uses stitches to strengthen the weakened vaginal tissue so that the vagina once again supports the bladder or the rectum. The procedure is done through an incision in the vagina, so recovery time is typically short. The surgery is successful in about 8 in 10 cases. Postsurgical complications may be similar to those of a fixation or suspension procedure.

Sacrocolpopexy and Sacrohysteropexy

Sacrocolpopexy is used to treat vaginal vault prolapse and vaginal wall prolapse. It can be done with an incision in the abdomen or with laparoscopy. Surgical mesh is attached to the front and back walls of the vagina. The ends of the mesh are then attached to the tailbone. This lifts the vagina back into place. Sacrocolpopexy is sometimes recommended for women younger than 60, women with overweight or obesity, or those who have more advanced prolapses or certain other health conditions. It is successful in 9 in 10 cases.

Sacrohysteropexy is used to treat uterine prolapse if you want to avoid hysterectomy. Surgical mesh is attached to the cervix and then to the tailbone, which lifts the uterus back into place. The hospital stay may be shorter than if you have a hysterectomy, and there may be fewer complications. In 9 in 10 cases, sacrohysteropexy cures prolapse symptoms for at least 3 to 5 years.

With either procedure, there is a risk of damage to the bowel. There is also a small risk that the mesh will wear through tissues and into the vagina or other organs, which is called exposure or erosion. Mesh erosion can cause scarring and long-lasting pain. Other complications may include pain during sex and damage to the bladder, bowel, ureters (the tubes that bring urine from the kidneys to the bladder), or blood vessels.

> **What type of mesh was banned by the FDA?**
>
> In 2019, the U.S. Food and Drug Administration banned mesh kits that required making an incision in the vagina to insert the mesh. These kits were used in surgery for anterior and posterior vaginal wall prolapse. This ban came in response to an increase in harmful side effects reported by women, including long-lasting pain. Women who have been treated with a transvaginal mesh product in the past do not need to see their ob-gyn unless they have complications such as vaginal bleeding, pelvic pain, or pain during sex. Surgical mesh placed in the abdomen may still be used safely to lift organs back into place (at the time of sacrocolpopexy or sacrohysteropexy) or to treat stress urinary incontinence (midurethral sling).
>
> –DR. CHARLES KILPATRICK

Hysterectomy

This is the removal of the uterus, which can treat uterine prolapse and other conditions. Combining a hysterectomy with sacrocolpopexy can reduce the risk of vaginal vault prolapse in the future. Women who choose a hysterectomy may have a lower risk of uterine and cervical cancer as well as lower risk of some other health issues in the future.

Hysterectomy can come with complications. In a U.S. study, women who had a hysterectomy during prolapse repair were four times as likely to have problems around the time of surgery compared to women who had a sacrohysteropexy. In addition, hysterectomy does not strengthen the pelvic ligaments that are involved in prolapse. Hysteropexy (uterine suspension procedure) can also be done using no mesh and attaching the uterus to your own ligaments in the pelvis. A hysteropexy procedure is often combined with other procedures to correct anterior and posterior vaginal prolapse.

Vaginal Closure Surgery

This surgery, also called obliterative surgery, treats advanced prolapse. The walls of the vagina are stitched together to shorten or close the vagina in order to support the organs above. This may be an option for women who do not want to have vaginal intercourse in the future. It is an effective treatment for prolapse, with a success rate just shy of 100 percent and high patient satisfaction. The surgery can be done using *general anesthesia* or *regional anesthesia*, so it can be a safer procedure for women with some health conditions. The surgery is often combined with another procedure to reduce the risk of stress urinary incontinence in the future.

Risks and Recovery

For most surgeries, you will need to take a few weeks off from work. During this time, you should avoid vigorous exercise, lifting, straining, and *sexual intercourse*. Surgery done via the vagina usually has a shorter recovery time than surgery done via the abdomen.

Surgery for prolapse comes with some risk, including the risk of bleeding, *urinary tract infection (UTI)*, or difficulty fully emptying the bladder or bowel (this usually is short-term). With any surgery there's also a risk of blood clots and reactions to *anesthesia*. Other complications may include the following.

Another Prolapse

This can affect up to 3 in 10 women who have surgery, though most studies place the number lower. The rate of repeat surgery for prolapse is 1 in 10 women, since the new prolapse is often less severe compared to the original prolapse. A repeat prolapse is more likely if you are younger than 60, have obesity, had an advanced prolapse when it was first treated, had vaginal surgery for prolapse, or had a prolapse of the front vaginal wall. A repeat prolapse is less likely if surgery included suspension of the uterus or top of the vagina.

It is not known whether anything can be done to keep prolapse from coming back after surgery. Avoiding pressure inside the abdomen for the first several weeks after surgery may help. Controlling weight, avoiding constipation, and not lifting heavy objects may also help.

Stress Urinary Incontinence

The risk of stress urinary incontinence is lower if you have a procedure for urinary incontinence at the same time as the prolapse repair. Adding the procedure to help treat stress urinary incontinence may increase the risk of postsurgical complications but prevent worsening leakage. Stress urinary incontinence can also be treated later.

Pain During Sex

In a study looking at women 2 years after surgery, painful sex affected 1 in 6. This is more likely after surgery done via the vagina. Treatment may include the use of vaginal estrogen and vaginal dilators.

Organ Injury

Rarely, there can be injury to the bladder, bowel, or urinary tract. A procedure called *cystoscopy* allows a surgeon to see the urinary tract during surgery. This viewing may reduce the risk of bladder or urethra injury or allow the surgeon to repair it immediately.

Complications From Surgical Mesh

Studies show more complications from surgical mesh than native tissue repair. These may include pelvic or vaginal pain, vaginal bleeding, and pain with intercourse. In addition, after surgery with mesh there is a small risk that the mesh will wear through tissues and into the vagina. If this happens, additional surgery may be needed to remove the mesh.

Abdominal Issues

Abdominal incisions carry a small risk of damage to the intestines or pelvic tissues sticking together (called adhesions). Adhesions may require another procedure to correct.

RESOURCES

Bladder Diary
niddk.nih.gov/health-information/urologic-diseases/bladder-control-problems/diagnosis

This tool from the National Institute of Diabetes and Digestive and Kidney Diseases helps you track your urinary symptoms.

Voices for PFD: Fact Sheets and Downloads
voicesforpfd.org/resources/fact-sheets-and-downloads/

Fact sheets from the American Urogynecologic Society covering pelvic diagnoses and treatment options, including pelvic organ prolapse, pessaries, sacrocolpopexy, vaginal closure surgery, vaginal hysterectomy for prolapse, surgeries using mesh, vaginal suspension surgery, constipation, cystoscopy, fistulas, and more. In English and Spanish.

Patient Guides to Incontinence
urologyhealth.org/educational-resources

Website from the American Urological Association including a patient guide to incontinence, and additional guides addressing overactive bladders, stress urinary incontinence, women's health and menopause, topical estrogen treatment, and more.

PT Locator
aptapelvichealth.org/ptlocator

A directory that helps patients find licensed physical therapists and physiotherapists who specialize in pelvic floor health and physical therapy.

Surgery for Prolapse
voicesforpfd.org/pelvic-organ-prolapse/surgery/

Webpage from the American Urogynecologic Society on types of prolapse surgery, preparing for surgery, and surgical mesh.

Understanding Pelvic Organ Prolapse
acog.org/POPvideos

Videos from ACOG showing the types of prolapse and how some pessaries are inserted.

My Menopause
acog.org/MyMenopause

Web resource from ACOG with information on the menopause transition, signs and symptoms, treatments, and self-care. Includes the latest information from the experts in ob-gyn care, menopause stories from real women, expert columns on how to manage symptoms, Q&A articles, videos, and more.

CHAPTER 14

Weight and Menopause

In her early 50s, Jane had aching joints and a hip problem. Pain led to less activity—her daily step count dropped to 1,000—and she gained 20 pounds in 18 months. She talked with her doctor about ways to relieve pain that would help her get moving again, and this conversation led to Jane having a hip replacement and getting a steroid injection in her knee. Now she's comfortable and back up to 7,000 steps a day, plus she does some bike riding. She's lost 14 pounds and plans to join a gym. "It's harder to lose weight at this age," Jane says. "I want to focus on weight loss now to avoid getting diabetes and other health problems later."

Society often judges people, especially women, by their weight. For those whose bodies don't fit an ideal, the stigma can be painful and affect quality of life. Regardless of weight, everyone has a right to respectful, high-quality health care that's delivered without judgment. But there are times when carrying extra pounds can create current and future health problems, and the *menopause transition* is one of those times.

Changes in weight are common during the transition. Women in midlife gain an average of 1½ pounds a year. Over time, this added weight increases the risk of chronic health conditions. Weight gain can happen even if you're eating and working out pretty much the same as you always have. And while gaining weight in midlife isn't always a problem, menopausal changes can influence how much weight you gain and how this increase affects your ability to stay healthy.

Gaining weight during the menopause transition isn't like gaining weight in your teens and 20s. During the transition there's an increase in fat mass and a decrease in lean body mass, often muscle. Lean body mass includes bones, muscles, ligaments, and tendons. Almost all women going through the menopause transition see an increase in waist size. For some, there's only a small change in the waist, but it can still be bothersome.

Obstetrician–gynecologists (ob-gyns) are increasingly focused on helping women maintain a healthy weight in midlife. They also aim to support those whose excess weight has already put them at risk of health problems. Your annual checkups may now include a discussion of diet and physical activity. You may also hear the term *body mass index (BMI)*. This is a score based on your height and weight. There is not a BMI cutoff at which a person crosses from being healthy to unhealthy, but a high BMI—which usually signals overweight or *obesity*—can predict health issues that affect quality of life, including:

- More symptoms of *menopause*—In a U.S. study of women in the menopause transition, those with obesity (a BMI of 30 or higher) were more likely to report *hot flashes*, vaginal and urinary problems, mood issues, and lowered sex drive, compared to those without obesity.

- Increased risk of serious health conditions—Overweight and obesity contribute to *sleep apnea*, *diabetes*, *high blood pressure*, heart disease, and *stroke*. Added weight is also linked to some cancers, cognitive decline, and conditions affecting the muscles, joints, nerves, and connective tissues.

- Social and emotional pressures—A changing body shape may contribute to a loss of self-confidence and sexual activity. In a U.S. study, 3 in 5 women who had been through menopause said concerns about their weight negatively affected their lives.

The reasons for weight gain are complex, and maintaining or losing weight is complex, too. The good news is that you don't need to get back to a specific weight. Even a small amount of weight loss has health benefits. In a U.S. study, losing just 3 to 5 percent of body weight over time was linked to reduced risk of heart disease and stroke. For a person who is 150 pounds, this might mean a loss of 4½ to 7½ pounds. In another study of women with overweight after menopause, those who lost an average of 10 pounds lowered their risk of breast cancer. And research shows that starting to exercise in midlife may offset or even reverse the previous years of inactivity, with substantial health benefits.

You and your ob-gyn can work together to help you reach and maintain a healthy weight during the menopause transition and beyond. Together you can talk about eating healthy food, adding daily exercise, and maintaining muscle mass. The goal should be fitness and good health now and in the future.

Midlife Changes and Weight Gain

Many factors combine to cause weight gain during midlife, including aging, *hormone* changes, reduced physical exercise, injuries, stress, *depression*, and lack of sleep.

Let's start with aging and hormones. *Estrogen*, *progesterone*, and other hormones affect *metabolism* and the biology of the digestive system. These influence how fat is stored and distributed in the body. The natural process of aging along with hormonal changes of menopause lead to two significant changes: 1) less muscle mass and 2) more fat that is stored around the belly and heart. As muscle is lost, your body uses fewer calories, so if your calorie intake stays the same as you approach midlife, you may gain weight. And the shift in fat to the middle of the body can lead to a higher risk of heart disease and lower quality of life.

Next is reduced physical activity. Many people become less active with age. When this happens and food intake stays the same, weight gain is inevitable. You may be inactive or less active because of midlife responsibilities. When you're overwhelmed with work commitments and family demands, it's easier to fall out of the exercise habit.

Midlife is also a time when chronic conditions become more common. For example, a large U.S. study of women in the menopause transition found that limitations in physical functioning affected 1 in 5 women between 40 and 55 and half of women between 56 and 66. Conditions like arthritis, painful joints, and injuries can lead to less activity, which then can lead to weight gain and more joint pain.

Stress and mental health have a powerful effect on weight distribution. Stress hormones are linked to eating more and storing more body fat—especially in the midsection. Depression and anxiety, which tend to peak during the menopause transition, can make it harder to get up or get out. And anxiety, like stress, generates higher levels of the stress hormone that is linked to accumulated belly fat. For more information, read Chapter 20, "Managing Stress," and Chapter 8, "Mood and Memory."

Sleep problems and weight gain have a strong link. Sleep helps regulate the hormones that influence the appetite and fat storage, so poor sleep is linked to changes in metabolism that contribute to weight gain. Poor sleep also increases the risk of diabetes and can cause you to slow down or stop exercising altogether. All of these make weight gain more likely. A small U.S. study showed that after three nights of disturbed sleep, women's bodies used less fat, potentially causing weight gain during the menopause years. Plus, an increase in weight is linked to disordered breathing during sleep as well as sleep apnea. If you're struggling to sleep well, read Chapter 9, "Sleep Problems."

Managing Fitness and Weight in Midlife

With these changes and forces working together to cause weight gain, what's the answer to managing weight? The better question may be, how can you stay fit with all the changes taking place in your body? Being fit in midlife has big benefits regardless of how much weight a person might lose. So we'll look at fitness first—even if it doesn't result in weight loss—and then talk about approaches that may help with weight loss itself.

> **Can hormone therapy help me lose weight?**
>
> The estrogen used in hormone therapy may change where fat is stored in the body, but hormone therapy by itself won't lead to weight loss. However, hormone therapy may help with night sweats that interrupt sleep. We know that poor sleep can lead to weight gain over time, so better sleep achieved with hormone therapy may help with weight control. Ultimately, when it comes to weight loss, the advice we've heard for years about healthy eating and regular exercise remains true now and as we get older.
> —DR. ESTHER EISENBERG

How to Get (or Keep) Moving

Some research suggests that physical activity needs to *increase* in midlife, to offset changes in metabolism, body fat, and **blood pressure**. Instead, people tend to become more sedentary, which leads to health problems. Fitness solutions sound a lot like what you've probably heard before: Keep moving. Be consistent. Use apps or smart devices to remind you to get up and exercise. For many people, committing to fitness is the start and weight management sometimes follows. But note that exercise alone isn't likely to address substantial weight gain.

Exercise in midlife has many health benefits, even if you are just starting. These may be similar to the effects of lifelong physical activity. In a UK study, inactive adults 40 and older who started exercising for 2½ hours a week were less likely to die over the next 20 years. The more active they became, the less likely they were to die during that period. People with serious health conditions at the start, like cancer and heart disease, also benefited.

Physical activity can feel daunting if you're not used to it. Being active can become more enjoyable as you adjust and if you do it with friends. Planning and scheduling your physical activity is a key to success. Research has shown that small increases in the time you spend being active add up to valuable health benefits. Base your physical activity around these guidelines:

- Find activities that build stamina and endurance. Walking is great exercise. So are bike rides, running, dancing, workout classes, and swimming. The bonus with all is that you'll likely sleep better being active in some way every day.

- Add activities that build strength, flexibility, and balance. Strength training is vital for maintaining muscle mass and bone health. This can be done with resistance bands, weights, or your own body weight (as in yoga). Flexibility and balance are important for sustaining your function and range of motion. Tai chi, yoga, or Pilates can help with this.

- Every week, aim to get *at least* 2½ hours of moderate activity, or 1¼ hours of vigorous activity. As you become more used to it, aim to be active for an average of 1 hour every day. Add two sessions of strength training on different days.

- Add 2 hours of strength training per week as well. This means working on all major muscle groups—abdomen, arms, back, chest, hips, legs, and shoulders. You can train with resistance bands, free weights, or weight machines. If you want to use machines, talk with your ob-gyn first, especially if you have been diagnosed with boss loss of the spine.

Cross-training is a strategy that is helpful to adopt in middle age. Since injuries become more common with aging, some activities you used to do when younger become more challenging and may be off-limits while you are rehabilitating a pulled muscle or sprain. Having a backup activity provides more full-body conditioning and allows you to maintain activity and continue training even if you are injured.

How to Eat Well (or Better)

Talking about food in midlife may mean a shift in thinking. Many women struggle for years trying to reach an idealized body type and end up in cycles of weight loss, weight gain, and fad dieting. Frequent dieting and disordered eating habits don't work and aren't healthy. It's also well-known that most people don't follow new diets for the long term and often regain the weight lost when they started a diet. This may include some of the latest approaches, like intermittent fasting (see the box "Key Facts About Intermittent Fasting").

Now is the time to reset expectations and focus on healthy, sustainable eating habits. Find an approach that you can stick with for the rest of your life. These principles can help:

- Eat larger portions of some foods—It's a green light for foods that are low in fat and calories, such as vegetables, salads, and broth-based soups. In one U.S. study, women who reduced their energy intake from fats lost the most weight.

- Avoid foods you could not create in your own kitchen—Ultra-processed foods are made from parts of whole foods, like fat, starch, and sugar, and they usually have a long list of other ingredients. These items—frozen meals and pizzas, sausages, instant noodles, energy bars, chips, cookies, and more—are cheap and easy, but they're consistently linked to weight gain and chronic diseases. Some processing may be unavoidable, like a can of tuna in water or cut fruit in syrup, but skipping ultra-processed foods is smart for long-term health. Choose fresh vegetables over veggie burgers. Choose whole apples instead of apple pie. Choose plain water over energy drinks and sodas.

> **Key Facts About Intermittent Fasting**
>
> **What is it?** Intermittent fasting is an alternative approach to losing or maintaining weight. It focuses less on what you eat and more on when you eat. There are different approaches, but the most common is to eat within specific, regular times and not eat at other times of day or night. The theory is that after hours without food, the body has used up the calories you ate in your last meal and begins burning fat.
>
> **How is it done?** Some plans involve eating only within a 6- to 8-hour window each day. Others involve eating just one meal 2 days a week and eating normally the other 5 days. You can enjoy a range of healthy foods. When you're not eating, you can drink as much water and zero-calorie beverages, such as black coffee and tea, as you like.
>
> **Does it work?** People using intermittent fasting tend to lose weight. Experts don't yet agree on whether this approach works better than traditional calorie restriction or has additional health benefits, but studies are underway. This is partly because it is difficult to study the effects of diets in the real world.
>
> **What else should I know?** In a small U.S. study, one group practiced intermittent fasting, and another worked with calorie restriction. Over the course of a year, people in both groups experienced similar calorie reduction (cutting 400+ calories a day) and weight loss (about 11 pounds). A reviewer suggested that the key to their success was not what time of day they ate. Participants formed support groups, met with a dietitian once a week, reduced their calories, and were weighed once a week. It's possible that these benefits helped them stick with their weight loss programs.
>
> **What's the takeaway?** It may be best to find a dietary approach that you can sustain long-term. Talk with your ob-gyn about different evidence-based approaches to weight loss and control, and then choose one that works best with your lifestyle.

- Create plant-based meals—Plant-based eating is linked to less weight gain during the menopause transition and lower risk of heart disease and stroke. You can start by flipping what you consider a main dish into a side dish and vice versa. For example, at dinner a veggie medley might become your main dish while lean chicken becomes a side. At lunch, build your meal around a salad. For dessert, opt for fruit. You can find tips for healthy eating, meal planning, and more at the MyPlate.gov website from the U.S. Department of Agriculture.

- Reduce calories—Total calorie intake needs to be reduced to lose weight. But everyone is different when it comes to food preferences. Talking with a registered dietitian may help you find a way of eating fewer calories while still enjoying your daily meals.

- Seek support—Consider joining a group that shares tips and encouragement. Virtual support and counseling are also effective. Some fee-based apps offer personalized guidance around weight loss, healthy eating, and other lifestyle habits along with tracking, coaching, and community support. You can also research the best low-cost or free apps for health coaching. Your ob-gyn might have recommendations, too.

- Step on a scale once week—The idea is to do this often enough that you're aware of how you're maintaining or losing weight, but not so often that you get discouraged. Weigh yourself first thing in the morning, before you eat.

When to Talk With Your Ob-Gyn

There's a lot of advice online for eating better, exercising more, and losing weight. But note that the diet and exercise industries are crowded with plans that make promises that fail to deliver. Look for reliable sources of information, which include sites from government agencies and nationally known medical centers. You can also look for sites that promote weight loss research, including the National Weight Control Registry. You can find links to some trusted sites in the Resources section at the end of this chapter.

If you've tried different approaches and can't reach your goals, talk with your ob-gyn. Remember that these are common concerns. Your ob-gyn should listen and talk with you respectfully about your weight and overall health. If past doctors blamed you for weight gain or did not give you enough time and attention to talk things through, it's important to seek out better care now.

When you discuss your weight with your ob-gyn or any doctor, they should ask about your medical history, diet, and physical activity, and your family history of obesity and conditions linked to it. They may do a physical exam. They may screen you for signs of disease linked to overweight and obesity. A doctor can help you manage your weight in several ways, including:

- Addressing conditions that keep you from physical activity—Joint pain and stiffness make it harder to get moving. You may need to address health conditions that cause discomfort or pain when you try to exercise more.

- Referring you to additional support—If you are having difficulty maintaining dietary changes, ask for a referral to a registered dietitian. For more on this, read Chapter 5, "Choosing Your Menopause Care Team." You can also ask about support groups for weight loss and other resources, some of which are available online.

- Prescribing medication to help you lose weight—Several types of weight loss medications are available. These work in different ways and can have side effects. If you have a BMI of greater than 30, or a BMI of at least 27 with certain medical conditions such as diabetes or heart disease, medications may help you lose weight. Some studies have shown that a diabetes medication called metformin can help people lose weight, especially when they are using it along with a weight loss plan.

Other Medications for Weight Loss

You may have heard of medications called ***GLP-1 receptor agonists***. They were developed to treat type 2 diabetes, but in studies of people with obesity who did not have diabetes, GLP-1s were found to help with weight loss. So now GLP-1s are used to treat overweight and obesity, too. When added to dietary changes and physical activity, GLP-1 medications can help with weight loss by

- slowing the movement of food through your stomach, so smaller amounts of food feel satisfying
- signaling to the brain that your stomach is full, which decreases appetite

In the trials for one of these drugs, people lost up to 15 percent of their body weight over 17 months. In a person weighing 250 pounds at the start, this would be a 37-pound weight loss. These medications can also improve blood sugar levels and blood pressure, and they offer benefits for the heart and kidneys. In addition, losing weight alone can lower the risk of multiple diseases.

> **How can I respond when people talk about my weight?**
>
> Sometimes people, including family members, comment on weight, thinking they are being helpful. They may mean well, but words can be hurtful. To cope with comments, remember that your weight and health are your private concerns. Other people don't know what you or your doctor may have talked about or what your weight goals may be. A well-timed reply, such as "Thank you for your concerns" or "My doctor thinks I'm doing fine," can let your questioner know their comments are off-limits.
>
> –DR. NANETTE SANTORO

Side effects of GLP-1 drugs may include nausea, vomiting, and diarrhea. These medications are expensive and not always covered by health insurance. When people stop taking these medications, much of the lost weight returns, and researchers are still learning what the long-term effects may be. Talk with your ob-gyn if you have questions about GLP-1 medications and whether they may be right for you.

Metformin is far less expensive than GLP-1s, but you and your ob-gyn should discuss the risks and benefits of any medication taken for weight loss.

Surgery for Weight Loss

For some people with obesity, *bariatric surgery* can be an effective long-term solution for weight management. Bariatric surgery also improves metabolic health and lowers the risk of dying from heart disease, diabetes, and cancer. This surgery may be an option if you

- have a BMI of 40 or more
- have a BMI of 35 to 39 and have major health issues linked to obesity

Bariatric surgery seeks to reduce the size of the stomach or change the way food moves through the bowel. It's usually done with *laparoscopy* by a surgeon who specializes in obesity treatment. There are three types of surgery. Note that the amount of weight lost and how quickly it comes off depend on the type of procedure and body weight before surgery.

Restrictive Surgery

This makes the stomach smaller and reduces how much food it can hold. The surgeon may use a gastric band, stapling, or a gastric sleeve procedure that removes a large part of the stomach. Weight loss after this surgery tends to be slow and steady.

Malabsorptive Surgery

This approach bypasses segments of the bowel, which changes the way food is absorbed through the intestines. Weight loss usually happens fast after this surgery and is easier to maintain.

Combination Surgery

This uses aspects of both restriction and malabsorption surgeries. It includes the Roux-en-Y gastric bypass, the most common weight loss procedure worldwide. Combination surgery may take longer than other surgeries, but the average weight loss is typically greatest with this approach. For example:

- Studies around the world involving more than 150,000 women between 40 and 65 showed that the greatest weight loss occurred in people with a BMI of 40 or higher who had Roux-en-Y gastric bypass. People in these categories tended to continue losing weight for at least 5 years.
- In a Portuguese study, 140 midlife women with obesity underwent Roux-en-Y gastric bypass or sleeve gastrectomy. The women with the most body fat had the greatest weight loss and the biggest improvements in certain

health conditions (diabetes, high blood pressure, and high cholesterol). Far more women were physically active after their surgery than before.

- In one international study, people lost about half their initial body weight and were able to keep it off for at least 10 years after gastric sleeve surgery.

But while the outcomes can be highly successful, there are risks with bariatric surgery. These risks may include

- leaking of stomach fluid into the abdomen
- injury to other organs, such as the spleen
- wearing away of the band or staples used in the surgery
- digestive issues, such as food intolerance
- infection or *complications* from *anesthesia*
- vitamin deficiencies

If you're thinking about bariatric surgery or have had it in the past, let your ob-gyn know so their records are up to date.

RESOURCES

The 7 Components of a Successful Weight Loss Plan
sbm.org/healthy-living/the-7-components-of-a-successful-weight-loss-plan
Article from the Society of Behavioral Medicine outlining the keys to weight management: realistic goals, preferred foods, physical activity, tracking, accountability, and support.

About the Mayo Clinic Diet
diet.mayoclinic.org/us/the-program/about-the-mayo-clinic-diet/
This fee-based plan from the Mayo Clinic includes diet plans, personalized weight loss programs, and unlimited group coaching.

Healthy Weight and Growth
cdc.gov/healthy-weight-growth/losing-weight/index.html
Tips from the Centers for Disease Control and Prevention on creating a weight loss plan.

How to Eat Healthy with MyPlate
myplate.gov
This interactive website from the U.S. Department of Agriculture helps you explore healthy food choices. Can be customized to fit your dietary tastes, needs, cultural traditions, and budget. Includes a quiz and additional tools.

Tips for Getting and Staying Active as You Age

nia.nih.gov/health/exercise-and-physical-activity/tips-getting-and-staying-active-you-age

Website from the National Institute on Aging covering how much activity you need, how to get going, how to set fitness goals, how to plan your workouts, and what to ask your doctor.

Mediterranean Diet

my.clevelandclinic.org/health/articles/16037-mediterranean-diet

Webpage from the Cleveland Clinic with easy-to-follow guidance to this healthy eating approach. Includes foods, serving goals, serving sizes, serving tips, suggested meals, and what to avoid.

National Weight Control Registry: Research Findings

nwcr.ws/Research/published%20research.htm

Links to studies on weight loss strategies that have proven successful.

My Menopause

acog.org/MyMenopause

Web resource from ACOG with information on the menopause transition, signs and symptoms, treatments, and self-care. Includes the latest information from the experts in ob-gyn care, menopause stories from real women, expert columns on how to manage symptoms, Q&A articles, videos, and more.

CHAPTER 15

Bone Health

Joan was 54 when she fell off her bike and fractured one of the small bones in her spine. A bone density scan showed osteopenia and osteoporosis at different points in her spine, and she started treatment right away. "I achieved much better bone density after several years of medication," she says. "My osteoporosis isn't 'cured,' but my bone density was more in line with other women my age. I have not had any side effects, so in my case, it's been a good thing. I also try to walk a couple of miles at least 5 days a week and eat more dairy products than I used to."

The *menopause transition* can be especially rough on bones. From midlife on, the risk of bone loss increases significantly. Bones probably won't break without a cause, like a fall—but fractures can happen unexpectedly, even in the 50s, among those with thinning bones. Typically, bones start weakening without any symptoms. Many people are not aware of bone loss until it's well advanced.

This is important to know because later in life half of women will eventually experience a fracture that is related to bone thinning. As people age, the likelihood of breaking bones is higher than it was in youth. After *menopause*—the last *menstrual period*—one fracture tends to lead to another. Changes related to aging make it harder for bones to heal, with increasingly severe consequences for health, mobility, and lifespan.

Bone density refers to the amount of minerals in the bones. High bone density means you have strong bones, and low bone density means your bones have weakened. In this chapter we'll look at what causes bone loss, when it is treated, and what treatment involves. We'll also look at the roles of *calcium*, vitamin D, and physical activity in protecting your bone health. And we'll discuss how you can talk with your *obstetrician–gynecologist (ob-gyn)* about your risk of bone loss. Midlife is the time to focus on maintaining as much bone density as you can.

How Bone Is Formed

Bones are made of protein, *collagen*, phosphate, and calcium. There are two types:

- Compact bone, which is the hard, solid outside part of a bone
- Spongy bone, which is found inside bones and filled with tiny holes, like a sponge

Each bone in the body has a compact outside and a spongy inside. And these bones change constantly throughout life. Old bone is removed through a process called resorption. New bone is built in a process called formation.

During childhood and the teen years, bone forms faster than it breaks down. This increases bone density and strength.

During early adulthood, the amount of bone formed is about equal to the bone that is broken down. This means bone density remains stable. **Estrogen** helps with this stability. But in midlife, when estrogen levels begin to decline, this process starts to reverse: bone breaks down faster than it is made. The period of fastest bone loss starts 1 year before the final menstrual period and lasts for about 3 years after. Studies suggest that over a period of 10 years, it's possible to lose around 10 percent of bone density.

Bone loss can get worse with age. When bone loss is mild, it's called *osteopenia*. When bone loss is advanced, it's called *osteoporosis*. In osteoporosis, the outside walls of compact bone become thinner, and the holes in spongy bone become larger. This causes the bones to become weaker, more brittle, and more prone to fractures.

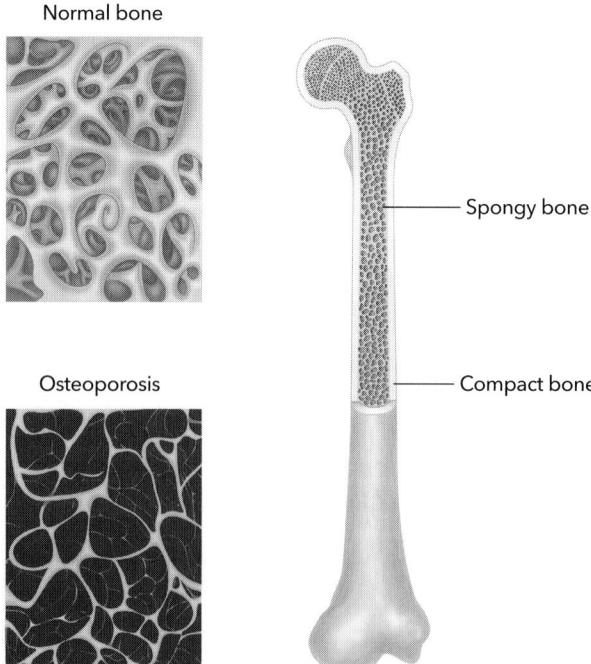

Effects of osteoporosis. Cross-sections show normal bone (top) and bone with osteoporosis (bottom). With osteoporosis, inner spongy bone becomes less dense and outer compact bone thins.

Having osteopenia in midlife is common, and it does not automatically mean osteoporosis will develop. But among people over 50, osteoporosis affects 1 in 5 women, and half of women over 50 and with osteoporosis will break a bone at some point. Breaking a hip or a bone in the spine is a leading cause of disability in older people.

Osteopenia and osteoporosis are called silent conditions. Osteoporosis may not cause any symptoms for years or even decades. The first signs of osteoporosis are seen in bones that already have a lot of spongy bone tissue. These include the hips, wrists, and spine.

For example, as the spinal bones (*vertebrae*) weaken, they can fracture. Fractures in the front part of the spinal bones can cause loss of height or a slight curving of the spine. This type of fracture often causes no pain. Other fractures of the spine can cause pain that travels from the back to the sides of the body. Among much older people, spinal fractures can happen even with minor incidents, like bumping against furniture or lifting a heavy suitcase.

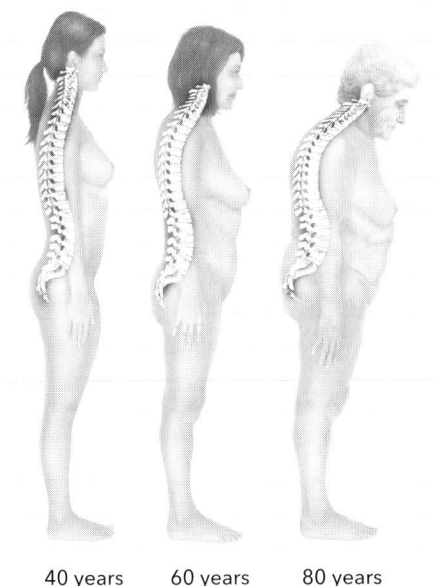

40 years   60 years   80 years

Osteoporosis of the spine. When the bones of the spine weaken and fracture, the spine can compress and curve over time.

> **Does osteopenia need to be treated?**
>
> Maybe. In some cases, your ob-gyn may recommend medication to reduce your risk of developing osteoporosis, especially if you've already broken a bone. If your osteopenia is stable and you haven't broken a bone, the most important things you can do are outlined in this chapter: increasing weight-bearing and other forms of exercise, eating well with a focus on recommended daily amounts of calcium and vitamin D, and avoiding smoking and limiting alcohol use. Some doctors also recommend switching to decaf coffee and soda because caffeine may cause a loss of bone density.
>
> –DR. ANDREW KAUNITZ

What Increases the Risk of Bone Loss

Though the decline in estrogen happens to all women, some are more likely than others to have bone loss and fractures. Factors that may contribute to osteoporosis and fractures include

- smoking
- alcohol use (more than one drink a day)
- early menopause (between 40 and 45) or *premature menopause* (before 40)
- family history of hip or spine fractures
- being underweight (having a *body mass index* or BMI that's less than 20 or weighing less than 127 pounds)

Racial background also affects the risk of osteoporosis. Research shows that in the United States, White and Hispanic women have the highest rates of fracture, followed by Native American, Asian, and Black women.

Certain medications may increase the risk of osteoporosis. These include

- some *corticosteroids* (used to treat *rheumatoid arthritis*, *inflammatory bowel disease*, allergies, and *autoimmune disorders*)
- *antidepressants* called *selective serotonin reuptake inhibitors (SSRIs)*
- antiseizure medications
- some medications used to treat *endometriosis* and other reproductive disorders
- thyroid medication
- some medications used for acid reflux or cancer treatment

And some medical conditions have also been linked to osteoporosis, including

- rheumatoid arthritis
- *diabetes*
- *kidney disease*
- *anorexia nervosa*
- *human immunodeficiency virus (HIV) infection*
- *acquired immunodeficiency syndrome (AIDS)*
- *primary ovarian insufficiency*

How Bone Loss Is Diagnosed

Routine screening can find osteopenia and osteoporosis. At an ob-gyn office visit, your doctor should review your medical history and measure your height. Losing height can indicate a fracture of a bone in your spine.

Your ob-gyn may use an online screening tool called FRAX (Fracture Risk Assessment Tool) to assess your risk of a fracture within the next 10 years. This tool uses several factors to calculate your risk, including your sex, age, height, weight, history of previous fracture, family history of hip fracture, use of steroid medication, smoking and alcohol use, and medical history. The U.S. version of FRAX also has calculations for White, Black, Asian, and Hispanic groups.

A bone mineral density test may be recommended if you are 65 or older, or you are younger than 65, past your last period, and at increased risk of osteoporosis. Screening is done using a DEXA scan (also called dual energy X-ray absorptiometry or DXA). This is a quick, painless imaging test that uses very low levels of X-rays. It identifies bone loss and helps assess your risk of fracture. You lie on a table and the scanner measures bone density at certain parts of your skeleton, usually the lower back and hips. Results will be given a T-score as shown in Table 15-1, "T-Scores and What They Mean."

Table 15-1 T-Scores and What They Mean

T-Score	Meaning	Examples
−1.0 or higher	Normal bone density	0.8, 0, −0.7
Between −1.0 and −2.5	Low bone density (osteopenia)	−1.1, −1.7, −2.4
−2.5 or lower	Osteoporosis	−2.6, −3.2, −3.7

A T-score of −2.5 or lower is diagnostic of osteoporosis. (Lower numbers might mean −2.6, −3.2, or −3.7.) If you are 50 or older and have had a fracture of the spine, hip, wrist, shoulder, rib, or pelvis, you probably have osteoporosis. Sometimes a T-score of −2.5 or lower can indicate a bone disease other than menopause as the cause of the osteoporosis. Your ob-gyn or another doctor can evaluate for this.

After your first DEXA scan, talk with your ob-gyn about when you should be tested again. Depending on the result, retesting every 2 to 3 years may be recommended. It may make sense to screen sooner, depending on your previous results, risk factors, and any treatment you start.

When and How to Treat Bone Loss

If you have a high risk of fracture, your ob-gyn may talk with you about treatment. The lifestyle changes used to prevent osteoporosis—physical activity and eating well—are also helpful when treating osteoporosis. Preventing falls also takes center stage after a diagnosis. Read the box "How to Avoid Falls" for more information.

How to Avoid Falls

With age, the combination of bone loss and the risk of falling becomes increasingly hazardous. Among seniors, falls are the leading cause of injuries leading to disability or death, especially among women. These approaches can reduce your risk of falling:

- Remove throw rugs or use rugs with nonskid backing.
- Use nonskid wax on hardwood floors.
- Eliminate clutter from the floor and stairs.
- Move cords and cables away from high-traffic areas.
- Make sure rooms are well lit and use a night light.
- Use handrails by stairs and in the bathroom.
- Store items at a height that does not require a step stool.
- Check and correct any vision problems.
- In winter weather, fit your boots with ice spikes or ice cleats. When walking on ice, bend forward slightly, walk flat-footed with your weight over your feet, and take shorter steps to maintain balance.

It's also important to review medications for side effects that may affect stability. If you have issues with balance or dizziness, talk with your ob-gyn. Depending on the cause, a physical therapist might be able to help. You can also consider having an occupational therapist assess your home for safety and fall risks.

Your ob-gyn may recommend that you see a doctor who specializes in treating osteoporosis. This could be an endocrinologist, a rheumatologist, a geriatrician, or a reproductive endocrinology and infertility (REI) specialist, an ob-gyn with training in disorders related to *hormones*. For more on REI doctors, read Chapter 5, "Choosing Your Menopause Care Team."

Medication cannot completely prevent bone fractures, but it can reduce the risk. Some medications slow bone loss. Others help rebuild bones. Osteoporosis medications differ in how they work, how they are taken, and how often they are taken. They can be given by mouth, with an injection, intravenously (through an IV), in a nasal spray, or as a skin patch. Some are taken daily. Others are taken weekly, monthly, yearly, or a few times a year. If you have (or are at risk of) blood clots, heart disease, or *stroke*, this may affect your medication options. Table 15-2, "Common Medications for Postmenopausal Osteoporosis," compares commonly prescribed medications.

Table 15-2 Common Medications for Postmenopausal Osteoporosis

Name of Medication	Used for Treatment or Fracture Prevention	How It Works	How It Is Given
Bisphosphonates	Different drugs at different dosages can be used for treatment, prevention, or both	Prevents resorption of bone	• A tablet taken by mouth daily, weekly, for a few days a month, or monthly • Through an IV once a year or a few times a year
Denosumab	Treatment, prevention, or both	Prevents resorption of bone	Injection every 6 months
Raloxifene	Treatment and prevention for women at increased risk of breast cancer	Prevents resorption of bone	A tablet taken by mouth daily
Hormone therapy	Prevention in women who meet specific criteria	Prevents resorption of bone	• A tablet or tablets taken by mouth daily or for a few days a month • Skin patch applied weekly or twice weekly

(continued)

Table 15-2 Common Medications for Postmenopausal Osteoporosis (continued)

Name of Medication	Used for Treatment or Fracture Prevention	How It Works	How It Is Given
Calcitonin (most often used when other treatments cannot be given; has a small risk of cancer)	Treatment for women 5 years past their last menstrual period	Prevents resorption of bone Promotes formation of new bone	• Nasal spray daily • Injection every other day
Abaloparatide or teriparatide	Treatment for up to 2 years in women at very high risk of fracture or who have fractures or high bone loss while taking other medications	Promotes formation of new bone	Injection every day
Romosozumab (should not be used if there is an increased risk of cardiovascular disease or stroke)	Treatment for up to 1 year in women at very high risk of fracture who have not had success with other medications	Prevents resorption of bone Promotes formation of new bone	Two injections each month

If osteoporosis is severe, or if the commonly used medications are not working, you may be offered medication that increases bone formation in your body. This medication is a synthetic form of parathyroid hormone that stimulates the growth of new bone and increases bone mineral density. It is taken daily as an injection underneath the skin, usually in the abdomen or thigh, and may be used for up to 2 years.

Hormone therapy may be an option for reducing fracture risk. You and your ob-gyn may consider this treatment if all of the following apply to you:

- Age younger than 60 or within 10 years of menopause
- Low risk of blot clots, breast cancer, and heart disease
- Having bothersome menopausal symptoms (**hot flashes**, night sweats)
- Cannot use other osteoporosis medications

Among those who stop taking hormone therapy, bone loss can be rapid unless another medication is used.

DEXA scans are used to monitor treatment. It usually takes at least 18 months of treatment to see an improvement in the DEXA score. If you're taking your medication consistently, a stable DEXA result—meaning no loss or gain of bone density—may be normal. If your treatment is going well, after several years your ob-gyn may recommend taking a break ("drug holiday") from your medication. This allows your body to get the benefits of the medication while minimizing possible side effects.

Lifestyle and Bone Loss

It's much better to prevent osteoporosis, or to prevent fractures if you already have the condition, than to treat them after they happen. Your lifestyle plays a key role in both. Consistent physical activity and getting enough calcium and vitamin D should be the cornerstones of your bone health plan.

> **Do I need a second opinion?**
>
> In the first year after having a broken bone, only 1 in 4 women who are 60 and older receives osteoporosis treatment. Researchers have found that Black women are less likely to get DEXA scans and receive medication than White and Hispanic women. Black women also have higher rates of poor outcomes after certain types of fracture. More research is needed to understand and address why some groups get different care than others. For now, if you've had a fracture or think you're at high risk and you are questioning your care, consider getting another doctor's advice.
>
> —DR. ESTHER EISENBERG

Best Activities for Bone Health

Being physically active increases bone density before menopause and slows bone loss after menopause. To protect your bones, it's extremely important to make time every week for focused exercise like the following:

- Weight-bearing activities—These include anything you do while standing or moving, so your muscles and bones work against gravity. Try brisk walking, running, dancing, racket sports, and jumping rope. (If you have osteoporosis, check with your doctor before doing activities that involve running or jumping.)

- Non-weight-bearing exercises—Tai chi, yoga, and Pilates can build endurance and improve your balance, flexibility, and posture. These can help sustain your physical function as you get older and reduce your risk of falls. Some studies suggest that yoga poses can improve bone density at the thigh bone and spine in women with osteopenia and osteoporosis.

More research needs to be done, but it's possible that the gentle pulling of different muscles may provide resistance that helps bone retain its density. But keep in mind that those with osteoporosis should avoid full-forward bends, back bends, and spinal twists.

- Strength training—Your muscles and bones are strengthened by resisting weight, such as your own body, exercise bands, weighted balls, dumbbells, or other strength-training equipment.

Be mindful of avoiding falls as you exercise. For example, consider walking or running on flat or paved trails. Wooded trails raise the risk of tripping on roots or rocks. Some physical activities, like rock climbing, cycling, hockey, and skiing, have a higher risk of injuries.

Calcium and Bones

You need enough calcium in your diet to help your bones stay healthy. Aim to get all or most of your calcium from foods rather than dietary supplements. Using supplements alone to meet your daily calcium needs does not reduce the risk of bone fractures. Also, supplements in excess can slightly increase the risk of kidney stones and, possibly, heart disease.

Before the final menstrual period, most women need 1,000 milligrams (mg) of calcium a day. After this, when they are *postmenopausal*, women need more calcium: 1,200 mg per day. Those with certain health conditions, such as kidney disease, should talk with their ob-gyn about how much calcium they need.

Many people do not get enough calcium from food. To increase your daily intake, eat a variety of calcium-rich foods. Skim milk, yogurt, and cheese are all high in calcium. Tofu, spinach, broccoli, bok choy, kale, almonds, and seeds are good sources of calcium. Adding sardines or anchovies with the bones to your diet can also increase your calcium intake. Many foods are fortified with calcium, too, including orange juice. You can also find fortified nondairy milks and yogurt, but they may be highly processed. Read the labels for added sugars, thickening agents, and other ingredients you might want to avoid.

Vitamin D and Bones

The body relies on vitamin D to help the gut absorb calcium. Until the age of 70, most people need 15 micrograms (mcg) of vitamin D a day. Sometimes this is described as 600 international units (IU) a day. People who are older than 70 should aim for 20 mcg (800 IU) daily.

Vitamin D is naturally found in a few foods, including fatty fish, egg yolks, and mushrooms. Many foods have vitamin D added, including cow's milk, nondairy milks, and cereal. Vitamin D can also be made in the body through exposure to sunlight. But most people do not get enough from sunlight alone, especially if you use sunscreen. If your ob-gyn thinks you may have low levels of vitamin D, a test can check the level in your blood. If it's below normal, you may need a supplement.

Other Nutrients and Bones

Protein and potassium are also needed to maintain bone health. Potassium, a mineral, helps the body process calcium. Many fruits and vegetables contain potassium. Most Americans already get enough protein in their diets.

RESOURCES

Bone Density Scan (DEXA or DXA)
radiologyinfo.org/en/info/dexa

DEXA information from the Radiological Society of North America, including a video guide.

Bone Health and Osteoporosis
niams.nih.gov/health-topics/bone-health-and-osteoporosis

Website from the National Institute of Arthritis and Musculoskeletal and Skin Diseases on what bone health means for you, bone density tests, the importance of calcium and vitamin D, and exercising for your bone health.

Bone Health and Postmenopausal Women
endocrine.org/patient-engagement/endocrine-library/menopause-and-bone-loss

Webpage from the Endocrine Society covering menopause and osteoporosis. Includes a guide to medical terms, information about medications, and a guide that can be downloaded.

My Menopause
acog.org/MyMenopause

Web resource from ACOG with information on the menopause transition, signs and symptoms, treatments, and self-care. Includes the latest information from the experts in ob-gyn care, menopause stories from real women, expert columns on how to manage symptoms, Q&A articles, videos, and more.

Part III

MANAGEMENT OF SYMPTOMS

CHAPTER 16

Lifestyle Changes and Alternative Approaches

Carole had no health problems until her 52nd birthday. Then her hot flashes began, first a few times a week and then every few hours over the next 6 years. "They caused an anxious feeling, like a mini panic attack," she says, and she was routinely waking up throughout the night. She tried plant-based supplements for a few months, but they didn't help. So she looked for other strategies. "Yoga has helped me," she says. "It calms my mind. I've also recently tried a meditation technique called yoga nidra. It's 90 minutes of yoga meditation while lying on my back. After the first time I tried it, I slept 6 hours straight."

Each woman experiences the *menopause transition* differently. Your individual needs and symptoms will affect the choices that you and your *obstetrician–gynecologist (ob-gyn)* make to help you feel better, but everyone can start with making lifestyle changes. This can include increasing exercise, eating healthy foods, quitting smoking, limiting caffeine and alcohol, prioritizing sleep, and trying calming techniques. In this chapter, we'll talk about self-care for menopausal symptoms and offer tips everyone can try.

For some people, nonprescription and over-the-counter products may provide relief. But keep in mind that many products sold online and in stores make claims that don't stand up to scientific testing. This chapter will also talk about which products work and what to watch out for when evaluating promises that seem too good to be true.

Self-Care as a Starting Point

We've said it before, and it bears repeating: Many of the lifestyle changes you're reading about in this book are the same things you've been hearing about your whole life. They may not be exciting, but they work for millions of women going through the menopause transition. In other words, there's no magic wand that will address any or all of your menopausal symptoms. But focusing on improving your overall health is likely to bring some relief and help you live longer.

Increase Physical Activity

Getting and staying active has profound benefits for your health and well-being. Regular physical activity lowers the risk of heart disease, **stroke, diabetes, bone loss**, dementia, and other chronic conditions. For some, these include relief from some menopausal symptoms.

- *Hot flashes* and night sweats—Some (but not all) research shows that aerobic exercise may reduce hot flashes. This is exercise that gets the lungs working and blood flowing, like brisk walking, running, swimming, and cycling. Keep in mind that exercise may trigger hot flashes for some women. If this happens to you, consider exercising in a cool environment, like an air-conditioned gym or yoga studio, and wear clothing that wicks moisture. Staying hydrated is also important during exercise. Remember that any physical activity, even if it causes hot flashes in the short term, has long-term benefits. It's possible that over time aerobic exercise helps the body better control core temperature and ease the sensation of hot flashes.

- Mood, anxiety, and stress—Physical activity is known to lessen the severity of *depression*, agitation, and stress, which become more common during the menopause transition. Exercise can also lower the risk of developing depression. One study found that just 2½ hours of walking per week lowers the risk of depression by 25 percent.

- Sleep—Studies have found that aerobic exercise during the menopause transition reduces *insomnia* and improves sleep quality. In a study involving women in *perimenopause*, three or more sessions a week of fitness qigong was especially beneficial for sleep. Qigong is a traditional Chinese practice involving posture, movement, and breathing.

- Weight—We know that exercise plays a key part in maintaining a healthy weight in midlife. Reducing weight by even a small amount can in turn reduce the risk of many conditions, such as heart disease, diabetes, and some cancers. Losing weight also decreases the risk of *pelvic organ prolapse*, which affects 1 in 4 women in their 40s and 1 in 3 in their 60s. You can read more about this condition in Chapter 13, "Pelvic Organ Prolapse."

- Sexual health—Growing evidence suggests that physical activity is linked to improved self-image and sexual health, especially in women. Regular exercise may help some people maintain or even resume sexual activity through midlife and beyond.

Quit Smoking

The benefits of quitting smoking may include relief from menopausal symptoms. Plus, freeing yourself from cigarettes is critically important for your health and well-being.

- Hot flashes and night sweats—Smoking increases the risk of hot flashes. In a multiyear study of more than 750 women aged 45 to 51, those who quit smoking were less likely to have hot flashes, including severe ones, than women who continued to smoke. Women who quit also had fewer hot flashes. But those who smoked were more likely to have hot flashes than women who had never smoked. The takeaway? To reduce hot flashes, stop smoking or just don't start.

- Mood, anxiety, and stress—It's possible that smoking increases the risk of mental health conditions. For example, the more people smoke, the higher their risk of depression. Similarly, smoking increases the risk of anxiety symptoms and anxiety disorders. The good news is that quitting is linked to lower rates of depression, especially as time goes on.

- Sleep—Smoking is linked to more severe insomnia and reduced sleep time. It's also related to breathing problems during sleep. In a study of more than 1,000 smokers and nonsmokers, smokers had a harder time falling asleep, staying asleep, and sleeping for long periods. Their sleep problems were even worse when smoking within 4 hours of bedtime.

- Pelvic organ problems—Women who smoke are at increased risk of **stress urinary incontinence** and pelvic organ prolapse, especially when smoking causes chronic coughing. Tobacco is a bladder irritant, which may increase the urge to urinate. And women who smoke are more likely to have **complications** following surgery for prolapse.

Menopausal and midlife concerns aside, quitting smoking is one of the most powerful actions you can take to prevent chronic disease and improve your future health. Quitting lowers your risk of many types of cancer, bone loss, mental health disorders, heart and lung diseases, stroke, dementia, and early death.

You may wonder if vaping is any better. The impact of vaping on menopause timing and symptoms is unknown, but we know that vaping is harmful to health. Though it doesn't use tobacco, vaping contains addictive *nicotine* and toxic chemicals. If you don't smoke, don't start vaping, either. If you're considering using vaping as a step toward quitting or reducing your use of cigarettes, here's what you need to know:

- Vape devices have fewer dangerous substances than traditional cigarettes and are thought to be less harmful to your health. But that doesn't mean they're safe. Vaping has been linked to lung disease, including asthma, and some research suggests that vaping raises the risk of heart disease and stroke. Also, the long-term effects of vaping on health are unknown.

- Most people should use proven ways to quit smoking. These include nicotine replacement products such as patches and gum, behavioral therapies and support, and medication. For some people in some circumstances—such as those who have not been successful with other quitting methods—vaping may be part of their efforts to quit smoking, but it's best to talk with your ob-gyn about this approach before you try it.

> **Can acupuncture help with my symptoms?**
>
> Studies have shown that 6 weeks of acupuncture may relieve hot flashes and night sweats with no side effects. Some people also use acupuncture to improve overall relaxation and well-being. From a doctor's perspective, there's little downside to acupuncture, so it may be worth trying if your symptoms are bothering you.
>
> –DR. CARRIE ANN TERRELL

Step Away From Caffeine

Caffeine may worsen some symptoms of menopause. Also, many people become more sensitive to the effects of caffeine as they age. If you have bothersome hot flashes or other menopausal symptoms, it's worth experimenting with limiting or avoiding coffee and other caffeinated beverages and products, like tea and caffeinated soda. You can also switch to decaf versions and see how you feel.

- Hot flashes and night sweats—Caffeine can expand the blood vessels and raise the heart rate, which can trigger hot flashes. A study of more than 1,800 women found that hot flashes were more than twice as likely during or after caffeine use.

- Mood, anxiety, and stress—Caffeine raises the risk of anxiety and can make anxiety symptoms worse. It can activate the body's stress responses and increase blood pressure. Some people are better able to tolerate caffeine, so take note of how that morning cup of fully caffeinated coffee or lunchtime soda makes you feel. If you notice changes, especially in anxiety level, try a week without caffeine as a test.

- Sleep—Caffeine intake makes insomnia worse and may also cause fragmented sleep. In several studies, people who abstained from caffeine all day had improved sleep quality and longer sleep times. It's worth avoiding caffeine from the afternoon onward and possibly even earlier in the day.

- *Urinary incontinence*—Caffeine is a bladder irritant and a **diuretic** and, like smoking, can make you feel like you need to urinate more often. In studies, caffeine intake is linked to **urgency urinary incontinence** (a sudden need to urinate along with leakage). Try herbal or caffeine-free teas instead to see if this helps symptoms.

Limit or Quit Alcohol

Doctors have long known that alcohol intake can affect some menopausal symptoms. And although small amounts of alcohol were once thought to be protective, current evidence now suggests this is unlikely. It's possible that any amount of alcohol, even the occasional glass of wine, is harmful for overall health.

- Hot flashes and night sweats—Though the research isn't clear, many women report that alcohol triggers hot flashes. Since the reasons aren't known, it's best to avoid alcohol altogether if you discover it makes your hot flashes worse.
- Mood, anxiety, and stress—Reducing drinking can lessen depression symptoms and stress and in turn improve quality of life. Alcohol use disorder and depression can happen together, with each condition raising the risk of the other. Drinking is also linked to a higher risk of anxiety.
- Sleep—Although alcohol may seem to help some people fall asleep sooner, it disrupts sleep during the second half of the night and people often wake up not feeling rested.
- Urinary incontinence—The evidence on alcohol as a cause of urinary incontinence is mixed. That said, alcohol is also a known bladder irritant and diuretic.
- Sexual health—A review of seven studies found that for women, drinking large amounts of alcohol was linked to problems with sexual stimulation, arousal, and reaching *orgasm*, as well as painful sex.

Back to the latest concerns about even small amounts of alcohol: The World Health Organization noted in 2023 that alcohol is toxic and causes at least seven types of cancer, including breast cancer and colorectal cancer. Alcohol use is also linked to heart disease, stroke, diabetes, and disorders of the liver, digestive system, and nerves. And it's associated with dementia and shortened lifespan. Reducing alcohol intake is a smart move, and quitting altogether is even better.

Practice Mind-Body Techniques

Mind–body approaches make use of the ways that the brain, feelings, body, and behaviors affect each other and influence your health. Techniques include meditation-based practices, breathing exercises, and related activities like yoga and tai chi. Various approaches to talk therapy are effective, too, whether in person or online.

- Hot flashes and night sweats—In many studies, mind–body practices have been shown to help relieve hot flashes. These include breathing slowly and deeply ("paced respiration") and mindfulness-based stress reduction. *Cognitive behavioral therapy (CBT)* designed for menopausal symptoms and hypnotic relaxation therapy have also shown promise. These interventions do not necessarily reduce the frequency or severity of hot flashes but may make them less bothersome. They may also improve other symptoms during the menopause transition, like anxiety, stress, and sleep disruption.

- Mood, anxiety, and stress—Various forms of talk therapy are proven treatments for depression, anxiety, trauma, and stress. Meditation, yoga, and relaxation practices can also be effective.

- Sleep—Cognitive behavioral therapy for insomnia, also called CBT-I, combines talk therapy strategies and behavioral changes and is a proven treatment for insomnia. Other approaches include relaxation techniques, meditation and mindfulness practices, yoga, and tai chi.

- Sexual health—Talk therapies, including couples counseling and sex therapy, are recommended approaches in some circumstances. Studies have shown success with mindfulness-based therapy and CBT for improving sexual desire in women. For support with sexual health issues in midlife, read Chapter 10, "Sexual Health."

In terms of long-term health, there's evidence that mind–body techniques help people manage pain and improve quality of life. Approaches that relieve stress and negative emotions may prevent **high blood pressure** and other health risk factors. Mind–body techniques can also be used in the treatment of chronic conditions, such as heart disease, **obesity**, cancer, diabetes, pain, and more.

Sleep Better

Sleeping a solid 7 to 9 hours a night may relieve certain symptoms of menopause. In addition, getting enough sleep is critical for your current and long-term health and quality of life. Poor quality sleep is common during the menopause transition, thanks mainly to hormonal changes, and the effects can be wide-ranging.

- Hot flashes and night sweats—Many studies have found a link between how often or how severely women experience hot flashes and the quality or duration of their sleep. It's unclear whether night sweats disrupt sleep, or whether disrupted sleep makes you more likely to notice night sweats. It's possible that taking steps to improve your sleep will make night sweats less bothersome, and vice versa.

- Mood, anxiety, and stress—Not getting enough sleep hurts women's emotional health and makes them vulnerable to stress. In a U.S. study, sleeping less than 6 hours a night was linked to frequent mental distress. Sleep is vital for relieving the brain fog of menopause, too. Without enough sleep, you're likely to struggle with learning, memory, and problem solving.

- Weight management—Sleep plays a crucial role in regulating appetite, *metabolism*, and weight. One study found that after just a few nights with disturbed sleep, women's bodies burned less fat, potentially contributing to weight gain.

- Sexual health—High-quality and sufficient sleep may be key to ongoing intimacy. A U.S. study found strong links between sleep duration, sexual activity, and sexual satisfaction.

Long-term, poor sleep raises the risk of dementia, diabetes, infection, heart disease, and stroke. Addressing sleep problems in the menopause transition can set you up for better sleep for the rest of your life. Read Chapter 9, "Sleep Problems," for recommendations.

> **Is chiropractic care an option for my symptoms?**
>
> There's no evidence that spinal adjustments done by a chiropractor can reduce hot flashes, night sweats, insomnia, or other symptoms of menopause. If your midlife concerns include things like lower back pain, chiropractic care may be able to help. Serious effects of chiropractic adjustment are rare, but people with *osteoporosis*, numbness or tingling in a limb, and higher risk of stroke should avoid spinal manipulation. For some aches and pains, massage may be a good option.
>
> —DR. ANDREW KAUNITZ

Nonprescription Products and Supplements

You may be wondering whether plant-based supplements or other so-called natural products can help with your menopausal symptoms. "Natural" sounds appealing, but it doesn't necessarily mean "safe." Dietary supplements and so-called "natural" health products are not tested by the U.S. Food and Drug Administration (FDA) or any other government authority. This means there's no way to know whether they contain the exact type or amount of ingredients needed to be safe or effective, or even the amount listed on the label. It's also hard to know whether the key ingredient has the benefits that are advertised. Some products are unlikely to help at all, while others have known risks. And some interact with medications and make them less effective.

Menopause is a major marketing opportunity for retailers and manufacturers. If you're active on social media, you may come across ads for products that claim to ease hot flashes, vaginal dryness, mood shifts, brain fog, weight gain, and more. Unfortunately, many product claims are misleading or false.

It's important to differentiate between supplements you take by mouth and products you use on the skin. Below, we'll discuss what's known about some heavily marketed supplements for hot flashes and brain health, and then we'll look at topical remedies for vaginal dryness. As always, let your ob-gyn know if you're using or considering any nonprescription product so they can confirm safety and effectiveness.

Supplements and Hot Flashes

The following products have been marketed for the relief of hot flashes, but currently there's no evidence to support using them for this purpose—and there is evidence that they are not effective. Fortunately, this has been a major area of research, so ob-gyns are clear that these supplements don't work.

- Soy and red clover (isoflavones or phytoestrogens)—Soybeans, some soy products, and red clover products contain high amounts of isoflavones. Isoflavones are similar to *estrogen* and come from plants. They are also known as phytoestrogens (plant estrogens). They act like a weak form of estrogen in the body.

    Many studies have investigated whether soy or red clover products relieve hot flashes. An analysis of 30 trials concluded that plant estrogens are likely of no benefit. These products do not seem to have significant side effects, but there is little to no evidence of their long-term safety. Women with an increased risk of *hormone*-sensitive cancer should avoid soy products altogether.

- Black cohosh—This North American plant has been marketed as a treatment for hot flashes, sleep disorders, and depression. Currently, the evidence does not show that it reduces symptoms. It does not appear to help with vaginal dryness either. Worse, some products labeled as black cohosh have been linked to liver damage, in some cases with severe outcomes.

There's also research looking at black cohosh and other therapies. A 1-year study of 351 women aged 45 to 55 who had two or more vasomotor symptoms per day compared black cohosh and black cohosh combinations (with herbs and soy) with **hormone therapy** and a placebo. Only the hormone therapy group showed improvement in menopausal symptoms. The group receiving herbs, including soy, had more intense symptoms after 1 year of treatment.

- Dong quai—Although this Chinese herbal medicine has been used to treat hot flashes, a study found it was not effective for reducing or relieving this symptom. Its side effects include increased sensitivity to sunlight (a higher risk of sunburn) and an increased risk of bleeding in people taking blood thinners. Limited evidence suggests that another Chinese herb, dang gui bu xue tang, may help with mild hot flashes.

- Ginseng—Ginseng is a plant used in Chinese medicine. The evidence for using ginseng to relieve menopausal symptoms is limited and based on small studies. While these have suggested ginseng may elevate mood and sense of well-being, this plant has not been found to relieve hot flashes.

- Vitamin E—In one study, vitamin E supplements were linked to one less hot flash a day. Very little evidence exists for the effectiveness of other vitamin supplements in the treatment of hot flashes.

Supplements and Brain Health

Despite what you may read and see on commercials, no dietary supplement has been shown to preserve thinking skills, improve brain function, or delay or prevent dementia in adults 50 and over. Doctors and researchers say the best nutrients for brain health come from aerobic exercise and a healthy diet.

- Cannabis and CBD—Many women report that cannabis and CBD improve anxiety, mood, and sleep. This makes sense because cannabis helps the brain calm down. But there's no long-term research on the effectiveness or side effects of using cannabis for any menopausal symptoms. And a recent study showed that cannabis use did not make hot flashes better.

- Kava—The root of the kava plant is sometimes used for anxiety, stress, or restlessness. The evidence on its effectiveness for anxiety is limited and mixed. The FDA has issued a warning that kava is associated with liver damage. It has also been linked to other severe side effects. There is no evidence that kava helps relieve hot flashes.

- Ashwagandha, also marketed for anxiety, is not proven to improve menopausal symptoms, and it may cause liver damage.

- St. John's wort may help some people with mild depression, but the evidence is mixed and it has potential interactions with commonly used prescription medications.

Read Chapter 8, "Mood and Memory," for ways to address mood and memory changes during the menopause transition.

Vaginal Moisturizers and Lubricants

Vaginal dryness and thinning of the vaginal lining is caused by reduced estrogen and can lead to genital discomfort and pain during sex. Unfortunately, unlike hot flashes, menopausal vaginal changes do not resolve on their own over time, so it's worth trying vaginal moisturizers and lubricants to find out what works for you. Some nonhormonal vaginal moisturizers and lubricants can be very effective.

Vaginal moisturizers trap moisture in and around the vagina to relieve dryness. They may reduce itching, irritation, and pain. Vaginal lubricants relieve friction and sexual pain related to vaginal dryness. You can buy vaginal moisturizers and lubricants over the counter. If anything you use seems to irritate the genital area, switch to something else.

An over-the-counter vaginal moisturizer that has shown promise is hyaluronic acid. This substance is made in the body and can be found in tablets or gels that are inserted into the vagina. Studies have found that hyaluronic acid products relieve vaginal dryness, itching, and burning. They can also improve lubrication and relieve pain during sex.

Some people use cooking oils, particularly coconut and olive oil, for lubrication during sex. While they may make intercourse more comfortable, they can't be used with latex condoms or dental dams, as oil can damage the latex. And some oils can disrupt vaginal pH and increase the risk of infection. Petroleum jelly can weaken condoms and is linked to increased bacteria in the vagina. Always talk with your ob-gyn if you're looking at oils for help with vaginal dryness. Silicone- and water-based lubes might be alternatives.

You may also have seen wild yam promoted for vaginal dryness. This is typically a cream used on the skin (not in the vagina). Wild yam can act like a weak estrogen in the body, but there's no evidence that it can improve vaginal or other menopausal symptoms.

We also don't have enough evidence to know whether herbal remedies or soy products are safe or useful for treating vaginal symptoms. The most effective approach continues to be estrogen therapy that's applied directly inside the vagina. For more information on this therapy, read Chapter 17, "Hormone Therapies."

Finally, compounded bioidentical hormones are sometimes touted as safer and more natural than prescription hormone therapy, especially for vaginal dryness. Compounded products are made by compounding pharmacies using a prescription, but they are not approved or monitored by the FDA, which is why health insurance usually does not cover them.

Note that FDA-approved, naturally occurring hormones are available in a wide range of prescription doses and delivery systems. FDA-approved hormones include oral micronized progesterone, oral and vaginal estradiol, and DHEA. This means "bioidentical" hormones are available to most women without the need for compounding. ACOG and the National Academies of Sciences, Engineering, and Medicine recommend FDA-approved hormone therapy and discourage the use of compounded hormone therapy. For more on bioidentical hormone therapy, read the box "Bioidentical Hormone Therapy" in Chapter 17, "Hormone Therapies."

Evaluating Product Claims

If the FDA hasn't approved a product and the manufacturer is making claims, how do you know what to think? Ob-gyns have a few suggestions.

Rule #1: Regardless of what's being claimed—rapid weight loss, rapid regrowth of hair, stopping hot flashes cold—if it sounds too good to be true, it probably is. And be wary of any claim that a product contains "a secret ingredient your doctor doesn't want you to know about." The products that really work to address symptoms are already well known to ob-gyns.

Rule #2: If a doctor or other person, well known or otherwise, promotes a treatment that is sold under their name, beware. This is a potential conflict of interest and should raise a red flag.

Rule #3: When evaluating research claims, look for the results, not just mention of the studies. Look for randomized controlled trials, which are studies where participants are randomly assigned to groups to test the effects of different treatments. The random grouping of people helps ensure the focus will stay on the product itself. And make sure the study has a comparison placebo group, meaning a group that uses a product with none of the ingredients being tested.

For more tips on evaluating product research claims, read the column "Making Sense of Ads That Cite Clinical Studies" at the ACOG website (see the Resources section for a link).

When What You're Trying Isn't Working

When you're suffering with symptoms, it's tempting to try almost anything that sounds like it might work. If you find a topical product that really improves symptoms, like an over-the-counter vaginal moisturizer, you can keep using it. But if your symptoms start interfering with daily life—your mood swings are challenging, or you regularly wake up clammy from night sweats—it's OK to check in with your ob-gyn and start talking about prescription options. There are many options to choose from, including estrogen-free and FDA-approved hormone medications. You don't have to suffer in silence.

RESOURCES

Finding and Evaluating Online Resources
nccih.nih.gov/health/finding-and-evaluating-online-resources

Webpage from the National Center for Complementary and Integrative Health with tips on how to evaluate alternative medicine information found on social media and mobile apps. Includes tips on what to ask about a site's claims, how to determine if you're reading an ad or news, and how to protect yourself from fake news sites.

How Safe Is This Product or Practice?
nccih.nih.gov/health/how-safe-is-this-product-or-practice

Webpage from the National Center for Complementary and Integrative Health listing more than 100 supplements and practices with links to find safety information, including side effects.

Making Sense of Ads That Cite Clinical Studies
acog.org/ClinicalStudies

Eight ways to learn if a product's research claims are based in good science.

Over-the-Counter Medicines: What's Right for You?
fda.gov/drugs/choosing-right-over-counter-medicine-otcs/over-counter-medicines-whats-right-you

Webpage from the U.S. Food and Drug Administration offers advice on using unregulated products and how to understand the labels. It also addresses what to avoid when you have certain health conditions and how to reduce your risk of an over-the-counter product interacting with medications.

My Menopause
acog.org/MyMenopause

Web resource from ACOG with information on the menopause transition, signs and symptoms, treatments, and self-care. Includes the latest information from the experts in ob-gyn care, menopause stories from real women, expert columns on how to manage symptoms, Q&A articles, videos, and more.

CHAPTER 17

Hormone Therapies

At 51, Anna was having hot flashes and felt anxious. When she talked with her ob-gyn, she learned that systemic hormone therapy could curb the hot flashes and possibly help with her mood. Her ob-gyn offered hormone patches, pills, or cream. "The patch seemed by far the easiest," she says. Anna started a combined patch that releases estrogen and progestin through the skin. She changes the patch twice a week, and almost immediately she saw improvement. "Within two days of using it, I felt better and the anxiety was gone." Anna plans to stay on hormone therapy for as long as it can safely relieve her symptoms.

Few topics related to the *menopause transition* have gotten as much attention as *hormone therapy*. In the past, this therapy for menopausal symptoms was called "hormone replacement therapy," but the word "replacement" has been dropped in recent years. Hormone therapy is not meant to fully replace the *estrogen* levels that are in the bloodstream during the reproductive years. The goals of therapy are to take enough estrogen to curb symptoms and improve quality of life while managing any risks.

When taken for *hot flashes* and night sweats, *hormones* are typically taken as a pill or absorbed through the skin. This is called systemic hormone therapy. The hormones enter the bloodstream and are distributed around the body. Once in the body, hormones act on key tissues via the estrogen receptor. This means systemic hormone therapy may also help with other symptoms, like vaginal dryness.

Topical treatment for vaginal dryness and vulvar irritation, usually in the form of estrogen suppositories or creams, is called local hormone therapy. "Local" means the estrogen works only in nearby tissues and does not go to other places in the body.

Hormone therapy works well for most women, though *obstetrician–gynecologists (ob-gyns)* recommend taking the lowest dose of hormone that works for the shortest time needed. And hundreds of studies have shown that this therapy is safe and effective for most women. In this chapter we'll talk about the benefits and risks of hormone therapy and how it's used. Your decision to use it will depend on your symptoms and medical history as well as your preferences. Talking with your ob-gyn is a good place to start.

Hormone Therapy: History and Controversy

In the 1990s, a section of the National Institutes of Health launched the Women's Health Initiative (WHI). The initiative included trials to study whether estrogen or an estrogen–*progestin* combination could help prevent heart disease and other diseases in *postmenopausal* women, whether or not they had bothersome symptoms. The research did not look at hormone therapy's effectiveness for treating menopausal symptoms. The 13-year WHI Hormone Therapy Trials included more than 27,000 women between the ages of 50 and 79.

In 2002, WHI researchers stopped their work, saying that hormone therapy used in the trials was linked to an increased risk of serious health problems, including blood clots, *stroke*, and breast cancer. This news was picked up by the media, and many midlife women immediately stopped using hormone therapy.

This negative reaction has been long-lasting and unfortunate. The primary purpose of the trials was to focus on heart disease because, at that time, it was widely believed that hormones might be used to prevent heart disease. For this reason, many participants were in their 60s and 70s, when heart disease is more common and when any positive effects of treatment might be seen. We now know that hormone therapy generally should not be started after 60 because the risks outweigh the benefits.

As for the medications used, researchers chose a specific combination of estrogen and progestin that was commonly used in the 1990s. These particular hormones are much less likely to be used in hormone therapy today. It's possible that some types of estrogen or progestin that were not used in the study might have produced different results.

Now, more than two decades later, we have many studies showing that hormone therapy can be used safely and effectively for menopausal symptoms. Plus, we have very precise assessments of its risks. When WHI researchers looked at results by age to learn how younger midlife women responded, they determined the benefits tend to outweigh the risks for women between 50 and 59.

Having said that, there are still some small but increased risks, including the risk of some types of cancer (see below), for some women. So any conversation about the use of this therapy should include a review of your health status and medical history. The bottom line? Hormone therapy isn't all bad, and it's not all good. A decision to use this therapy to improve menopausal symptoms and quality of life is best determined by understanding your unique situation and talking with your ob-gyn.

How Systemic Therapy Works

Systemic therapy releases hormones into the bloodstream. The estrogen part of the therapy can be delivered in different ways, including

- as a pill taken by mouth
- in a patch worn on the skin that is changed once or twice a week

- as gels or sprays applied to the skin
- as a vaginal ring that is inserted every 3 months and slowly releases estrogen into the bloodstream

Estrogen alone increases the risk of **endometrial cancer**. If you have had a **hysterectomy**, you can safely use systemic estrogen by itself. But if you still have your **uterus**, your ob-gyn will prescribe progestin. This medication helps keep the lining of the uterus thin, so cancer is less likely to develop. Progestin can be delivered in different ways, including

- as a pill taken by mouth
- as tablets or gels you place in the **vagina**
- in an **intrauterine device (IUD)**—the same as the IUD used for **birth control**—that releases progestin in the uterus

Progestin can also be combined with estrogen in the same pill or patch.

Estrogen-only therapy is taken daily. There are two ways to combine estrogen and progestin for women who still have a uterus:

- Continuous-combined therapy: Both estrogen and progestin are taken every day.
- Cyclic therapy: Estrogen is taken daily. Progestin is added for 10 to 14 days each month (usually as a pill).

You and your ob-gyn can discuss the approach that works best for you and your lifestyle.

If you are past your final period and have a uterus, you have another option. Estrogen therapy can be combined with a medication called bazedoxifene. This is in a class of medications called **selective estrogen receptor modulators (SERMs)**. Bazedoxifene is a SERM that stops estrogen from thickening the lining of the uterus. This reduces the risk of endometrial cancer in the same way that progestin does. Estrogen combined with bazedoxifene treats hot flashes and night sweats and helps prevent bone loss and osteoporosis. It is taken by mouth as a single tablet once a day.

> **Should I have hormone testing before starting hormone therapy?**
>
> Hormone testing isn't recommended before starting hormone therapy. Hormone levels change a lot during the menopause transition, so testing likely would not offer any useful information. Your ob-gyn should be able to recommend hormone therapy based on your symptoms, menstrual changes, and medical history.
>
> –DR. ANDREW KAUNITZ

Benefits of Systemic Hormone Therapy

Hormone therapy has a range of positive effects on menopausal symptoms. Medications can directly address some symptoms while indirectly addressing others.

Relief From Hot Flashes and Night Sweats

Systemic hormone therapy is the most effective treatment for hot flashes and night sweats. An analysis of research involving more than 3,300 women found that systemic therapy reduced the number of hot flashes by an average of 75 percent. For example, those who had 40 hot flashes a week before treatment had about 10 hot flashes a week while on treatment. Hormone therapy also makes hot flashes milder.

Relief From Vaginal Dryness

Systemic therapy can relieve vaginal and vulvar dryness and irritation, increase vaginal lubrication, and restore the structure of vaginal tissue. But if dryness and irritation are your only symptoms, your ob-gyn may recommend local estrogen therapy instead. You can read more on this later in the chapter.

Improved Sexual Health

If vaginal symptoms improve on systemic therapy, sexual functioning may also improve. Increased vaginal lubrication can help reduce pain and tissue tearing caused by *sexual intercourse*. It's not clear whether taking estrogen improves sexual desire, but there are medications approved by the U.S. Food and Drug Administration (FDA) that can help with desire. You can read about them in Chapter 10, "Sexual Health."

Better Bone Health

Systemic estrogen protects against the bone loss that happens early in the menopause transition. Estrogen is not prescribed solely for bone loss prevention, but it's a positive side effect for those who are taking systemic therapy for hot flashes and night sweats.

Improved Sleep

Systemic therapy can relieve sleep disruption linked to night sweats and insomnia during the menopause transition. It can improve sleep quality, help you fall asleep sooner, and reduce nighttime wakefulness. Estrogen taken through the skin may be more beneficial for sleep than estrogen pills.

Lower Risk of Depression

Systemic therapy may help with mood symptoms. In a U.S. study, 1 year on estrogen patches and oral progestin helped prevent depressive symptoms in women during *perimenopause* and after their last period. Sometimes estrogen is used alongside an *antidepressant*. It's unclear whether hormone therapy helps with anxiety.

Improved Joint Pain, Skin, and Hair

In one U.S. study, systemic estrogen used after menopause was linked to a small reduction in joint pain that lasted several years. Meanwhile, there is little evidence that skin and hair benefit from hormone therapy, though some women and doctors believe this is true. Estrogen therapy may improve the texture, appearance, thickness, and elasticity of skin.

It's also important to note that hormone therapy should not be expected to be an effective weight loss treatment. If you have questions about weight changes in midlife, read Chapter 14, "Weight and Menopause."

Side Effects and Risks of Systemic Therapy

Many women are able to take systemic hormone therapy with few problems. Possible side effects include

- vaginal spotting or bleeding, which usually stops within 6 months
- temporary breast soreness
- bloating (fluid retention)
- headaches

Talk with your ob-gyn if these side effects trouble you or last longer than expected. In most cases, a lower dose of estrogen can help symptoms without causing these problems. If you're using estrogen pills, switching to a patch or gel may stop these side effects.

You and your ob-gyn should also talk about the risks of using systemic therapy. Generally, therapy may increase the risk of certain health problems, including breast cancer, blood clots, and heart disease. The overall risk is lower when hormone therapy is started within 10 years of the last period.

Risk may also depend on what form of estrogen therapy you use. This is because the body processes different forms of medication in different ways. For example, pills are processed by the liver, so women with liver disease may want to avoid oral medication. Patches send estrogen through the skin straight to the bloodstream, so the medication bypasses the liver. Specific health risks are outlined below.

Breast Cancer

Combined therapy—taking estrogen and progestin together—is linked to a small increased risk of breast cancer, especially when therapy is used for more than 5 years. In contrast, among women who have had a hysterectomy, estrogen-only therapy does not increase breast cancer risk and may even reduce breast cancer risk. If you have a history of hormone-sensitive breast cancer, your ob-gyn will likely recommend trying hormone-free therapies, rather than systemic hormone therapy, to treat hot flashes, night sweats, and other symptoms. Women who have had their breast tissue removed to reduce their risk of breast cancer may be able to safely take systemic therapy.

> **Can testosterone be used for any menopausal symptoms?**
>
> The hormone testosterone has been studied for menopausal symptoms. There's currently no evidence that testosterone can help with hot flashes. It's also not FDA approved to treat low sexual desire in women, in part because of the risks. These include cholesterol problems, excess hair growth, and acne. There also are no long-term studies that look at the effects of testosterone use on future breast cancer or cardiovascular disease. But there is some evidence that testosterone can help those with sexual interest or arousal disorders. You can read more about this in Chapter 10, "Sexual Health."
>
> —DR. NANETTE SANTORO

Blood Clots

Estrogen used with or without progestin is linked with a small risk of blood clots and stroke. This risk increases with age and other factors, including heart disease, kidney disease, and *obesity*. Patches, sprays, and rings appear to pose less risk than pills.

Heart Disease

Starting estrogen and progestin after age 60 may increase the risk of heart attacks. Some research suggests that therapy with estrogen and progestin might protect against heart attacks in women who start when they are younger than 60 or within 10 years of their last period. But other studies do not support this finding. More research is needed. For more information on lowering your risk of heart disease, read Chapter 19, "Heart Disease and Diabetes."

Gallbladder Disease

There is a small increased risk of gallbladder disease associated with estrogen therapy with or without progestin. This risk is greatest with pills.

When talking about risks, remember that many are related to your health and family history. It's clear that some women should not use systemic hormone therapy. You should talk with your ob-gyn about hormone-free treatments for your menopausal symptoms if you've ever had

- breast cancer, endometrial cancer, stroke, or heart disease
- a higher risk of blood clots (for example, if you have *factor V Leiden*, an inherited blood clotting disorder)
- meningioma, a type of tumor in the brain or spinal cord
- active liver disease

- untreated *high blood pressure*
- porphyria cutanea tarda, a rare skin disorder

You also should not start hormone therapy if you are or think you might be pregnant.

How Long to Stay on Hormone Therapy

Many women who start systemic therapy experience great relief of symptoms. Reducing hot flashes and night sweats and the benefits that come with it—better sleep and mood—can improve quality of life so much that women naturally ask how long they can keep it going.

When to stop hormone therapy is an individual decision. You and your ob-gyn should talk every year about your symptoms and any changes in your health. If your hot flashes and night sweats are controlled and your health is stable, you may continue therapy. Some women stop within 5 years or when their symptoms stop being bothersome. Most women will no longer have hot flashes by 7 to 10 years after their final *menstrual period*. But others continue to use it after their 50s to relieve symptoms. Use of hormone therapy should always be based on the risks, benefits, and symptoms of each person.

Women who experience early menopause (between 40 and 45) or *premature menopause* (before 40) and who do not have a history of breast cancer often take hormone therapy at least until 51, the average age of the last period. Doing so helps manage menopausal symptoms and reduces the risk of health conditions caused by early or premature menopause.

Coming off hormone therapy can cause symptoms to come back. For hot flashes, the return of symptoms can be temporary and last a few weeks to months, or they may come raging back as bad as they were when treatment was first started. Studies show this affects half of women, regardless of their age and how long they were using hormone therapy. It's not clear if stopping hormone therapy suddenly or gradually makes a difference. Symptoms such as vaginal dryness should be expected to get worse when systemic therapy is stopped, which underscores the importance of local (vaginal) hormone therapy.

Local Hormone Therapy

Changes in estrogen levels often affect the vagina, *vulva*, and *urinary tract* during the menopause transition. Over time, the vaginal lining can get thinner, dryer, and less elastic. This can lead to vaginal and vulvar discomfort and pain or bleeding with sexual intercourse. The decrease in estrogen may also thin the lining of the urinary tract and lead to urinary symptoms. In contrast with hot flashes, vaginal symptoms caused by estrogen loss do not get better over time.

Vaginal estrogen directly relieves dryness and irritation and helps restore thickness and elasticity to the vaginal lining. Vaginal estrogen also can ease irritation of the urinary tract, reduce urinary frequency, and improve incontinence. And vaginal estrogen may reduce postmenopausal **urinary tract infections (UTIs)**.

Vaginal estrogen is available in rings, capsules, tablets, and creams. A very low dose of estrogen is used, which means you don't need to take progestin, even if you have a uterus. Local hormone therapy might be a good option if you have

- vaginal burning and itching
- decreased lubrication and pain during sex
- bleeding or spotting after sex
- more frequent vaginal infections and UTIs
- frequent urination

If you have these symptoms but also want to treat bothersome hot flashes or night sweats, systemic hormone therapy may be a better choice for you. Some women use both systemic and local therapy.

Side Effects of Local Hormone Therapy

Side effects of local therapy are uncommon and may ease as you adjust to the medication. Talk with your ob-gyn if you have

- breast tenderness
- itching or redness of the genital area
- headache
- nausea
- vaginal itching or discharge

Low-dose local estrogen does not appear to raise the risk of endometrial cancer. If you have a history of breast cancer, discuss vaginal estrogen with your ob-gyn and oncologist. Most doctors recommend using nonhormonal treatments. That said, research shows that there's very little absorption of low-dose and ultra-low-dose vaginal estrogen. Any serious impact on health is unlikely, including for women who have had breast cancer and are at low risk of it coming back. Still, your oncologist should be your guide.

Compounded bioidentical hormones are sometimes touted as safer and more natural than prescription hormone therapy, especially for vaginal dryness. Compounded products are made by compounding pharmacies using a prescription, but they are not approved or monitored by the FDA, which is why health insurance usually does not cover them. There are other concerns with their use, and ACOG and the National Academies of Sciences, Engineering, and Medicine do not recommend them. You can read more in the box "Bioidentical Hormone Therapy."

Bioidentical Hormone Therapy

Bioidentical hormones are chemically the same as hormones produced by the body. They are usually made from plants. Many bioidentical hormones have been FDA approved in prescription form. These include oral micronized progesterone, oral and vaginal estradiol, and DHEA.

Other bioidentical hormones are compounded preparations. These hormone treatments are made by a compounding pharmacist using a prescription. They are available in various forms. They may be taken by mouth, through the skin, as implants or injectables, or as tablets placed in the vagina. Here's what you should know:

- We have much less information about the safety of compounded bioidentical hormones than we do about standard hormone medications, including FDA-approved bioidentical formulations.

- Compounded drugs are not approved or regulated by the FDA. This means that most compounded preparations have not been thoroughly tested for safety or effectiveness. For this reason, compounded drugs are often not covered by health insurance. Compounded drugs also vary in strength and purity. You can take too little or too much of a hormone without knowing it.

- Studies have not shown any benefit to compounded bioidentical hormones over standard hormone therapy. And because we don't have the same level of information about the safety and effectiveness of bioidentical compounded treatments, standard therapy is the safer option. While the FDA monitors for and reports on health problems caused by medication, there is no such monitoring system for compounded hormones.

In some specific cases, compounded medications may be appropriate. For example, a person who is allergic to peanuts would not be able to take micronized progesterone if the capsule contains peanut oil. A customized treatment might be created instead. This would involve working with the compounding pharmacist to address concerns about the strength and purity of the medication.

Talking With Your Ob-Gyn

Hormone therapy is a very effective option for treating menopausal symptoms. It's especially useful if you have symptoms in addition to hot flashes, like vaginal dryness, mood changes, and issues with memory. But starting hormone therapy is an individual decision and depends in part on your health status and medical history. It may not be the best option for you. To find out, talk with your ob-gyn about your symptoms.

Fortunately, there are other effective ways that menopausal symptoms can be treated for those who don't want or cannot take hormone therapy. If you're looking for information on nonhormonal treatments, read Chapter 18, "Estrogen-Free Medical Therapies."

RESOURCES

Hormone Replacement Therapy
medlineplus.gov/hormonereplacementtherapy.html
Summary page from the National Library of Medicine that includes links to statistics, research, and journal articles on menopausal hormone therapy.

Menopause: Medicines to Help You
fda.gov/consumers/free-publications-women/menopause-medicines-help-you
Information from the U.S. Food and Drug Administration with details on different hormone medications, including details on different brands and how they work.

Menopause Topics: Hormone Therapy
menopause.org/patient-education/menopause-topics/hormone-therapy
Webpage on hormone therapy from The Menopause Society.

My Menopause
acog.org/MyMenopause
Web resource from ACOG with information on the menopause transition, signs and symptoms, treatments, and self-care. Includes the latest information from the experts in ob-gyn care, menopause stories from real women, expert columns on how to manage symptoms, Q&A articles, videos, and more.

CHAPTER 18

Estrogen-Free Medical Therapies

When Sheila was 53, she started having up to 30 hot flashes a day. She tried herbal remedies marketed for menopause but nothing changed. Her doctor mentioned venlafaxine, an antidepressant that's also used to treat hot flashes. This treatment option appealed to Sheila, partly because the dose could easily be adjusted. "Within 36 hours of starting venlafaxine, my hot flashes had reduced in frequency and intensity by 75 percent," she says. Also, she hasn't had any side effects. "The improvement has continued to be amazing. I'm 58 now and still take the medication. I get some hot flashes, but I'm past the peak."

If lifestyle changes and over-the-counter products haven't helped your menopausal symptoms and you want to avoid therapies that use *estrogen*, here's good news: There are safe and effective estrogen-free medications to reduce *hot flashes* and night sweats. There are also estrogen-free treatments for vaginal dryness, which can cause painful sex during the *menopause transition*.

Estrogen-free options are vital for women who can't use *hormone therapy* for health reasons. For example, those with current or past breast cancer may struggle with early *menopause* induced by *chemotherapy*, and their cancer treatments may worsen menopausal symptoms. Their hot flashes may be more severe and continue longer than average. And there's a possibility that estrogen treatment could increase the risk of breast cancer coming back.

But wanting to avoid hormone therapy isn't limited to those with medical conditions. Some women just prefer the idea of not using estrogen to manage symptoms during the menopause transition. They may also want to avoid the possible health risks of hormone therapy, which increase with age. In this chapter, we'll look at the estrogen-free medications that you and your *obstetrician–gynecologist (ob-gyn)* can consider. We'll cover their benefits, risks, and side effects, as well as who can benefit most from them.

If you decide to try a medication discussed here, you may find that it improves your quality of life along with relieving your menopausal symptoms. If you also want to consider hormone therapy and why ob-gyns consider it safe for many women, read Chapter 17, "Hormone Therapies." In any case, the decision to use medication should be made in partnership with your ob-gyn. Together you can find what will work best for your symptoms and goals for treatment.

Medications for Hot Flashes and Night Sweats

Estrogen-free medications for hot flashes and night sweats can be very effective. They may not work as well as hormone therapy, but some treatment may be better than no treatment, especially if your symptoms disrupt sleep. Two medications are approved by the U.S. Food and Drug Administration (FDA) for menopausal symptoms.

There also are medications for hot flashes and night sweats that are used "off-label." When a medication is FDA approved for a condition and becomes available, doctors can prescribe it for other conditions if they judge that it is appropriate. This is called off-label use. Doctors might recommend off-label use of a medication when evidence from clinical studies suggests it can help treat a disease or symptom. One popular example is **GLP-1 receptor agonists,** which were developed to treat type 2 *diabetes* but are now widely used for weight loss. Doctors might also recommend off-label medication use when other FDA-approved medications haven't worked.

Off-label use of some medications is common during menopause because they can be very effective for symptoms. But you and your ob-gyn should always talk about the benefits and risks for your situation. For a comparison of the following medications, see Table 18-1, "Estrogen-Free Medications for Menopausal Symptoms."

Fezolinetant

This FDA-approved medication treats moderate to severe hot flashes and night sweats. It works in the part of the brain that helps control body temperature. In international trials, more than 500 women aged 40 to 65 who took a high dose of fezolinetant saw their hot flashes cut in half. Those on a lower dose also had improvement. In addition, their hot flashes felt less severe. Women on fezolinetant woke up less often at night, had less distress related to hot flashes, and had improved quality of life.

Fezolinetant is taken as a pill at the same time every day. The most common side effect is headaches. Rarely, the medication can cause stomach pain, diarrhea, insomnia, and back pain. There's also a rare risk of liver injury with this medication. Your ob-gyn should check your liver function with a blood test before you start taking it. Blood tests should also be done at 1, 2, 3, 6, and 9 months of treatment.

Fezolinetant cannot be taken with certain other medications because it interacts with them. Be sure to tell your ob-gyn if anything new is prescribed for you or if you are starting a new over-the-counter medication. There are several medications in development that act similarly to fezolinetant. If you are unable to take it, it's possible that a newer medication will become available that will work for you.

Paroxetine Mesylate

Paroxetine mesylate is an *antidepressant* that's FDA approved for treatment of hot flashes. This medication is known as a *selective serotonin reuptake inhibitor (SSRI)*. It should be taken at the same time every day, usually at bedtime. The most common side effects are nausea, vomiting, drowsiness, dizziness, trouble sleeping, loss of appetite, weakness, dry mouth, sweating, blurred vision, and yawning. If side effects don't get better, talk with your ob-gyn right away.

Other Antidepressants

In addition to paroxetine mesylate, there are other antidepressants that are used for hot flashes and other menopausal symptoms. They are SSRIs and *selective serotonin–norepinephrine reuptake inhibitors (SNRIs)* used off-label. Sometimes they are taken at lower doses than the doses used for *depression*.

SSRIs and SNRIs are usually taken as a pill once a day. Side effects may include nausea, dizziness, dry mouth, nervousness, constipation, sleepiness, sweating, and sexual difficulties such as reduced sexual desire or even the inability to have an orgasm. These side effects often go away with time or when the dosing is adjusted. The medications venlafaxine, desvenlafaxine, fluoxetine, and escitalopram appear to be effective for hot flashes.

Gabapentin

Gabapentin is used to treat seizures and nerve pain. It is not FDA approved for treatment of hot flashes, but studies have shown that it reduces their frequency and severity. In a U.S. trial of women taking gabapentin, almost half had fewer hot flashes, and more than half reported that their hot flashes were less severe.

Gabapentin is taken as a pill up to three times a day, with or without food. The starting dose usually is taken at night because it can cause sleepiness. Your ob-gyn may have you work your way up to three doses per day, or if your worst hot flashes occur only at night, you can limit use to nighttime dosing only. Side effects may include dizziness, swelling in the lower legs or hands, and possibly nightmares.

Oxybutynin

Oxybutynin is approved to treat overactive bladder. Used off-label it can also relieve hot flashes and night sweats. One U.S. study looked at the effects of oxybutynin on women in the menopause transition. Study participants reported 28 or more hot flashes per week, and 2 in 3 were receiving treatment for breast cancer. Over 6 weeks, oxybutynin significantly reduced the number and severity of their hot flashes. But some research also suggests that long-term use in those older than 55 may increase the risk of cognitive decline. Talk with your ob-gyn about this risk.

Oxybutynin is taken as a pill at the same time every day, usually on an empty stomach. It also comes as a skin patch that is applied every 3 or 4 days. Side effects may include dry mouth, stomach pain, or difficulty urinating.

Clonidine

Clonidine treats **high blood pressure**. It can also be used off-label to treat hot flashes, though most studies have shown only small benefits. Clonidine is used as a pill or skin patch. Side effects may include dry mouth, insomnia, sleepiness, and constipation.

Pregabalin

Pregabalin is another medication that controls seizures. In studies of off-label pregabalin for menopausal symptoms, women reported fewer hot flashes and improved mood. Pregabalin is taken as a pill twice a day. Side effects may include dizziness, sleepiness, and difficulty concentrating. These side effects were less common with a lower dose. When taking pregabalin or gabapentin, it's important not to drive or operate machinery at first until you know how your body reacts to the medicine.

Table 18-1   Estrogen-Free Medications for Menopausal Symptoms

Medication (Type)	FDA Approved or Off-Label Use*	Common Side Effects
Hot Flashes and Night Sweats		
Fezolinetant (selective neurokinin-3 receptor antagonist)	FDA approved†	Headaches
Paroxetine mesylate (SSRI antidepressant)	FDA approved	Nausea, dizziness, dry mouth, nervousness, constipation, sleepiness, sweating, and reduced sexual desire
Venlafaxine, desvenlafaxine, fluoxetine, and escitalopram (other SSRI and SNRI antidepressants)	Off label	Nausea, dizziness, dry mouth, nervousness, constipation, sleepiness, sweating, reduced sexual desire, and inability to have an orgasm
Gabapentin (antiseizure medication; the medication pregabalin may have similar side effects)	Off label	Sleepiness, dizziness, swelling in the lower legs or hands, and possibly nightmares

(continued)

Table 18-1 Estrogen-Free Medications for Menopausal Symptoms (continued)

Medication (Type)	FDA Approved or Off-Label Use*	Common Side Effects
Oxybutynin (overactive bladder medication)	Off label	Dry mouth, stomach pain, or difficulty urinating
Clonidine (high blood pressure medication)	Off label	Dry mouth, insomnia, sleepiness, and constipation
Painful Sex and Vaginal Dryness		
Ospemifene (selective estrogen receptor modulator [SERM])	FDA approved	Hot flashes, vaginal discharge, muscle spasms, or increased sweating
Prasterone (DHEA)	FDA approved	Vaginal discharge

*Notes whether medication is FDA approved for the symptoms listed or commonly used off-label to treat those symptoms.

†There is a rare risk of serious liver injury with the use of fezolinetant.

> **Does taking an antidepressant for menopausal symptoms mean I have depression?**
>
> While antidepressants have long been used for mood and anxiety disorders, taking one for hot flashes or night sweats does not mean you have depression. Antidepressants include many different categories of medications. Some antidepressants can help the brain better regulate body temperature, and some are taken in doses that are lower than typical doses for depression treatment. If you've had depression or been treated for it in the past, you may have an increased risk of depression coming back during the menopause transition. You may want to discuss this with your ob-gyn.
>
> —DR. ESTHER EISENBERG

Medications for Vaginal Symptoms

Low-dose vaginal estrogen is the most effective treatment for vaginal symptoms of menopause. These estrogen products are placed in the vagina, where they help restore the natural thickness and elasticity of the vaginal lining and relieve dryness and irritation.

Although the very low doses of estrogen used in vaginal tablets or creams do not appear to raise the risk of *endometrial cancer*, you should talk with your ob-gyn if you have any abnormal bleeding. If you're looking for estrogen-free treatments for vaginal symptoms, there are two prescription options. (You can also read Chapter 16, "Lifestyle Changes and Alternative Approaches," for details on helpful over-the-counter remedies for vaginal symptoms.)

Prasterone

Prasterone is a vaginal insert that's FDA approved for moderate to severe painful intercourse. It's made of DHEA, a steroid naturally found in the body. When prasterone is placed in the vagina, the tissues convert it into *androgens* and estrogen, which restore lubrication and ease dryness and itching. This medication is not linked to endometrial cancer.

Prasterone has been studied as a treatment for women with a history of breast cancer, who are at higher risk of severe vaginal dryness. In one U.S. study, more than 450 women with a history of breast or gynecologic cancer used one of three vaginal treatments: a low dose of DHEA, a higher dose of DHEA, or a plain moisturizer. All reported improvements in vaginal dryness and painful sex. But the group using a higher dose of DHEA reported even better sexual functioning. Still, more studies are needed to learn if DHEA is completely safe for use after breast cancer recovery.

Prasterone vaginal inserts are used daily. The most common side effect is vaginal discharge.

Ospemifene

Ospemifene is FDA approved for painful sex and moderate to severe *postmenopausal* vaginal dryness. It's in a class of drugs called *selective estrogen receptor modulators (SERMs)*. These medications stimulate certain tissues that respond to estrogen, but not others. In one study, using ospemifene for 12 weeks to 1 year was linked to improved vaginal health and fewer reports of painful intercourse.

Studies do not link ospemifene to an increased risk of breast cancer or endometrial cancer, but you should tell your ob-gyn about any abnormal bleeding or other new symptoms. Before taking it, tell your ob-gyn if you have a history of *stroke*, blood clots, high blood pressure, high *cholesterol*, diabetes, heart disease, or *lupus*.

Ospemifene is taken as a pill once a day. Side effects may include hot flashes, vaginal discharge, muscle spasms, and increased sweating.

When to Talk About Estrogen-Free Medications

A personal history of *hormone*-related cancer is not the only reason to talk about estrogen-free medications for hot flashes and vaginal dryness. For example, if you are 60 or older or more than 10 years out from your last period, it is generally recommended that you not start systemic hormone therapy (though vaginal estrogen products are OK). Starting hormone therapy this far out from your last period may increase the risk of heart disease, stroke, blood clots, and dementia.

You should also avoid hormone therapy if you have health conditions that are worsened with estrogen, such as *endometriosis* or lupus. Estrogen-free medications are safer alternatives.

> **How long does medication for hot flashes work?**
>
> Usually, medications for hot flashes can work for as long as you take them. But as with most medications, everyone's response is different. Keep in mind that it can take a few weeks to see the full benefit. Your ob-gyn may need to adjust the dosage or try different medications to find what works best for you. It's important to have regular follow-ups with your ob-gyn to monitor the effectiveness and adjust the treatment as needed.
>
> –DR. MARY ROSSER

Talking With Your Ob-Gyn

Lifestyle changes and over-the-counter products don't work for everyone. If this describes you, and you want to avoid estrogen-based therapies, talk with your ob-gyn about the medications discussed in this chapter. Remember, this is a personal decision that should be made with your ob-gyn based on your health and risk factors.

Also, you may not need medication forever. No matter what type of medication you try, you and your ob-gyn should talk each year about any new risk factors you may have or new information that may emerge about that medication.

RESOURCES

Managing Urogenital and Vulvovaginal Atrophy in Breast Cancer Survivors Receiving Endocrine Therapy
consultqd.clevelandclinic.org/managing-urogenital-and-vulvovaginal-atrophy-in-breast-cancer-survivors-receiving-endocrine-therapy

Information from the Cleveland Clinic on the safest ways to treat vaginal symptoms after having breast cancer.

Menopause Topics: Hot Flashes
menopause.org/patient-education/menopause-topics/hot-flashes

Information on treatments for hot flashes and night sweats from The Menopause Society, including alternatives to hormone therapy.

Nonhormonal Treatments for Menopause
health.harvard.edu/womens-health/nonhormonal-treatments-for-menopause

Article from Harvard Medical School outlining various nonhormonal approaches. Includes mind–body approaches, medications, weight loss, over-the-counter products, lifestyle changes, and vaginal moisturizers and lubricants.

Understanding Unapproved Use of Approved Drugs "Off Label"
fda.gov/patients/learn-about-expanded-access-and-other-treatment-options/understanding-unapproved-use-approved-drugs-label

Article from the U.S. Food and Drug Administration that explains off-label use of medications and when they might be recommended.

My Menopause
acog.org/MyMenopause

Web resource from ACOG with information on the menopause transition, signs and symptoms, treatments, and self-care. Includes the latest information from the experts in ob-gyn care, menopause stories from real women, expert columns on how to manage symptoms, Q&A articles, videos, and more.

Part IV

STAYING HEALTHY IN MENOPAUSE AND BEYOND

CHAPTER 19

Heart Disease and Diabetes

Judith was diagnosed with diabetes at 40. She made lifestyle changes, including joining a weight management program and walking with friends, and dropped more than 80 pounds. Several years later, after the death of her mother and the start of perimenopause, she developed high blood pressure. An advanced practice nurse recommended medications to control her blood pressure and they have been effective. As she has taken control of each diagnosis, Judith has focused on the future. "I hope managing my blood pressure and diabetes means I'll have a longer, fitter life," she says.

Changes in heart health, blood sugar, and other health markers are common during midlife. Some changes come naturally with age or are linked to family history, but others have a link to the *menopause transition*. It's important to know your numbers—blood pressure, *cholesterol*, blood sugar, and weight—and keep an eye on them so you can manage and keep them in the healthy range. Increases in all can set the stage for serious illness in the future.

Heart disease and *stroke* become far more common among women from midlife on. In fact, they are the leading cause of death in women. One in every 2 or 3 women dies of heart disease or stroke. And 9 in 10 women have at least one risk factor for heart disease and stroke. This is why midlife is a critical time to ensure that your lifestyle and behaviors are helpful to your health, rather than harmful.

It's worth the effort. Heart disease is preventable in the vast majority of cases. When you take steps to protect your heart, you'll also reduce your risk of other serious illnesses. **Obesity, high blood pressure**, high cholesterol, and *diabetes* make heart disease and stroke more likely. They also increase the risk of dementia and cancer. Lifestyle choices, such as diet and exercise, and routine health care can make a dramatic difference in this risk.

Obstetrician–gynecologists (ob-gyns) are a key resource in protecting long-term health. Their expertise goes far beyond women's reproductive needs. You and your ob-gyn can work together on your nutrition, physical activity, and other health goals.

What to Know About Heart Disease

In midlife, more people start to develop diseases and conditions that affect the heart and blood vessels. Together these are called *cardiovascular disease (CVD)*. Some common conditions stem from *atherosclerosis*, a buildup of *plaque* in *arteries*. This buildup can narrow the arteries and block blood flow, which in turn can lead to a heart attack or stroke.

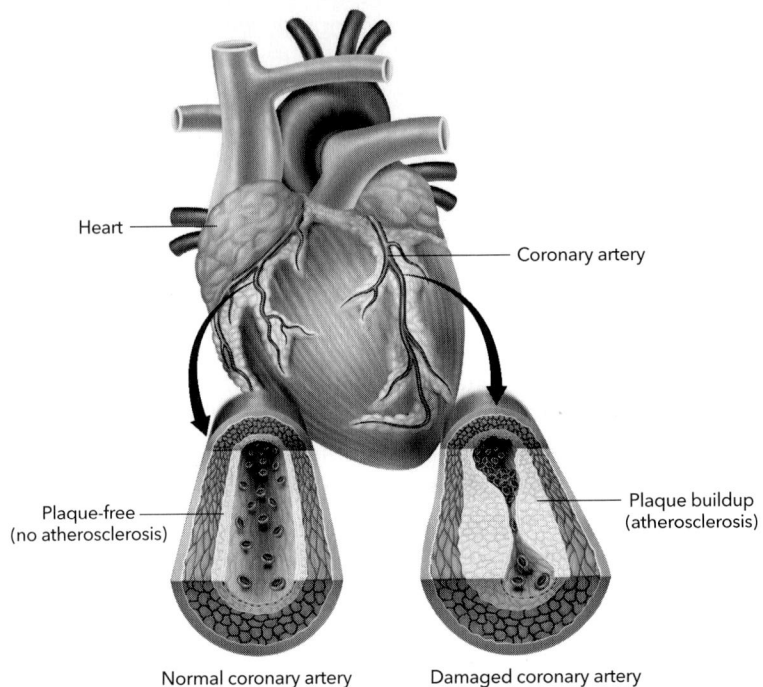

Atherosclerosis. This condition develops when arteries are narrowed and hardened by plaque buildup. When atherosclerosis affects the coronary arteries, it is called coronary artery disease.

A heart attack happens when blood flow to part of the heart is blocked. This can happen when plaque that has broken open forms a blood clot. A blockage causes damage to heart muscle and sometimes leads to death. Many people survive a heart attack, but changes to diet, lifestyle, and medications are essential to supporting heart health after the first heart attack.

A stroke happens when a blood vessel to the brain is blocked by a blood clot. It can also happen when high blood pressure causes a blood vessel in the brain to burst. Strokes can cause damage to brain tissue. This can cause disability, which may be temporary or lifelong. Rehabilitation therapy is needed after a stroke to help restore function to the affected part of the body.

Heart failure happens when the heart can't pump blood well enough to deliver *oxygen* to the rest of the body. This condition develops over time and can get worse if it's not treated. Another name for this condition is congestive heart failure.

There are other conditions under the umbrella of CVD, including

- arrhythmia, a condition that causes the heart to beat too fast, too slow, or in a different pattern than normal
- heart valve problems, including leaking of the valves
- peripheral artery disease, a condition that causes narrowing or blockages in the blood vessels of the arms, legs, and major organs

Among men, the risk of CVD rises in the 30s and 40s. Among women, risk rises between 55 and 64, the years following the last period. This is partly because *estrogen* plays a key role in the health of blood vessels and the heart. As your estrogen level declines during the menopause transition and as you age, these protective benefits are lost.

For example, lower estrogen levels in the run-up to a woman's last period are linked to a higher risk of plaque forming in the arteries. Some symptoms of menopause, especially *hot flashes*, may signal vulnerability to heart disease or brain disease in the future. By about age 75, the CVD risk for all adults—men and women—is nearly the same.

Research about women's hearts is improving, and we have learned that, in fact, heart disease in women is different than in men. Sometimes, the symptoms of a heart attack are different as well. Women having a heart attack may feel pain in the neck, jaw, upper back, or shoulder. They may have shortness of breath, sweating, fatigue, and heartburn. You can read more about symptoms at the website of the American Heart Association (see Resources). It's important to call 911 if you suspect a heart attack, and to fully explain what's happening to emergency department nurses and doctors.

> **Do I need vitamins or supplements for my heart health?**
>
> Great question. Many people take vitamins and supplements believing they will support their heart health. But there's no evidence that the most common supplements can prevent heart disease. There is a small chance that supplemental folate and B vitamins reduce the risk of stroke, but they should not be taken for this reason alone. The best way to support heart health is to eat a plant-based diet and cut back on foods that harm overall health, including foods high in saturated fat, salt, and preservatives. A balanced diet that contains lots of whole grains, fruits, and vegetables provides all the vitamins you need.
>
> —DR. MARY ROSSER

Who's at Highest Risk of CVD

Many people have risk factors for CVD. Some of these can't be changed, including

- age 55 and older (age 45 if you have diabetes)
- family history of heart attacks or heart disease
- personal history of certain conditions during pregnancy, including high blood pressure, *preeclampsia*, or *gestational diabetes*
- *premature menopause* (last period before 40) or early menopause (last period between 40 and 45)
- *primary ovarian insufficiency*
- surgical removal of the *ovaries*
- certain *autoimmune disorders*, including *lupus* and *rheumatoid arthritis*
- past cancer treatments, including *chemotherapy* and *radiation*

But there are other CVD risk factors that you can address, often with the help of a doctor. These include

- high blood pressure
- high cholesterol and *triglycerides*
- *depression* or sleep disorders in midlife
- smoking or drinking
- lack of physical activity
- overweight and obesity

This brings us back to awareness of your numbers—blood pressure, cholesterol, blood sugar, and weight—and reminds us that lifestyle can play a big role in preventing CVD.

A Guide to High Blood Pressure

Blood pressure is the force of blood pushing against the walls of the arteries. The arteries carry blood from your heart to your lungs, where the blood picks up oxygen to deliver to organs and tissues via the arteries in your vascular system. The organs and tissues use the oxygen to power their activities. *Veins* then bring the now oxygen-poor blood back to the heart and lungs.

As people age, blood vessels become stiffer. This means the heart needs to work harder to move blood through the arteries, and blood pressure rises as a result. When blood pressure is too high (a condition called *hypertension*), the increased force can damage the walls of your blood vessels. Those damaged areas are where plaque tends to form. High blood pressure is a major risk factor for heart disease and stroke. It can also damage the blood vessels in your eyes and *kidneys*.

Your blood pressure reading has two numbers that are separated by a slash: 110/75, for example. You may hear this referred to as "110 over 75." The first number is the pressure against the artery walls when the heart contracts. This is called *systolic blood pressure*. The second number is the pressure against the artery walls when the heart relaxes between contractions. This is called *diastolic blood pressure*. The box "Reading Your Blood Pressure" explains what the numbers mean.

Reading Your Blood Pressure

The American Heart Association and American College of Cardiology recommend the following blood pressure guidelines for adults 18 and older. The first number is the systolic reading. This is the pressure in the arteries when the heart contracts to send blood into the body. The second number is the diastolic reading. This is the pressure in the arteries when the heart is resting between beats. Results are reported in millimeters of mercury (mm Hg).

Normal:	Less than 120/80 mm Hg
Elevated:	Systolic between 120 and 129 mm Hg **and** diastolic less than 80 mm Hg
Stage 1 hypertension:	Systolic between 130 and 139 mm Hg **or** diastolic between 80 and 89 mm Hg
Stage 2 hypertension:	Systolic at least 140 mm Hg **or** diastolic at least 90 mm Hg
Hypertensive crisis:	Systolic over 180 mm Hg and/or diastolic over 120 mm Hg

Blood pressure in the hypertensive crisis range increases your risk for stroke.

Your blood pressure can change daily and throughout the day. It may be influenced by physical activity, caffeine, anxiety, and other factors.
A single reading is not enough to diagnose high blood pressure. That's why your ob-gyn may take your blood pressure reading more than once and track changes over time.

Before 45, more men than women have high blood pressure. In midlife, women start to close the gap as blood pressure increases with age. During *perimenopause*, signs and symptoms linked to heart disease—including high blood pressure—become more common. After 65, high blood pressure is more common among women than men.

Your ob-gyn should check your blood pressure once a year, but you can also check it at home. Most pharmacies sell blood pressure cuffs for home use. They can give you a good idea of your average pressure if you monitor periodically. To check your monitor's accuracy, bring it to your next ob-gyn visit and see how the reading compares to the reading done by your nurse or doctor.

A Guide to Triglycerides and Cholesterol

Triglycerides are the most common form of fat in the body. They provide energy to power the body's activities. Cholesterol is a building block for cells and hormones. Most of the cholesterol in your body is made by the liver. A small amount comes from food, such as meat and dairy products. There are two kinds of cholesterol:

1. High-density lipoprotein (HDL or "good cholesterol") helps prevent heart disease. It picks up cholesterol in the bloodstream and takes it to the liver, where it is broken down.

2. Low-density lipoprotein (LDL or "bad cholesterol") can collect in the walls of blood vessels. Too much LDL in the walls of the arteries can trigger a response by the body's *immune system* called inflammation. Inflammation can lead to a buildup of plaque in the arteries and eventually to atherosclerosis.

High blood levels of total cholesterol, LDL, and triglycerides are risk factors for CVD in both men and women. Estrogen is thought to protect women from heart disease by naturally increasing the levels of HDL. But during the menopause transition, LDL may start to go up. And although reducing LDL levels can help prevent CVD, it does not appear to help women as much as it helps men.

Your ob-gyn can order a blood test that measures your levels of triglycerides and cholesterol. The National Heart, Lung, and Blood Institute recommends that women 55 to 65 be screened for high cholesterol every 1 to 2 years. After 65, annual screening is recommended. If you have type 2 diabetes or other known risk factors for CVD, start screening earlier than 55. The box "Reviewing Cholesterol Testing Results" explains what the numbers mean.

What to Know About Diabetes

Diabetes is a disease in which the body does not make enough of a hormone called *insulin* or does not use it as it should. Normally, your body changes most of the food you eat into *glucose*. Glucose is then carried to the body's cells with the help of insulin. If your body does not make enough insulin, or the insulin does not work as it should, the glucose cannot enter the body's cells. Instead, glucose builds up in the blood. This makes your blood sugar level too high.

Reviewing Cholesterol Testing Results

The American Heart Association and American College of Cardiology recommend the cholesterol guidelines listed below. Results are reported in milligrams per deciliter (mg/dL).

Total Cholesterol

Normal:	Less than 200 mg/dL
Borderline high:	200 to 239 mg/dL
High:	At or above 240 mg/dL

LDL (Bad) Cholesterol

Optimal:	Less than 100 mg/dL
Near optimal:	100 to 129 mg/dL
Borderline high:	130 to 159 mg/dL
High:	160 to 189 mg/dL
Very high:	190 mg/dL and higher

HDL (Good) Cholesterol

Level at or above 60 mg/dL is ideal

Triglycerides

Normal:	Less than 150 mg/dL
Borderline high:	150 to 199 mg/dL
High:	200 to 499 mg/dL
Very high:	Above 500 mg/dL

It's important that your ob-gyn or other doctor interpret your results. Based on your risk factors for heart disease or diabetes, your ob-gyn may recommend that you focus on diet, lifestyle, medications, or all three to lower any numbers that are too high.

There are two types of diabetes:

Type 1—People with type 1 diabetes need to take insulin to survive because the body makes little or no insulin on its own.

Type 2—In people with type 2 diabetes, insulin is produced, but it does not work as it should. The body becomes resistant to the effects of insulin and produces more insulin to keep glucose levels normal. Over time, the body cannot maintain high enough levels to keep the glucose levels normal, blood sugar levels rise, and diabetes develops. Type 2 diabetes may also develop as a result of other diseases or as a side effect of certain medications.

People with type 2 diabetes may be able to control blood sugar levels with diet, medication, or both. In some cases, people with type 2 diabetes may need to take insulin to control blood sugar.

Over the past 20 years, the rate of type 2 diabetes has risen more quickly among women of reproductive age than among the general adult population. Many women are unaware of the diabetes risk, which rises again around the time of menopause. Part of this is related to weight gain, which can lead to insulin resistance. If you have diabetes and don't get treatment, heart disease and other serious health problems become much more likely. Luckily, most cases of type 2 diabetes among women in midlife are preventable.

The American Diabetes Association recommends diabetes screening every 3 years if you are 35 or older. It also recommends that adults with overweight or obesity and at least one other risk factor for diabetes (see below) be screened. The box "Understanding Blood Sugar Testing" explains what screening results mean.

Understanding Blood Sugar Testing

A fasting glucose test can tell you if your blood sugar is in a normal range or if you have **prediabetes** or diabetes. Fasting means you have not had anything to eat or drink (other than water) for at least 8 hours before the blood test. The following guidelines from the American Diabetes Association can help you understand your numbers. Glucose testing results are reported in milligrams per deciliter (mg/dL). Fasting blood glucose levels are reported as follows:

Normal:	Less than 100 mg/dL
Prediabetes:	100 to 125 mg/dL
Diabetes:	126 mg/dL or higher

Another test that may be used is the hemoglobin A1C test. This measures what your average blood sugar has been for the past few months. You do not have to fast for this blood test. Results are listed as percentages.

Normal:	Less than 5.7 percent
Prediabetes:	5.7 to 6.4 percent
Diabetes:	6.5 percent or higher

Your ob-gyn or other doctor should review your results and discuss diet, lifestyle, or medications if your A1C is too high.

Prediabetes affects 1 in 3 adults in the U.S. and half of those 65 and older. Most people with prediabetes don't know they have it. But the good news is that for some people, lifestyle changes and sometimes medication may help return blood glucose levels to normal.

As many as 7 in 10 people with prediabetes develop diabetes. The longer you have untreated diabetes, the more likely it is that you will develop **complications**, like damage to the heart, blood vessels, kidneys, eyes, or nerves. After menopause, women with type 2 diabetes are three times more likely to have heart disease or stroke compared to women without diabetes. This is why it is so important to stick to the guidelines for screening.

Who's at Highest Risk of Diabetes

Many people have risk factors for developing type 2 diabetes. Some of these can't be changed, including

- age 35 or older
- family history of diabetes
- personal history of gestational diabetes or **polycystic ovary syndrome**

But there are other diabetes risk factors that you can address, often with the help of a doctor. These include

- overweight or obesity
- lack of consistent physical activity
- high cholesterol levels
- depression or sleep disorders in midlife
- smoking

Weight is the single most important factor related to developing type 2 diabetes. A person with overweight is seven times more likely to develop diabetes than someone with a healthy weight. A person with obesity is 20 to 40 times more likely to develop diabetes. Smoking also plays a significant role. People who smoke are more likely to develop type 2 diabetes and are at higher risk of serious complications of the disease.

And while anyone can develop type 2 diabetes, some people are affected more often than others. This includes people of African, Asian, Hispanic, Native American, and Pacific Islander descent.

Lifestyle Changes and Reducing Risk

It's important to understand the steps you can take to reduce your risk of heart disease, stroke, and diabetes. If you currently have a CVD or diabetes diagnosis, many of these lifestyle changes may be helpful, too. Some of the approaches below can also be found in the American Heart Association's Life's Essential 8. You can find the link in the Resources section.

Manage Your Weight

Overweight and obesity increase the risk of heart disease, stroke, high blood pressure, diabetes, and other serious illnesses. Extra fat in the belly (for women, a waist size of 35" or more) is more dangerous than extra fat in the hips and thighs. Even a small amount of weight loss—as little as 5 to 10 percent of body weight—can significantly reduce the risk of developing life-threatening diseases. Talk with your ob-gyn about a plan for nutrition and physical activity that can help you lose weight safely and effectively. For guidance, read Chapter 14, "Weight and Menopause."

Quit Smoking

Smoking is a major cause of heart disease and diabetes. The more you smoke and the longer you smoke, the higher your risk. If you smoke, it is difficult but important to quit. You can get help from your ob-gyn and from "quit lines" that have been set up in every state. Call 1-800-QUIT-NOW (784-8669) to find out how to access the quit line in your area.

Limit or Eliminate Alcohol

Keeping your alcohol consumption to no more than 1 drink a day or less may help reduce your risk of heart disease. Women's bodies do not break down alcohol as well as men's and are more sensitive to alcohol. More importantly, researchers now believe that drinking even modest amounts of alcohol may increase the risk of CVD, cancer, and other serious health problems. Heavy drinking may raise your risk of developing diabetes.

Stay Active

A sedentary lifestyle and lack of consistent physical activity raises your risk of CVD and diabetes. You don't need to become a triathlete. Walking briskly for half an hour a day, for example, can reduce your risk of type 2 diabetes. More challenging workouts bring even bigger health benefits. The Centers for Disease Control and Prevention recommend getting at least 2½ hours of exercise every week. That could mean 30-minute workouts on 5 days a week. A brisk walk at lunchtime will bring about many healthful benefits.

Improve Your Diet

There are many resources online to help plan healthful, nutrient-dense meals. Working with a registered dietitian can also help. These principles of eating well are key:

- Eat whole grains—Thanks to their high fiber content, whole grains help maintain a stable blood sugar level. Studies consistently show that people who routinely eat whole grains are less likely to develop diabetes than those who favor processed carbohydrates. Diets rich in whole grains—and fiber generally—also reduce your risk of heart disease, stroke, and some cancers.

- Eat fruits and vegetables—These are healthy, low-fat sources of nutrients and fiber. If the skin of fruits is edible, eat that, too. Beans, peas, lentils, and leafy vegetables like spinach and kale are great additions to your diet.

- Choose healthy protein sources—Plant-based eating reduces the risk of diabetes and CVD, especially when you do it consistently. Beans, nuts, and whole grains are healthy sources of protein. Low-fat dairy, poultry, and fish are also healthy choices. Avoid red meat (beef, lamb, and pork) and processed meat (hot dogs, deli meats, bacon). These raise your risk of CVD and diabetes, even if you eat modest amounts.

- Choose healthy fats—Unsaturated fats come mostly from plants, and include avocados, nuts, and seeds. Most plant oils (olive, canola, peanut, and sunflower) are unsaturated. Unsaturated fats are also available from fatty fish, like salmon, sardines, and tuna. Eating fish at least twice a week could reduce your risk of heart disease. Avoid trans fats and partially hydrogenated vegetable oils, which are linked to an increased diabetes and CVD risk.

- Cut down on sugars—Sugars are linked to diabetes, though the connection isn't fully understood. It's partly because diets high in sugar lead to weight gain. There are ways to cut down on sugar, including avoiding high-fructose corn syrup and sugar-filled sodas. Drink unsweetened water, coffee, or tea instead.

Are diet drinks a good choice when I cut out sugar?

Quitting regular, sugar-filled soda is a step in the right direction for better health. But diet drinks may not be the best alternative because artificial sweeteners may have negative health effects. Water is always recommended over other beverages, plus unsweetened tea or unsweetened water with flavor. An occasional diet drink may satisfy the craving for something sweet, but sodas with caffeine and artificial sweeteners should not be a big part of your daily hydration plan.

–DR. ESTHER EISENBERG

Limit Sodium Intake

Aim for less than 2,300 milligrams (mg) of sodium a day. That's a little under 1 teaspoon of table salt. High-sodium diets can lead to high blood pressure. Managing your sodium intake means reading labels to check sodium content per serving, avoiding processed foods, and not routinely adding salt when cooking.

Limit Cholesterol Intake

Aim to stay below 200 mg of cholesterol a day. You'll likely go over that if you routinely eat high-fat dairy products, liver, and egg yolks.

Avoid Ultra-Processed Foods

This is a big one. Ultra-processed foods are everywhere in the American diet. They include fast foods, sugary drinks, most frozen meals, and many breakfast cereals and breads. Ultra-processed foods are linked to a higher risk of CVD, as well as overweight and obesity, high blood pressure, and diabetes. The more servings of ultra-processed foods eaten daily, the higher the risk of CVD.

Options for Medication

If lifestyle changes are not enough, or if you are at high risk of CVD or diabetes, your ob-gyn may monitor your blood pressure, cholesterol, and blood sugar more often. They may recommend medication if you have risk factors for CVD or diabetes. Your ob-gyn may also recommend that you see a cardiologist, a doctor who specializes in heart health.

Heart Disease Medications

Many different medications are used to prevent or treat heart disease. Decisions about heart medications depend on your current health and your future risk. Treatment options may include medications that

- lower blood pressure, including angiotensin-converting enzyme (ACE) inhibitors, angiotensin II receptor blockers (ARBs), beta-blockers, calcium channel blockers, and *diuretics* (water pills)
- thin the blood to prevent blood clots, including anticoagulants and antiplatelets
- lower cholesterol, including statins that can also reduce plaque buildup in arteries and lower triglycerides

Diabetes Medication

Medication for type 2 diabetes includes metformin, which can help prevent or delay the onset of diabetes in people with prediabetes, those at high risk of the disease, and people with obesity.

Weight loss may also help prevent both type 2 diabetes and CVD in people with overweight or obesity. Weight-loss treatment may include

- medications that make weight loss easier, including **GLP-1 receptor agonists** that can also reduce blood sugar levels in people with type 2 diabetes
- *bariatric surgery* options

To learn about these drugs and procedures and their benefits and risks, read Chapter 14, "Weight and Menopause." And remember, midlife is the time to take care of yourself, make changes to improve your quality of life, and focus on living well for a long time. Knowing your numbers and how to keep them in a healthy range will go a long way toward maintaining health in and beyond the menopause transition.

RESOURCES

Cholesterol: The Good and the Bad
heart.org/en/health-topics/cholesterol/hdl-good-ldl-bad-cholesterol-and-triglycerides
Video from the American Heart Association that explains HDL, LDL, cholesterol, and triglycerides.

Life's Essential 8
heart.org/en/healthy-living/healthy-lifestyle/lifes-essential-8
Webpage from the American Heart Association that discusses eight key areas to focus on when taking care of your heart health.

Menopause and Women's Health
goredforwomen.org/en/know-your-risk/menopause
Go Red website from the American Heart Association on heart health and menopause. Covers early menopause, hormone therapy, beyond menopause, symptoms of heart attack and stroke, and more.

National Diabetes Prevention Program
cdc.gov/diabetes-prevention/lifestyle-change-program/index.html
Webpages from the Centers for Disease Control and Prevention on the National Diabetes Prevention Program. This includes the lifestyle change program that helps people delay or prevent type 2 diabetes. Participants work with a lifestyle coach online or in person.

The Heart Truth

nhlbi.nih.gov/health-topics/education-and-awareness/heart-truth

Website from the National Heart, Lung, and Blood Institute about heart-healthy living. Includes sections on women and heart disease, resources for managing blood pressure, fact sheets on heart disease among various racial and ethnic groups, a guidebook on lowering cholesterol, and lifestyle changes that lower your risk of CVD.

Your Game Plan to Prevent Type 2 Diabetes

niddk.nih.gov/health-information/diabetes/overview/preventing-type-2-diabetes/game-plan

Webpages from the National Institute of Diabetes and Digestive and Kidney Diseases with guidance on how to reduce your diabetes risk. Includes setting goals, ways to stick to your plan, working with your health care team, and support with healthy eating and physical activity.

My Menopause

acog.org/MyMenopause

Web resource from ACOG with information on the menopause transition, signs and symptoms, treatments, and self-care. Includes the latest information from the experts in ob-gyn care, menopause stories from real women, expert columns on how to manage symptoms, Q&A articles, videos, and more.

CHAPTER 20

Managing Stress

As symptoms of perimenopause started, Alexandra faced rising pressures in her work and marriage. At 44, she was exhausted, anxious, and forgetful. "I felt I was falling apart at the seams," she says, and stress was overwhelming. Her husband suggested they meet with a couple's counselor, and Alexandra worked with her own therapist, who told her stress at this time of life is common. Now Alexandra manages stress with a whiteboard that organizes her day, and she takes "guilt-free mental health days." Breathing exercises are calming, and prescribed medication eases insomnia. Intimate time with her husband is also helpful for stress relief, as is keeping up with friends. "I highly recommend talking with other women who have similar concerns," she says.

For many women, the *menopause transition* happens at the same time that various life stressors converge. In a U.S. study of more than 500 midlife women, about 9 in 10 said they experienced significant stress during the 10-year span of the study. Most had to cope with multiple challenges—pressures relating to work, finances, health, aging parents, growing children, relationships, loss, and life transitions. With so many things happening during the same season of life, it's no wonder that midlife stress levels peak. The good news is that taking steps, even small ones, to reduce stress can lead to positive change.

If you feel overwhelmed over a long period of time, you may have chronic stress. Even if you seem fine to others, chronic stress is a barrier to relaxation, joy, and productivity. It also harms your physical and mental health and can cause or contribute to a range of health conditions even after the causes of stress are resolved.

You can reduce or prevent the harmful effects of chronic stress on your health. This comes in part from learning to control your reactions to stress. You have likely heard of resilience—successfully adapting to challenging circumstances. It can be empowering to develop tools and techniques to manage your response to stressful situations. Keep in mind that it is never too late to develop coping strategies.

It's also important to remember that chronic stress often stems from things that feel, or are, beyond our control. For example, money and the economy topped the list of worries for Americans aged 45 to 64 in the 2023 "Stress in America" survey from the American Psychological Association. Other common stressors include work responsibilities, ageism or other barriers in the workplace, and health issues. Americans also face chronic stress from unpaid caregiving, which falls largely on women. Recent research has linked the burden of caregiving to worse menopausal symptoms.

Stress is unevenly distributed in other ways, too. Overall, more than 1 in 4 adults who took the most recent "Stress in America" survey said discrimination was a source of stress in their lives. This concern was much more common among LGBTQ people, adults with disabilities, and Black and Hispanic Americans. Women in the survey had higher stress levels than men and were more likely to report family responsibilities and relationships as major life stressors.

In this chapter, we'll look at how chronic stress can affect your health. We'll cover ways that you can manage your response to stress, and we'll address when you may need to talk with your *obstetrician–gynecologist (ob-gyn)* about getting help. Women often beat themselves up when they feel like they are struggling at this time of life, thinking they should just be able to power through it. They can feel inadequate when they can't do it all. Now is the time to treat yourself with kindness and ask for help when you need it.

When Stress Is a Health Issue

Stress is the body's response to something happening to you or around you. Stress in short bursts causes normal reactions in the body and brain that can lead you to do something helpful, like meet a deadline or move out of the way of something dangerous. In the right doses, stress can be a pathway to growth and fulfillment. Life would be boring without any challenges, and the stress of a new challenge can help people find new paths in life.

But there's a tipping point at which it becomes harmful. When stress is very high or lasts a long time—what's called chronic stress—it can negatively affect the body and mind. So the goal is not to live a stress-free life but to recognize and manage stress that has become chronic and possibly harmful to your health.

What does chronic stress look like? You may experience intense worry or perceive threats related to work, family, or social expectations. You might turn problems over and over in your mind, feel stuck in anxiety and agitation, set yourself impossible goals, or lie awake at night. Chronic stress can affect multiple processes in your body and mind.

Nervous System

During the "fight, flight, or freeze" response, your body is flooded with stress *hormones* called adrenaline and cortisol. Your heart beats faster, your breathing quickens, and your *blood pressure* rises. The body also puts normal functions like digestion on hold to send energy to the stress response. Over time, these bodily reactions, if held for too long, can lead to wear and tear on your body.

> **Stress makes me feel so anxious now. Is this normal?**
>
> Yes. During the menopause transition, hormonal shifts can affect brain chemistry and trigger anxiety, especially when we're in stressful situations. Plus, night sweats can disrupt sleep, and not being well rested makes it harder to manage stress and anxiety. Some ways to combat both stress and anxiety during the menopause transition include exercise, deep breathing, and relaxing activities like reading, meditating, or gardening. But if you notice new anxiety or anxiety that seems out of proportion to the situation, talk with your ob-gyn. Together you can decide if you need therapy, medication, or other help to manage what's going on.
>
> —DR. GLORIA RÍCHARD-DAVIS

Thinking and Feeling

Chronic stress influences how you learn and make decisions. Stress can lead to anxiety and *depression* as well as feeling easily annoyed or angry, having trouble handling frustration, and feeling hyperactive or nervous. High levels of cortisol caused by chronic stress can impair memory.

Hormones and the Immune System

Hormonal responses to chronic stress are linked to the development of physical and mental health conditions. These include *obesity*, chronic fatigue, **high blood pressure**, *diabetes*, and depression. Stress may also lower the ability to fight infection. For example, stressed caregivers may spend more days out with a cold or flu than other people. Researchers also suspect that chronic stress contributes to the development of *autoimmune disorders* such as *Crohn's disease*, *lupus*, and *rheumatoid arthritis*. At the very least, managing stress is likely to help control the symptoms of an existing autoimmune condition.

Heart and Blood Vessels

Chronic stress can make people more prone to high blood pressure, blood clots, abnormal heartbeats, inflammation in blood vessels, and heart attacks. Levels of *estrogen* before the menopause transition may help women's blood vessels respond better during stress and thus protect against heart disease. In *postmenopause*, women have less estrogen and lose this natural level of protection for blood vessels.

Digestion

Stress can kill your appetite or make you hungrier. If you respond with stress eating, weight gain can follow and increase the risk of other health problems. Stress can affect your digestion in multiple ways. It can cause stomach pain, nausea, and bloating, and it can make you more likely to experience *inflammatory bowel disease* or *irritable bowel syndrome (IBS)*.

Muscles and Skeleton

Stress causes the muscles to tense up, sometimes for long periods. This can contribute to tension headaches, migraines, and chronic pain.

Breathing

Stress may cause shortness of breath and rapid breathing. This may trigger breathing problems, especially for people with asthma and other lung conditions, or those who are prone to panic attacks.

Managing Stress in Different Environments

The combined pressures of the workplace, home, and responsibilities as a caregiver can be intense. Consider each situation separately to help identify ways to reduce or manage the pressure.

Stress at Work

If you're working through *hot flashes*, brain fog, or depressive symptoms, it's no surprise that you may lose concentration at work. You might be uncomfortable through the day, tired or distracted, and anxious about your performance. You may have trouble reaching goals or achieving a tolerable life–work balance. Perhaps you could use time off but don't want to share the reason. It's common to feel this way. In a UK survey, 1 in 4 women reported that intense menopausal symptoms made them consider leaving the workforce.

If these issues are affecting you at work, consider talking with your manager about accommodations. You may also be able to get support via an employee assistance program. In an ideal world, companies would have staff trained in menopause who can help employees navigate symptoms and related issues. Many organizations aren't there yet. Even managers who understand the need for prenatal appointments or breastfeeding spaces are usually not as attuned to what the menopause transition may mean. But you can bring the issue forward. Reasonable accommodations for menopause might include

- adjusting the temperature and airflow of the workplace
- easing up on rules about uncomfortable uniforms or dress codes
- placing a desk or workstation next to an open window or fan
- making sure that cold water and bathrooms are easily accessible
- providing a quiet room for rest

- allowing flexible start and finish times and working from home
- adjusting roles within the company

Stress at Home

Many women come home from work and face a "second shift": managing the household and taking care of the people in it, including children of all ages. People with children often report higher stress levels than those without children. In the "Stress in America" survey, 3 in 5 women reported feeling overwhelmed by family responsibilities.

Partnerships add stress as well. More than 1 in 5 women between 45 and 64 say their relationship is a key source of stress. Some women may be supporting a partner or spouse through work struggles or health problems. (Taking care of spouses can be even more challenging than supporting children or aging parents, research shows.) For other women, midlife means facing divorce or the death of a spouse.

Menopausal symptoms can make it harder to cope with these stressors. This is a time to reduce the demands of your roles in any way that you can. Support groups and counseling can help you find practical and emotional solutions. It may help to know you're not alone when it comes to facing stressful circumstances. You can also read the "Stress in America" survey for more findings. The link to the study appears in the Resources section at the end of this chapter.

Stress in Caregiving

Often, midlife brings another set of responsibilities: caring for family members as they age. Usually, these are parents or in-laws, but some people also care for older aunts, uncles, and others. Many people spend part of their lives supporting elders through chronic illnesses and other disabilities.

Women are the people who most commonly provide unpaid care to others. Half of women caregivers have jobs outside the home. Most are also responsible for their own households and children. Caregiving is a mixed blessing. You may cherish the opportunity to spend more time with loved ones and ensure their safety and wellness. Even so, the tasks can be overwhelming: managing medications, giving injections, bathing and dressing an elder, cooking and cleaning, paying bills, driving to appointments, running errands, and responding to changes in an elder's mental health. Caregiving is especially stressful when it involves a person with dementia or another condition that needs constant supervision.

The stress of eldercare really can't be overstated. Intense caregiving limits the ability to find quiet time to recharge, interrupts family and social lives, and, in some cases, affects the ability to maintain work hours and earnings. Eldercare is also linked to caregiver mood swings and anxiety, which may show up as disrupted eating and sleep patterns.

> **Taking care of my parents is stressful. Where can I find help?**
>
> Eldercare is common—more than 37 million people in the United States take care of an aging family member or other person. That's a lot of caregivers, but when you're shouldering this burden, you can feel alone and isolated. Finding help is essential. Start with the Eldercare Locator at eldercare.acl.gov/home. This is a nationwide service that offers caregiver resources, a searchable directory of local services, and personalized online or phone support. You can also reach out to your elder's doctor or the social workers at their nearby hospital. Doctors and social workers often have lists of local in-home care agencies and other support services.
>
> —DR. MARY ROSSER

Remember that your health has to come before your care of others. When you're healthy and energized, you'll have more to give yourself and your loved ones. Consider the following:

- Keep up with your wellness checks and health screenings and keep an eye on your blood pressure with a home blood pressure cuff.

- Look for a support group. Your ob-gyn might be aware of nearby groups, and you can find support online as well.

- Think about seeing a therapist. You may need to learn or relearn stress management techniques. Talk therapy can be helpful for processing the challenges of caregiving.

- Seek out agencies that provide in-home eldercare or respite care. Agencies can help you shoulder the burden, and if needed, they can recommend assisted living or other living situations you can research. Also, think about relatives, friends, and neighbors who can lend a hand and relieve you of being a sole caregiver all the time.

Science-Based Self-Care Strategies

When you are taking care of your stress, you're benefiting your mind and body in multiple ways. That said, any list of lifestyle changes can feel daunting. Start with one or two tweaks that seem doable for now. All of these are effective for stress.

Get Up and Move

Physical activity is a proven way to reduce stress, anxiety, and depression and improve energy and well-being. Physical activity reduces levels of stress hormones and generates "feel-good" chemicals that relieve pain and improve mood. Walk the dog, run, bike, hike, swim, unroll your yoga mat in your backyard, or get to a dance class. Better still, do one of these activities with a friend or partner—social support is linked to more consistent physical activity. Just 20 to 30 minutes of aerobic exercise—walking, jogging, dancing, biking, and so on—helps relieve stress. For more on getting and staying active, read Chapter 14, "Weight and Menopause."

Move Into Nature

People's minds and bodies do better when they regularly visit green spaces. Spending 20 to 30 minutes in a park, backyard, or woods can help lower blood pressure and levels of stress hormones. Immersing yourself in the natural world for at least 2 hours a week is linked to better health and emotional wellness.

Talk About It

In the "Stress in America" survey, half of adults said they wished they had someone to turn to for advice and support. Adult friendships reduce the risk of mental health issues. Your blood pressure and heart rate are steadier when you talk or share tough tasks with supportive friends. People with friends they can confide in are less likely to die from heart problems and some other chronic diseases. Consider reaching out to a religious leader or someone else in the community. Explore local or online support groups.

Combat Loneliness

Everyone needs social support. Research suggests that people can make new friends at any age and that even minor social interactions are valuable. Developing interests and hobbies is a way to connect with others and keeps you from being isolated. Volunteer work can improve physical and mental health, reduce stress, build social networks, help you learn new skills, and restore your sense of purpose and self-esteem.

Nourish Your Body and Brain

Eat healthfully and regularly. Choose whole grains, lean protein, and lots of fruit and vegetables. Limit caffeine and alcohol and stay away from smoking, vaping, and other substances. To explore healthful eating, read Chapter 14, "Weight and Menopause," and Chapter 19, "Heart Disease and Diabetes."

Practice Good Sleep Hygiene

"Sleep hygiene" is the term for behaviors and environmental changes that can help you sleep better. Improvements in sleep hygiene can be very effective for most people. The focus should be on changing any habits that don't help—late-night scrolling on your phone, for example—and then developing bedtime routines and preparing your bedroom to promote good sleep. Most adults require 7 to 9 hours of sleep a night. For help, read Chapter 9, "Sleep Problems."

Explore Mind-Body Practices
Yoga, tai chi, qigong, and some other practices combine mental focus and body movements with the goal of improving well-being. Related techniques include guided imagery and meditation, deep breathing routines, and positive thinking exercises. These have not all been thoroughly studied, but some evidence indicates they have benefits for relieving stress.

Talking With Your Ob-Gyn

Self-care is essential for stress management, but everyone has times when it's not enough. For ob-gyns, talking about stress is an important part of the job. They are familiar with the challenges women face throughout their lives and often hear from patients who need help coping. Talk with your ob-gyn if you

- have mental health concerns, like mood issues or agitation that does not go away
- have physical signs of stress, like new heart palpitations, stomach pain, or headaches
- are using unhealthy ways to cope, like smoking, drinking, binge eating, binge-watching TV episodes, online gambling, and excessive online shopping
- are more irritable or short-tempered than usual or unable to focus on tasks
- have tried to cope on your own without success

Your ob-gyn can provide a confidential space for talking about the sources of stress in your life and your ability to cope. More importantly, they can

- talk with you about the possible effects of stress on your mental and physical health
- screen you for anxiety and depression, and for physical causes of your symptoms
- connect you with resources, such as support groups for people with similar experiences
- prescribe medication if needed, sharing the decision making with you
- refer you to a mental health specialist for counseling

Sometimes it helps to prepare for a conversation about what's going on and how it's affecting you. Start keeping a stress diary so you can identify how it shows up in your body and mind. This can be something as simple as notes on your phone or something you write out on paper. When you start talking with your ob-gyn, be honest. It will be easier for them to help you if they have the full picture. And ask questions. You and your ob-gyn are partners in your care. If they recommend something that doesn't make sense to you, keep talking.

Finally, find a doctor who understands you. You may be more comfortable talking with clinicians of a similar racial, ethnic, or religious background. LGBTQ people and those with disabilities may seek doctors who are allies to their community. If your stress is related to a traumatic experience, you may need your doctor and medical facility to be "trauma informed." This means the space and processes are designed to help you feel safe and in control.

Working With a Counselor

Therapy for stress management comes in different forms. Many people find success with talk therapy, which can be done alone or with family members and in person or virtually. For those dealing with more serious mental health challenges, like trauma responses, long-term therapy may be needed.

Talk Therapy

Cognitive behavioral therapy (CBT) is a structured talk therapy and one of the most effective treatments for stress. CBT focuses on the ways you think about difficult situations and how your thinking affects your feelings, behaviors, and physical reactions. CBT can relieve distress that interferes with your quality of life or daily functioning. The approach includes identifying "thinking traps," patterns of thinking that don't serve you well. It also involves challenging negative expectations. A course of CBT treatment typically lasts 2 to 4 months. It may be used alone or combined with medication or other interventions.

Mindfulness-Based Therapy

Mindfulness means observing the present moment without judgment. The therapy trains you to recognize how you react to stressors and shift those reactions. Mindfulness-based stress reduction usually involves eight sessions and home practice. Mindfulness-based cognitive therapy includes CBT techniques.

EMDR Therapy

EMDR, short for eye movement desensitization and reprocessing, is a therapy most often used by people who have experienced trauma. The World Health Organization has recognized EMDR as an effective therapy for *post-traumatic stress disorder (PTSD)*, but it can be done to address recent traumatic events like car accidents or home break-ins. The theory behind EMDR is that traumatic memories can get "stuck" in the brain and lead to physical problems and mood issues, including depression and anxiety. EMDR helps reprocess the memories and change their impact on you. If this form of therapy interests you, look for a therapist with specialized training in EMDR.

RESOURCES

All About Stress
psychcentral.com/stress/stress-overview
A comprehensive webpage from PsychCentral offering an in-depth overview of stress, including its definition, causes, symptoms, and effective strategies for stress management.

Family Caregiver Services by State
caregiver.org/connecting-caregivers/services-by-state/
Interactive website listing resources for caregivers and the people they care for, from the Family Caregiver Alliance. Includes best programs for caregiving, focusing on dementia services, webinars presenting tools for caregivers, and online support groups.

Menopause Workplace Resource Guide for Women
swhr.org/resources/menopause-workplace-resource-guide-for-women/
Free guide from the Society for Women's Health Research on how to navigate menopause in the workplace. Includes information on reasonable accommodation for various types of work and how to request one.

National Center for PTSD: Mindfulness Coach
ptsd.va.gov/appvid/mobile/mindfulcoach_app.asp#
Site that offers Mindfulness Coach, an app with mindfulness tools that can be used alone or along with therapy. While it is offered by the National Center for PTSD, the free app can be used by anyone who wants to use mindfulness to reduce stress and boost well-being. Note that Mindfulness Coach should not replace work with a therapist if it's needed.

Stress in America: A Nation Recovering From Collective Trauma
apa.org/news/press/releases/stress/2023/collective-trauma-recovery
The recent "Stress in America" survey from the American Psychological Association looks at stress in American life following the COVID-19 pandemic.

What Is EMDR Therapy and Why Is It Used to Treat PTSD?
apa.org/topics/psychotherapy/emdr-therapy-ptsd

Article from the American Psychological Association that explains how EMDR works for traumatic memories and who can benefit from it the most.

My Menopause
acog.org/MyMenopause

Web resource from ACOG with information on the menopause transition, signs and symptoms, treatments, and self-care. Includes the latest information from the experts in ob-gyn care, menopause stories from real women, expert columns on how to manage symptoms, Q&A articles, videos, and more.

CHAPTER 21

Screenings and Vaccinations After Menopause

At 45, Michelle is in perimenopause and looking ahead to preventive health care. Her health history includes screening for benign breast lumps and removal of polyps during a routine colonoscopy, so she understands how important health screenings can be. She now has annual mammograms and plans to continue them through her post-menopausal years. She also plans to keep up with vaccination after menopause, especially for shingles. "Shingles is a miserable illness, and I want to protect myself with the vaccine," she says.

This book is about empowering you to be as healthy as possible through your *menopause transition* and beyond. In this final chapter, we'll explore the screenings and vaccinations you need to maintain good health in the years after your final *menstrual period*. Moving forward from that last period, you are *postmenopausal*, and you may live decades longer. This makes taking care of your health now all the more important.

Fortunately, the *obstetrician–gynecologist (ob-gyn)* you relied on through other phases of life, including your transition through menopausal symptoms, can continue to guide you in your postmenopausal years. Your annual visits will change over time as your health needs change, but you and your ob-gyn can talk about many topics, including sex, *sexually transmitted infections (STIs)*, *urinary tract infections (UTIs)*, pelvic pain, *urinary incontinence*, and other conditions that become more common in midlife. Your ob-gyn can also help you track your cancer and other health screenings and maintain your vaccination record.

Annual Wellness Visits After Menopause

If you've been keeping up with your annual ob-gyn visits while you managed *hot flashes*, night sweats, vaginal dryness, or other menopausal symptoms, the transition to postmenopausal care should be seamless. You may continue to need *hormone therapy* or other medications for years after your last period if your symptoms continue to bother you. Your ob-gyn can help you decide how long that might be. But now is also the time to lean on your ob-gyn as you plan for your long-term health.

Some things about your annual visits will remain the same. Your ob-gyn will update your medical history, ask about any new symptoms, and recommend a physical exam. You will talk about whether a *pelvic exam*, *cervical cancer* screening, and breast exam are needed. You may also talk about your overall health, your weight, and how to manage other health conditions or your risk of developing them.

Pelvic Exam and Cervical Cancer Screening

You're likely familiar with the pelvic exam, in which an ob-gyn inserts a gloved finger into the *vagina* and presses on the abdomen to feel for the size and shape of the *uterus*, *ovaries*, and other pelvic organs. In the past, a pelvic exam was a routine part of an annual wellness check. Now, ACOG recommends that the decision to have a pelvic exam be based on a conversation between you and your ob-gyn. Having this exam may be important if you have new pelvic pain, urinary problems, pain during sex, or unexplained vaginal bleeding or discharge.

You may also have cervical cancer screening during your annual visit. Your ob-gyn will likely follow ACOG guidelines for this screening:

- Up to age 65, there are three options. You can have both a Pap test and a test for *human papillomavirus (HPV)* every 5 years. You can have a Pap test alone every 3 years. Or you can have HPV testing alone every 5 years.

- After 65, you can stop having cervical cancer screenings if you've never had abnormal cervical cells or cervical cancer, and you've had two or three negative screening tests in a row, depending on the type of test.

Note that there are some exceptions to these guidelines. You may need more screenings more often if you

- have a history of cervical cancer
- have *human immunodeficiency virus (HIV)*
- have a weakened *immune system*
- were exposed before birth to DES, a *hormone* given to pregnant women between 1940 and 1971

If you've had the HPV vaccine, you should still follow the screening guidelines. The *vaccine* doesn't protect against every type of HPV. You and your ob-gyn can talk through the guidelines and determine when you need your next cervical cancer screening.

Also, you may still need screening even if you had a *hysterectomy*. A total hysterectomy removes the *cervix*, along with the uterus, but women with a history of cervical cancer or precancer should continue screening. This is done by taking cells from the top of the vagina, which could still have some cervical cells. Another type of hysterectomy keeps the cervix in place, and in these cases, screening should also continue.

Sometimes an ob-gyn recommends a rectovaginal exam during an annual visit. Wearing gloves, your ob-gyn inserts one finger into the vagina and another finger into the *rectum* using the same hand. The other hand is used to press on the lower abdomen. This allows your ob-gyn to feel for lumps or other abnormal changes in both the rectum and vagina. They can check the size, shape, and position of the pelvic organs and the ligaments that hold the uterus in place.

Breast Exam

During your annual visit, your ob-gyn may recommend a clinical breast exam. This should be the same breast exam you've had in the past, with your ob-gyn checking for lumps in breast tissue and your underarm area. If you're 40 or older, at average risk of breast cancer, and do not have symptoms, you should have a clinical breast exam every year. If you are at increased risk of breast cancer, you may have this exam more often.

As part of your clinical breast exam, your ob-gyn may ask if you've noticed any changes in either breast, including

- a lump or hard area in the breast or underarm area
- change in shape, size, or color, especially if it happens on one breast only
- puckering, itchiness, or scaling of the breast or nipple
- new indentation or a changed position of your nipple
- sudden nipple discharge
- new persistent pain in one part of the breast

You may also talk about breast self-awareness, which is having a sense of what is normal for your breasts so you can tell if there are changes, even small ones.

> **Should I still be doing monthly self-exams of my breasts?**
>
> Ob-gyns don't recommend monthly breast self-exams anymore. For women at average risk, monthly self-exams weren't shown to reduce deaths from breast cancer. The focus now is on breast self-awareness. This means having a sense of what is normal for your breasts so that you can tell if there are changes—even small changes—and report them to your ob-gyn. If you notice breast changes such as pain, a lump, unexpected nipple discharge, or redness, make an appointment to see your ob-gyn.
>
> —DR. CARRIE ANN TERRELL

Breast Cancer Screening

You and your ob-gyn should discuss when and how often you will have breast cancer screening. In the United States, 1 in 8 women will develop breast cancer by age 75. Regular breast screening can help find cancer at an earlier and more curable stage. Screening can also find problems in the breasts that are not cancer.

Screening *mammography* is the primary tool used to screen for breast cancer and other breast problems. Mammography uses X-ray technology to view the breasts. The images created are called a *mammogram*, and a physician called a *radiologist* reads the images. Radiologists use a system called BI-RADS to report results. Your screening mammogram result will be given a score ranging from 0 to 5. Scores mean the following:

0—**More information is needed.** You may need another mammogram before a score can be given.

1—**Nothing abnormal is seen.** You should continue to have routine screening.

2—**Benign conditions, such as *cysts*, are seen.** You should continue to have routine screening.

3—**Something is seen that probably is not cancer.** A repeat mammogram should be done within 6 months.

4—**Something is seen that is suspicious for cancer.** You may need to have a *biopsy*.

5—**Something is seen that is highly suggestive of cancer.** You will need to have a biopsy.

Radiologists are also required to report on the density of breast tissue. Fibrous tissue and fat give breasts their shape. When breasts are dense, they have more fibrous tissue and less fat. Breast density is a common and normal finding on a mammogram. But dense breast tissue is a risk factor for breast cancer, and it can make cancer harder to see on a mammogram.

Standard mammograms provide a 2-dimensional image. Some mammograms use multiple breast X-rays to build a 3-dimensional image. Using 3D mammography may reduce the need for additional screening, especially in women with dense breasts. You and your ob-gyn can talk about how breast density may affect your cancer screenings. You can read more in the box "What to Know About Breast Density."

So how often should you have a mammogram? For women at average risk of breast cancer, screening mammography is recommended every 1 to 2 years beginning at 40. Screening should continue until at least 75. The main risk factors for breast cancer—being a woman and getting older—cannot be controlled. But you may be at high risk of breast cancer if you have

- a family history of breast cancer, *ovarian cancer*, or other inherited types of cancer
- *BRCA1 and BRCA2* or other genetic mutations
- a history of chest *radiation* treatments at a young age
- a history of high-risk breast biopsy results

Women without these risk factors are at average risk. Still, you and your ob-gyn should share information, talk about your wishes, and agree on when and how often you will have breast cancer screening.

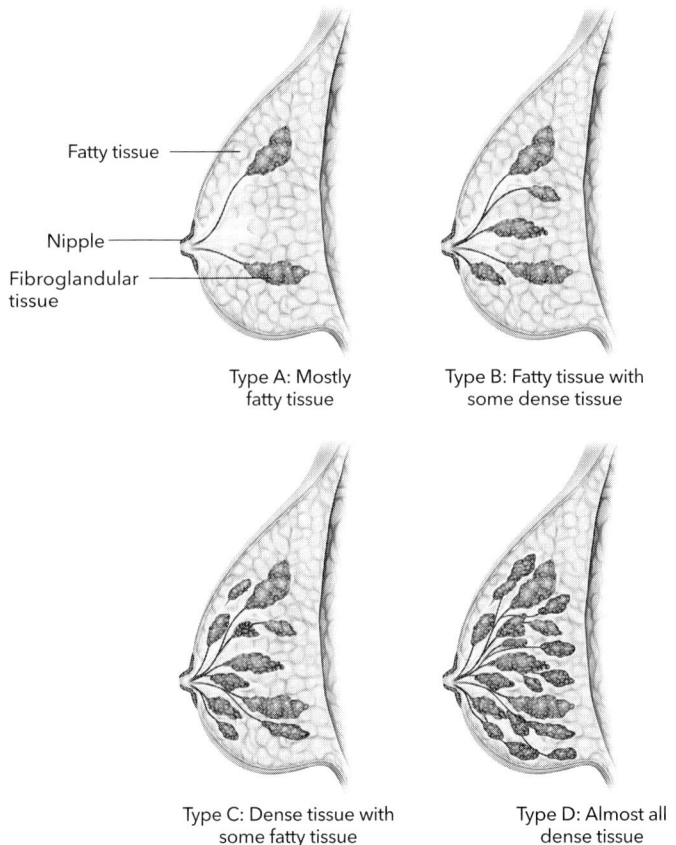

Breast density. Dense breast tissue is the term used when the breasts have more dense, fibroglandular tissue than fatty tissue. Dense breast tissue is seen on mammograms.

> **What to Know About Breast Density**
>
> If you have dense breast tissue, you're not alone. About half of women over 40 have dense breasts. This condition tends to run in families. And some women are more prone to dense breasts, including Black women, people with a low *body mass index (BMI)*, and those who continue to use hormone therapy after their last period.
>
> Women with dense breasts have a modestly higher risk of breast cancer than those without dense breasts. But dense breasts do not increase the risk of dying from breast cancer. For this reason, ACOG does not recommend extra screenings if you have dense breasts and no other risk factors for breast cancer. Research does not show that extra or different screening methods reduce breast cancer deaths for those with dense breasts.

Additional screening may be needed if your screening mammogram shows signs of a problem. This might include breast ultrasound, which uses soundwaves to create images of the inside of your breasts. An ultrasound can show whether a lump in your breast is solid (which could be a *tumor*) or a cyst filled with fluid. A breast biopsy removes a small piece of tissue so it can be checked in a lab for cancer or other abnormalities. Biopsy is often done with a special needle. Using ultrasound can help locate the right spot to take tissue from.

Other Health Screenings

The chance of developing certain diseases rises with age. For some health screenings, your ob-gyn can order tests. For others, your ob-gyn can refer you to specialists who can manage your testing. Each screening is an opportunity to prevent or delay disease and reduce its damage over time. Screening can also help diagnose diseases at an earlier stage—sometimes before you even have symptoms. This may help with treatment and increase your chance of a good outcome.

In previous chapters, we've discussed screening for mood disorders such as *depression* and anxiety (Chapter 8, "Mood and Memory"), *osteoporosis* (Chapter 15, "Bone Health"), and heart disease and *diabetes* (Chapter 19, "Heart Disease and Diabetes"). Here we'll talk about other screenings and how often they should be done.

Colon Cancer Screening

Colon cancer often begins as a *polyp*, a small clump of cells found in the lining of the *colon*. Routine screenings can help detect and remove polyps before they become cancer.

The American Cancer Society recommends that people at average risk of colon cancer start screening at 45. It may be done with a stool-based test that's mailed to a lab or with *colonoscopy* or other tests that look directly at the colon and rectum. Most mail-in tests should be done every year. If colonoscopy is used instead, it may be done every 10 years. Most people can continue screening through age 75. Between 76 and 85, screening decisions should be based on current health, past screening results, and a person's preferences. After 85, screening is no longer recommended.

Decisions about when to screen may also depend on your risk of developing cancer. You may be at increased risk of colon cancer if you have

- a personal history of colon cancer or certain types of polyps
- a family history of colon cancer
- a personal history of *inflammatory bowel disease (IBD)*, including ulcerative colitis or Crohn's disease
- confirmed or suspected hereditary cancer syndrome, such as *Lynch syndrome*
- a personal history of radiation to the abdomen or pelvic area to treat a prior cancer

If you've had a colonoscopy before, you know that it requires bowel prep—drinking a fluid that triggers bowel movements over a 12-hour period to clean out stool. The test itself requires sedation. A flexible tube with a camera is used to check the rectum and the lining of the large bowel. The doctor doing the procedure may take a tissue sample for testing or remove any polyps they find. Any tissue that is removed will be studied for cancer cells.

There's also testing called virtual colonoscopy. A *computed tomography (CT)* scan of the colon and rectum can reveal polyps and cancer. This can be combined with X-rays to produce 3D pictures. The procedure requires bowel preparation but not sedation. If your results are concerning, you will need a standard colonoscopy, too. A virtual colonoscopy may be repeated every 5 years.

Thyroid Function Screening

The *thyroid gland* is located at the base of your neck in front of your windpipe. The thyroid gland makes, stores, and releases two hormones—T_4 (thyroxine) and T_3 (triiodothyronine). These hormones help control your *metabolism*, which is the rate at which every part of your body works. When your thyroid gland is working in the way it should, your metabolism stays at a steady pace—not too fast and not too slow.

Certain disorders can cause the thyroid gland to make too much or too little hormone. This can lead to thyroid disease. And thyroid disease can harm more than your metabolism. Your heart, bones, energy, and mood can also be affected by thyroid problems.

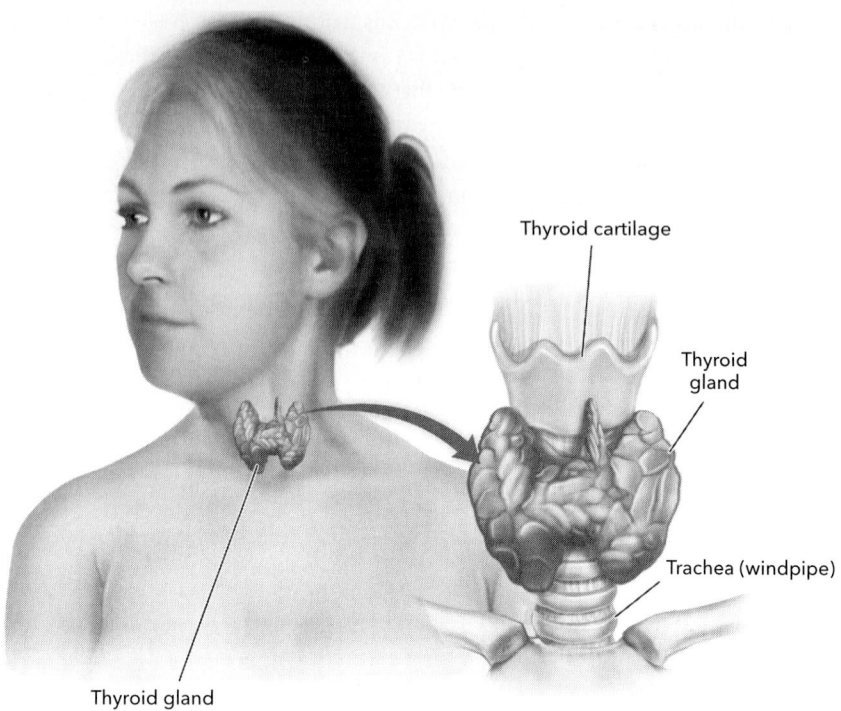

Thyroid gland. The thyroid gland is a butterfly-shaped organ at the base of the neck. It makes, stores, and releases hormones that help control metabolism. When your thyroid gland is working in the way it should, your metabolism stays at a steady pace—not too fast and not too slow.

The American Thyroid Association recommends checking thyroid function beginning at 35. The test should be repeated every 5 years, or more often for people with certain symptoms or risk factors. The American College of Physicians recommends screening women 50 and older who have symptoms that could be caused by thyroid disease. Talk with your ob-gyn or other doctor about when you need thyroid screening.

Screening for thyroid disorders typically starts with a blood test that checks your levels of certain hormones and *antibodies* (proteins that help protect you from disease). If the results are concerning, your doctor may recommend additional tests using ultrasound or scans. These can help investigate abnormalities and show whether your thyroid is too active or not active enough. Tests can help diagnose serious and disabling conditions, such as Graves disease and other forms of *hyperthyroidism*, *hypothyroidism*, Hashimoto disease, and thyroid cancer.

Dental Checkups

Dental care remains important in midlife and beyond. This is partly because dental problems are associated with a higher risk of disease. Inflammation of the gums (*gingivitis*) is linked to conditions affecting the lungs, blood vessels, and heart. Gum disease that leads to tooth loss is linked to a higher risk of dementia.

Dental problems also affect daily functioning. In a U.S. study, almost 2 in 5 adults between 50 and 64 reported they had dental problems that caused pain, difficulty eating, and missed work within the past 2 years. People who had regular dental cleanings and checkups were less likely to report these problems.

The American Dental Association (ADA) recommends regular dental visits for teeth cleaning and X-rays. This helps identify dental problems before they have a serious effect on your health and become more expensive to treat. For most people, the ADA advises a dental checkup once or twice a year throughout life.

Eye Exams

Eye exams become increasingly important from midlife on. With age you are more likely to need reading glasses. After 40, you are also more likely to develop eye diseases, though you may not have symptoms until later. By 65, 1 in 3 adults have an eye disease that affects their vision. Early diagnosis and treatment of cataracts, glaucoma, macular degeneration, and other conditions can help maintain your vision for longer. Maintaining vision may also be a key to avoiding future dementia. If you have *prediabetes*, diabetes, or **high blood pressure**, annual eye exams are even more important.

If you have not had your eyes checked in over a year, schedule an appointment. Based on your eye health and risk factors, your eye doctor will let you know how often you should be seen after this visit.

> ### How are vaccines approved?
>
> In the United States, vaccines are approved by the U.S. Food and Drug Administration (FDA) only after thorough research. Testing starts with animals and small groups of human volunteers. Later, vaccines are tested in large clinical trials with thousands of volunteers. If a clinical trial shows that a vaccine is safe and effective, there are a few other safety reviews. Then vaccine experts meet to review the testing results. Once a vaccine is licensed by the FDA, a committee at the Centers for Disease Control and Prevention (CDC) recommends how best to use it to control disease. This recommendation goes to the CDC director, who reviews and approves the recommendation.
>
> –DR. CHARLES KILPATRICK

Hearing Tests

Hearing tests are another key to maintaining your health and function as you get older. When hearing loss is untreated, it contributes to social isolation, loneliness, and lower levels of employment. Age-related hearing loss is also a warning for a higher risk of cognitive decline and dementia, possibly because of reduced mental stimulation. Adults with hearing difficulties are more vulnerable to balance problems and falls, hospitalizations, and earlier death than those with normal hearing.

The American Speech–Language–Hearing Association recommends that up until midlife, adults get screened for hearing loss every 10 years. After age 50, or sooner if you have risk factors for hearing loss, get screened every 3 years. If you have concerns at any age, see a doctor or audiologist who can do a hearing test. Some warehouse clubs also have hearing clinics where you can get your hearing tested. Be sure to get tested at least once by 65.

If you have hearing loss, don't delay getting a hearing aid. Current technology is better than ever. Some hearing aids are chargeable and can be personalized using your cell phone. This means you can adjust them to suit your environment.

Skin Cancer Self-Checks

Skin cancer becomes more common as people age. The American Cancer Society does not have guidelines for the early detection of skin cancer. But experts recommend that everyone do skin self-checks on a regular basis, usually once a month. This will help you spot any new growths, moles, or spots. Those at high risk of skin cancer may consider seeing a dermatologist once a year for a full-body skin check. Risk factors include having a lot of moles or other growths, lower immunity, or a personal or family history of skin cancer.

Vaccination for Midlife and Beyond

Vaccines help protect you from diseases that can be serious or even deadly. Many of these diseases are common, but vaccines can prevent them. And if you got routine vaccines on schedule as a younger person, you should continue the trend. This is because

- older adults are more likely to get certain diseases
- older adults are at higher risk for serious health problems caused by illnesses like COVID-19 or the flu
- protection from some vaccines can fade over time
- your vaccines protect others, too, which is especially important if you spend time with babies or people who have long-term health problems or weakened immune systems

You may need additional vaccines if you

- have a chronic health condition, such as diabetes or heart, lung, or liver disease
- did not get all your vaccines when you were a child
- have a health condition that makes it harder for your body to fight off infections, such as HIV or problems with your spleen
- smoke
- travel outside the United States
- work in certain places, like a hospital or nursing home

Some people should not get specific vaccinations—for example, if you previously had an allergic reaction to a particular vaccine. Discuss all vaccinations with your ob-gyn or other doctor. Read the Table 21-1, "Midlife Vaccination Guide," for details on which vaccines may be recommended for you.

Table 21-1 Midlife Vaccination Guide

The Centers for Disease Control and Prevention recommends the following vaccines for midlife and older adults. Other vaccines may also be recommended based on your age or health. Talk with your ob-gyn about whether you need other vaccines in addition to these.

Vaccine	Age	Doses and Timing	Notes
COVID-19	All adults	One shot every year of current vaccine	People 65 and older or with weakened immune systems may get additional doses
Flu (influenza)	All adults	One shot every year, ideally in September or October	
Hepatitis B	Adults through age 59	Two shots 1 month apart or Three shots 6 months apart	People 60 and older with risk factors may also get vaccinated
Pneumonia (pneumococcal disease)	Adults 50 and older	Type of vaccine and number of doses can vary by age and vaccination history	People younger than 50 with certain medical conditions or who have had their spleen removed may also get vaccinated

(continued)

Table 21-1 Midlife Vaccination Guide (continued)

Vaccine	Age	Doses and Timing	Notes
RSV (respiratory syncytial virus)	Adults 75 and older	One shot, ideally in late summer or early fall. Does not have to be repeated every year	People 60 to 74 and with increased risk of severe RSV may also get vaccinated
Shingles (herpes zoster)	Adults 50 and older	Two shots, 2 to 6 months apart	People with weakened immune systems may get the second dose 1 to 2 months after the first dose
Tdap (**tetanus, diphtheria**, whooping cough) or Td (tetanus and diphtheria)	All adults	Booster shot every 10 years. After a severe or dirty wound or burn 5+ years since the last booster, get another one	People who never received Tdap should get one now

Source: Centers for Disease Control and Prevention (CDC). For the most up-to-date information on when to have vaccines, visit the CDC page on Recommended Vaccinations for Adults at cdc.gov/vaccines/imz-schedules/adult-easyread.html.

Your ob-gyn may offer some vaccines in their office. You can also get vaccines at your local health center or pharmacy. For vaccines related to international travel, you may need to go to a travel medicine clinic.

Finally, as you think about your health after menopause, remember that knowing your own body and mind, watching for changes that may signal a health problem, and being actively involved in your health care are the keys to staying well. The goal is to avoid serious illness and disability through midlife and into your older years. Once you've navigated your menopause transition, there's so much more ahead, and you can be healthy and strong enough to enjoy it all.

RESOURCES

American Cancer Society Guideline for Colorectal Cancer Screening
cancer.org/cancer/types/colon-rectal-cancer/detection-diagnosis-staging/acs-recommendations.html
An ACS webpage explaining colon cancer screening for people at average risk and high risk.

Dental Exam
medlineplus.gov/lab-tests/dental-exam/

Webpage from the National Library on Medicine that explains dental exams, how to prepare for them, and how to keep your teeth and gums healthy.

Eye Exam and Vision Testing Basics
aao.org/eye-health/tips-prevention/eye-exams-101

Guide from the American Academy of Ophthalmology that explains when you should have an eye exam and what's involved in testing your vision.

Hearing Tests for Adults
medlineplus.gov/lab-tests/hearing-tests-for-adults/

Webpage from the National Library of Medicine that explains how hearing tests are done and what the results mean.

How to Do a Skin Self-Exam
cancer.org/cancer/risk-prevention/sun-and-uv/skin-exams.html

Step-by-step guide from the American Cancer Society to doing skin checks at home.

Mammography Facilities
accessdata.fda.gov/scripts/cdrh/cfdocs/cfMQSA/mqsa.cfm

Tool from the U.S. Food and Drug Administration to help you search for a certified mammography facility in your area.

Vaccines & Immunizations
cdc.gov/vaccines/index.html

Web resource from the Centers for Disease Control and Prevention that covers vaccine basics, vaccine schedules for adults and families, and more.

My Menopause
acog.org/MyMenopause

Web resource from ACOG with information on the menopause transition, signs and symptoms, treatments, and self-care. Includes the latest information from the experts in ob-gyn care, menopause stories from real women, expert columns on how to manage symptoms, Q&A articles, videos, and more.

Part V
RESOURCES

FOR MORE READING

Menopause: What Your Ob-Gyn Wants You to Know was developed using more than 750 documents as source material, including

- ACOG clinical guidance and recommendations
- randomized clinical trials that divide people into groups to compare different treatments
- systematic reviews that analyze existing scientific study results
- data-based reports from government agencies

Below are some of the most recent studies and articles you can use for more reading. This list can serve as a starting point as you do your own research on the menopause transition, treatments, and care recommendations.

Chapter 1: Understanding the Menopause Transition

Disparities in Reproductive Aging and Midlife Health Between Black and White Women: The Study of Women's Health Across the Nation (SWAN). Published in *Women's Midlife Health*, 2022 (Vol. 8), by Harlow SD et al. Available at womensmidlifehealthjournal.biomedcentral.com/articles/10.1186/s40695-022-00073-y

Impact of Violence Against Women on Quality of Life and Menopause-Related Disorders. Published in *Maturitas*, 2024 (Vol. 180), by Mendoza-Huertas L et al. Available at sciencedirect.com/science/article/pii/S0378512223005054

Menopause: Understanding the Implications of Society and Culture. Published in *Pre-Collegiate Global Health Review*, January 14, 2022. Available at pghr.org/post/menopause-understanding-the-implications-of-society-and-culture

Normalising Menopause. Published in *BMJ*, 2022 (Vol. 377), by Hickey M et al. Available at bmj.com/content/377/bmj-2021-069369

Self-Reported Menstrual Cycle Length During Reproductive Years in Relation to Menopausal Symptoms at Midlife in Project Viva. Published in *Menopause*, 2022 (Vol. 29, Issue 10), by Mínguez-Alarcón L et al. Available at journals.lww.com/menopausejournal/abstract/2022/10000/self_reported_menstrual_cycle_length_during.5.aspx

Chapter 2: Understanding Perimenopause

Management of Acute Abnormal Uterine Bleeding in Nonpregnant Reproductive-Aged Women. ACOG Committee Opinion No. 557. Published in 2013. Reaffirmed in 2024. Available at acog.org/clinical/clinical-guidance/committee-opinion/articles/2013/04/management-of-acute-abnormal-uterine-bleeding-in-nonpregnant-reproductive-aged-women

The Menopause Transition and Cognition. Published in *JAMA*, 2020 (Vol. 323, Issue 15), by Greendale GA et al. Available at jamanetwork.com/journals/jama/fullarticle/2763134

Understanding the Menopause Journey. Published in *Climacteric*, 2025, by Santoro N. Available at tandfonline.com/doi/10.1080/13697137.2024.2445303

Chapter 3: Understanding Early and Premature Menopause

Early Menopause in Acquired Immunodeficiency Syndrome. Published in *Journal of Research in Medical Sciences*, 2021 (Vol. 26, Issue 1), by Ahmed MH et al. Available at journals.lww.com/jrms/fulltext/2021/26000/early_menopause_in_acquired_immunodeficiency.122.aspx

Genetic Insights Into Biological Mechanisms Governing Human Ovarian Ageing. Published in *Nature* (Vol. 596), 2021, by Ruth KS et al. Available at nature.com/articles/s41586-021-03779-7

Trends and Predictors of Hysterectomy Prevalence Among Women in the United States. Published in *American Journal of Obstetrics & Gynecology*, 2022 (Vol. 227, Issue 4), by Harvey SV et al. Available at ajog.org/article/S0002-9378(22)00482-3/abstract

Chapter 4: Menopause Signs and Symptoms

An Online Survey of Perimenopausal Women to Determine Their Attitudes and Knowledge of the Menopause. Published in *Women's Health*, 2022 (Vol. 18), by Harper JC et al. Available at journals.sagepub.com/doi/10.1177/17455057221106890

Cognitive Decline in Early and Premature Menopause. Published in *International Journal of Molecular Sciences*, 2023 (Vol. 24, Issue 7), by Sochoka M et al. Available at mdpi.com/1422-0067/24/7/6566

Female Pattern Hair Loss: An Overview With Focus on the Genetics. Published in *Genes (Basel)*, 2023 (Vol. 14, Issue 7), by Ho CY et al. Available at mdpi.com/2073-4425/14/7/1326

Menopause and Sleep Disorders. Published in *Journal of Mid-Life Health*, 2022 (Vol. 13, Issue 1), by Tandon VR et al. Available at journals.lww.com/jomh/fulltext/2022/13010/menopause_and_sleep_disorders.8.aspx

Menopause, Skin and Common Dermatoses. Part 2: Skin Disorders. Published in *Clinical and Experimental Dermatology*, 2022 (Vol. 47), by Kamp E et al. Available at academic.oup.com/ced/article/47/12/2117/6966236

Perimenopausal Women's Voices: How Does Their Period at the End of Reproductive Life Affect Wellbeing? Published in *Post Reproductive Health*, 2023 (Vol. 29, Issue 4), by Ray E et al. Available at journals.sagepub.com/doi/full/10.1177/20533691231216162

Skin, Hair and Beyond: The Impact of Menopause. Published in *Climacteric*, 2022 (Vol. 25, Issue 5), by Zouboulis CC et al. Available at tandfonline.com/doi/full/10.1080/13697137.2022.2050206

Spouses' Perceptions of and Attitudes Toward Female Menopause: A Mixed-Methods Systematic Review. Published in *Climacteric*, 2020 (Vol. 23, Issue 2), by Zhang X et al. Available at tandfonline.com/doi/10.1080/13697137.2019.1703937

The Relationship Between Pelvic Floor Function and Sexual Function in Perimenopausal Women. Published in *Sexual Medicine*, 2021 (Vol. 9, Issue 6), by Zhou Z et al. Available at academic.oup.com/smoa/article/9/6/100441/6956814

Understanding Attitudes, Beliefs, and Behaviors Surrounding Menopause Transition: Results From Three Surveys. Published in *Patient-Reported Outcome Measures*, 2022 (Vol. 13), by Richard-Davis G et al. Available at dovepress.com/understanding-attitudes-beliefs-and-behaviors-surrounding-menopause-tr-peer-reviewed-fulltext-article-PROM

Women's Knowledge and Attitudes to the Menopause: A Comparison of Women Over 40 Who Were in the Perimenopause, Post Menopause, and Those Not in the Peri or Post Menopause. Published in *BMC Women's Health*, 2023 (Vol. 23), by Tariq B et al. Available at bmcwomenshealth.biomedcentral.com/articles/10.1186/s12905-023-02424-x

Chapter 5: Choosing Your Menopause Care Team

Caring for Patients Who Have Experienced Trauma. ACOG Committee Opinion No. 825. Published in 2021. Reaffirmed in 2024. Available at acog.org/clinical/clinical-guidance/committee-opinion/articles/2021/04/caring-for-patients-who-have-experienced-trauma

LGBTQIA+ Menopause: Room for Improvement. Published in *The Lancet*, 2022 (Vol. 400, Issue 10363), by Glyde T. Available at thelancet.com/journals/lancet/article/PIIS0140-6736(22)01935-3/fulltext

Positioning Psychiatric Pharmacists to Improve Mental Health Care. Published in *The Mental Health Clinician*, 2022 (Vol. 12, Issue 2), by Dopheide JA et al. Available at mhc.kglmeridian.com/view/journals/mhcl/12/2/article-p77.xml

Chapter 6: Hot Flashes and Night Sweats

Cardiovascular Risk and Midlife Cognitive Decline in the Study of Women's Health Across the Nation. Published in *Alzheimer's & Dementia*, 2021 (Vol. 17, Issue 8), by Derby CA et al. Available at alz-journals.onlinelibrary.wiley.com/doi/10.1002/alz.12300

Impact of Violence Against Women on Quality of Life and Menopause-Related Disorders. Published in *Maturitas*, 2024 (Vol. 180), by Mendoza-Huertas L. Available at sciencedirect.com/science/article/pii/S0378512223005054

Menopausal Vasomotor Symptoms and Risk of Incident Cardiovascular Disease Events in SWAN. Published in *Journal of the American Heart Association*, 2021 (Vol. 10), by Thurston RC et al. Available at ahajournals.org/doi/10.1161/JAHA.120.017416

Vasomotor Symptoms: More Than Temporary Menopausal Symptoms. Published in *Journal of Menopausal Medicine*, 2020 (Vol. 26, Issue 3), by Ryu KJ et al. Available at e-jmm.org/DOIx.php?id=10.6118/jmm.20030

Chapter 7: Abnormal Bleeding

When Racial Bias Is Embedded in Medical Norms: How Physicians Can Approach Patients' Uterine Cancer Risk and Care. Published August 10, 2022, by ACOG. Available at acog.org/news/news-articles/2022/08/racial-bias-in-medical-norms-how-physicians-approach-patients-uterine-cancer-risk

Chapter 8: Mood and Memory

ADHD Symptoms in Females of Childhood, Adolescent, Reproductive and Menopause Period. Published in *Materia Socio-Medica*, 2021 (Vol. 33, Issue 2), by Antoniou E et al. Available at ejmanager.com/mnstemps/16/16-1626210060.pdf?t=1740163366

Anxiety and Depression in Midlife Transition and Beyond: The Role of Estrogens. Published in *Current Opinion in Endocrine and Metabolic Research*, 2023 (Vol. 31), by Soares CN. Available at sciencedirect.com/science/article/abs/pii/S2451965023000248

Cannabidiol (CBD) in the Self-Treatment of Depression—Exploratory Study and a New Phenomenon of Concern for Psychiatrists. Published in *Frontiers in Psychiatry*, 2022 (Vol. 13), by Wieckiewcz G et al. Available at frontiersin.org/journals/psychiatry/articles/10.3389/fpsyt.2022.837946/full

Cognitive Decline in Early and Premature Menopause. Published in *International Journal of Molecular Sciences*, 2023 (Vol. 24, Issue 7), by Sochoka M et al. Available at mdpi.com/1422-0067/24/7/6566

Dementia Prevention, Intervention, and Care: 2020 Report of the Lancet Commission. Published in *Lancet*, 2020 (Vol. 396, Issue 10248), by Livingston G et al. Available at thelancet.com/journals/lancet/article/PIIS0140-6736(20)30367-6/fulltext

Does Menopause Elevate the Risk for Developing Depression and Anxiety? Results From a Systematic Review. Published in *Australas Psychiatry*, 2023 (Vol. 31, Issue 2), by Alblooshi S et al. Available at journals.sagepub.com/doi/10.1177/10398562231165439

Exercising Is Good for the Brain but Exercising Outside Is Potentially Better. Published in *Nature: Scientific Reports*, 2023 (Vol. 13), by Boere K et al. Available at nature.com/articles/s41598-022-26093-2

Menopause and Cognitive Impairment: A Narrative Review of Current Knowledge. Published in *World Journal of Psychiatry*, 2021 (Vol. 11, Issue 8), by Conde DM et al. Available at wjgnet.com/2220-3206/full/v11/i8/412.htm

Strategies to Cope With Stress and Anxiety During the Menopausal Transition. Published in *Maturitas*, 2022 (Vol. 166), by Stute P and Lozza-Fiacco S. Available at sciencedirect.com/science/article/pii/S0378512222001670

Systematic Review and Meta-analysis of the Effects of Menopause Hormone Therapy on Risk of Alzheimer's Disease and Dementia. Published in *Frontiers in Aging Neuroscience*, 2023 (Vol. 15), by Nerattini M et al. Available at frontiersin.org/journals/aging-neuroscience/articles/10.3389/fnagi.2023.1260427/full

The Interplay Among Natural Menopause, Insomnia, and Cognitive Health: A Population-Based Study. Published in *Nature and Science of Sleep*, 2023 (Vol. 15), by Shieu MM et al. Available at dovepress.com/the-interplay-among-natural-menopause-insomnia-and-cognitive-health-a--peer-reviewed-fulltext-article-NSS

The Therapeutic Impact of Plant-Based and Nutritional Supplements on Anxiety, Depressive Symptoms and Sleep Quality Among Adults and Elderly: A Systematic Review of the Literature. Published in *International Journal of Environmental Research and Public Health*, 2023 (Vol. 20, Issue 6), by Kamat D et al. Available at mdpi.com/1660-4601/20/6/5171

What Is the Impact of Nature on Human Health? A Scoping Review of the Literature. Published in *Journal of Global Health*, 2022 (Vol. 12), by Nejade RM et al. Available at jogh.org/2022/jogh-12-04099

Chapter 9: Sleep Problems

Association of Sleep Duration in Middle and Old Age With Incidence of Dementia. Published in *Nature Communications*, 2021 (Vol. 12), by Sabia S et al. Available at nature.com/articles/s41467-021-22354-2

Associations of Anxiety and Depression With Restless Leg Syndrome: A Systematic Review and Meta-analysis. Published in *Frontiers in Neurology*, 2024 (Vol. 15), by An T et al. Available at frontiersin.org/journals/neurology/articles/10.3389/fneur.2024.1366839/full

High Glycemic Index and Glycemic Load Diets as Risk Factors for Insomnia: Analyses From the Women's Health Initiative. Published in *The American Journal of Clinical Nutrition*, 2020 (Vol. 111, Issue 2), by Gangwisch JE et al. Available at sciencedirect.com/science/article/pii/S0002916522010188

Light at Night in Older Age Is Associated With Obesity, Diabetes, and Hypertension. Published in *Sleep*, 2023 (Vol. 46, Issue 3), by Kim M et al. Available at academic.oup.com/sleep/article/46/3/zsac130/6608953

Oral Magnesium Supplementation for Insomnia in Older Adults: A Systematic Review & Meta-analysis. Published in *BMC Complementary Medicine and Therapies*, 2021 (Vol. 21), by Mah J and Pitre T. Available at bmccomplementmedtherapies.biomedcentral.com/articles/10.1186/s12906-021-03297-z

Psychological and Physical Approaches for Sleep Disorders: What the Science Says. Published in *NCCIH Clinical Digest*, 2024, by National Center for Complementary and Integrative Health. Available at nccih.nih.gov/health/providers/digest/psychological-and-physical-approaches-for-sleep-disorders-science

Quantity of Melatonin and CBD in Melatonin Gummies Sold in the US. Published in *JAMA*, 2023 (Vol. 329, Issue 16), by Cohen PA et al. Available at jamanetwork.com/journals/jama/fullarticle/2804077

Re-considering the Role of Sleep Hygiene Behaviours in Sleep: Associations Between Sleep Hygiene, Perceptions and Sleep. Published in *International Journal of Behavioral Medicine*, 2023 (Vol. 31), by McAlpine T et al. Available at link.springer.com/article/10.1007/s12529-023-10212-y

The Association of Pet Ownership and Sleep Quality and Sleep Disorders in United States. Published in *Human–Animal Interactions*, 2023, by Medlin K and Wisnieski L. Available at doi.org/10.1079/hai.2023.0005

The Effects of Cannabinoids on Sleep. Published in *Journal of Primary Care & Community Health*, 2022 (Vol. 13), by Kolla BP et al. Available at journals.sagepub.com/doi/10.1177/21501319221081277

The Impact of Bedtime Technology Use on Sleep Quality and Excessive Daytime Sleepiness in Adults. Published in *Sleep Science*, 2022 (Vol. 15, Issue S 02), by AlShareef SM et al. Available at thieme-connect.de/products/ejournals/abstract/10.5935/1984-0063.20200128

Time Spent in Outdoor Light Is Associated With Mood, Sleep, and Circadian Rhythm-Related Outcomes: A Cross-Sectional and Longitudinal Study in Over 400,000 UK Biobank Participants. Published in *Journal of Affective Disorders*, 2021 (Vol. 295), by Burns AC et al. Available at sciencedirect.com/science/article/abs/pii/S0165032721008612

Chapter 10: Sexual Health

Compounded Bioidentical Menopausal Hormone Therapy. ACOG Clinical Consensus No. 6. Published in 2023. Available at acog.org/clinical/clinical-guidance/clinical-consensus/articles/2023/11/compounded-bioidentical-menopausal-hormone-therapy

Declines in Sexual Activity and Function Predict Incident Health Problems in Older Adults: Prospective Findings From the English Longitudinal Study of Ageing. Published in *Archives of Sexual Behavior*, 2020 (Vol. 49), by Jackson SE et al. Available at link.springer.com/article/10.1007/s10508-019-1443-4

Factors Influencing the Quality of Sexual Life in the Older Adults: A Scoping Review. Published in *International Journal of Nursing Sciences*, 2023 (Vol. 10, Issue 2), by Zhang F et al. Available at sciencedirect.com/science/article/pii/S2352013223000285

International Society for the Study of Women's Sexual Health Clinical Practice Guideline for the Use of Systemic Testosterone for Hypoactive Sexual Desire Disorder in Women. Published in *Journal of Women's Health*, 2021 (Vol. 30, Issue 4), by Parrish SJ et al. Available at liebertpub.com/doi/full/10.1089/jwh.2021.29037

Predicting Changes to Sexual Activity in Later Life: A Longitudinal Study. Published in *Sexuality Research and Social Policy*, 2023 (Vol. 21), by Gore-Gorszewska G et al. Available at link.springer.com/article/10.1007/s13178-023-00853-9

Safety Assessment of Compounded Non-FDA-Approved Hormonal Therapy Versus FDA-Approved Hormonal Therapy in Treating Postmenopausal Women. Published in *Menopause*, 2021 (Vol. 28, Issue 8), by Jiang X et al. Available at journals.lww.com/menopausejournal/abstract/2021/08000/safety_assessment_of_compounded_non_fda_approved.6.aspx

Sex for Seniors: How Physicians Discuss Older Adult's Sexuality. Published in *Israel Journal of Health Policy Research*, 2020 (Vol. 9), by Gewirtz-Meydan A et al. Available at ijhpr.biomedcentral.com/articles/10.1186/s13584-020-00366-5

Sexual Activity of Older Adults: Let's Talk About It. Published in *The Lancet*, 2023 (Vol. 4, Issue 3), by Steckenrider J. Available at thelancet.com/journals/lanhl/article/PIIS2666-7568(23)00003-X/fulltext

Sexuality and Sexual Activity in Older Age: An Age Old Issue? Published in *The Lancet Regional Health*, 2023 (Vol. 39), by Grabovac I and McDermott DT. Available at thelancet.com/journals/lanwpc/article/PIIS2666-6065(23)00149-9/fulltext

Sexually Transmitted Infection Knowledge Among Older Adults: Psychometrics and Test–Retest Reliability. Published in *International Journal of Environmental Research and Public Health*, 2020 (Vol. 17, Issue 7), by Smith ML et al. Available at mdpi.com/1660-4601/17/7/2462

Women's Health: Sex, Intimacy, and Menopause. Published in 2022 (May/June) by the National Poll on Healthy Aging Team, Institute for Healthcare Policy and Innovation, University of Michigan. Available at healthyagingpoll.org/reports-more/report/womens-health-sex-intimacy-and-menopause

Chapter 11: Vaginal and Vulvar Conditions

A Randomized Trial on the Effectiveness and Safety of 5 Water-Based Personal Lubricants. Published in *The Journal of Sexual Medicine*, 2023 (Vol. 20, Issue 4), by Palacios S et al. Available at academic.oup.com/jsm/article/20/4/498/7035572

Exploring Relationships Between Genito-Pelvic Pain/Penetration Disorder, Sex Guilt, and Religiosity Among College Women in the U.S. Published in *The Journal of Sexual Medicine*, 2021 (Vol. 18, Issue 4), by Azim KA et al. Available at sciencedirect.com/science/article/abs/pii/S1743609521002447

Genitourinary Syndrome of Menopause: A Narrative Review Focusing on Its Effects on the Sexual Health and Quality of Life of Women. Published in *Cureas*, 2023 (Vol. 15, Issue 11), by Wasnik VB et al. Available at cureus.com/articles/184094-genitourinary-syndrome-of-menopause-a-narrative-review-focusing-on-its-effects-on-the-sexual-health-and-quality-of-life-of-women#!/

Hyaluronic Acid in Postmenopause Vaginal Atrophy: A Systematic Review. Published in *The Journal of Sexual Medicine*, 2021 (Vol. 18, Issue 1), by Dos Santos CCM et al. Available at academic.oup.com/jsm/article-abstract/18/1/156/6956009

Polycarbophil Vaginal Moisturizing Gel Versus Hyaluronic Acid Gel in Women Affected by Vaginal Dryness in Late Menopausal Transition: A Prospective Randomized Trial. Published in *European Journal of Obstetrics & Gynecology and Reproductive Biology*, 2022 (Vol. 270), by Cagnacci A et al. Available at ejog.org/article/S0301-2115(22)00030-6/fulltext

Lubricants for the Promotion of Sexual Health and Well-Being: A Systematic Review. Published in *Sexual and Reproductive Health Matters*, 2022 (Vol. 29, Issue 3), by Kennedy CE et al. Available at tandfonline.com/doi/full/10.1080/26410397.2022.2044198

The Genitourinary Syndrome of Menopause: An Overview of Recent Data. Published in *Cureas*, 2020 (Vol. 12, Issue 4), by Angelou K et al. Available at cureus.com/articles/29859-the-genitourinary-syndrome-of-menopause-an-overview-of-the-recent-data#!/

Chapter 12: Urinary Incontinence

Effects of Violence Against Women on Health During Menopause: A Systematic Review and Metanalysis. Published in *Clinical and Experimental Obstetrics & Gynecology*, 2021 (Vol. 48, Issue 6), by Mendoza-Huertas L et al. Available at imrpress.com/journal/CEOG/48/6/10.31083/j.ceog4806205/htm

Impact of Menopausal Status and Recurrent UTIs on Symptoms, Severity, and Daily Life: Findings From an Online Survey of Women Reporting a Recent UTI. Published in *Antibiotics*, 2023 (Vol. 12, Issue 7), by Sanyaolu LN et al. Available at mdpi.com/2079-6382/12/7/1150

The Investigation of Percutaneous Tibial Nerve Stimulation (PTNS) as a Minimally Invasive, Non-surgical, Non-hormonal Treatment for Overactive Bladder Symptoms. Published in *Journal of Clinical Medicine*, 2023 (Vol. 12, Issue 10), by McPhail C et al. Available at mdpi.com/2077-0383/12/10/3490

Chapter 13: Pelvic Organ Prolapse

Voices for Pelvic Floor Disorders. Surgery. Published in 2025 by the American Urogynecologic Society. Available at voicesforpfd.org/pelvic-organ-prolapse/surgery/

Chapter 14: Weight and Menopause

Beneficial Effects of Intermittent Fasting: A Narrative Review. Published in *Journal of Yeungman Medical Science*, 2023 (Vol. 40, Issue 1), by Song DK and Kim YW. Available at e-jyms.org/journal/view.php?doi=10.12701/jyms.2022.00010

Ethical Considerations for the Care of Patients With Obesity. ACOG Committee Opinion No. 763. Published in 2019. Available at acog.org/clinical/clinical-guidance/committee-opinion/articles/2019/01/ethical-considerations-for-the-care-of-patients-with-obesity

Long-Term Effects of Laparoscopic Sleeve Gastrectomy: What Are the Results Beyond 10 Years? Published in *Obesity Surgery*, 2021 (Vol. 31), by Kraljević M et al. Available at link.springer.com/article/10.1007/s11695-021-05437-3

Menopause Is Associated With Postprandial Metabolism, Metabolic Health and Lifestyle: The ZOE PREDICT Study. Published in *Lancet eBioMedicine*, 2022 (Vol. 85), by Bermingham KM et al. Available at thelancet.com/journals/ebiom/article/PIIS2352-3964(22)00485-6/fulltext

Metabolic Health, Menopause, and Physical Activity—A 4-Year Follow-Up Study. Published in *International Journal of Obesity*, 2022 (Vol. 46), by Hyvärinen M et al. Available at nature.com/articles/s41366-021-01022-x

Preventing Obesity in Midlife Women: A Recommendation From the Women's Preventive Services Initiative. Published in *Annals of Internal Medicine*, 2022 (Vol. 175), by Chelmow D et al. Available at acpjournals.org/doi/10.7326/M22-0252

Summary for Patients: Time-Restricted Eating Without Calorie Counting for Weight Loss. Published in *Annals of Internal Medicine*, 2023 (Vol. 176). Available at acpjournals.org/doi/10.7326/P23-0003

The Urgent Need for Disability Studies Among Midlife Adults. Published in *Women's Midlife Health*, 2020 (Vol. 6), by Karvonnen-Gutierrez CA and Strotmeyer ES. Available at womensmidlifehealthjournal.biomedcentral.com/articles/10.1186/s40695-020-00057-w

Ultra-processed Foods, Weight Gain, and Co-morbidity Risk. Published in *Current Obesity Reports*, 2022 (Vol. 11), by Crimarco A et al. Available at link.springer.com/article/10.1007/s13679-021-00460-y

What Makes Individuals Stick to Their Exercise Regime? A One-Year Follow-Up Study Among Novice Exercisers in a Fitness Club Setting. Published in *Frontiers in Psychology*, 2021 (Vol. 12), by Gjestvang C et al. Available at frontiersin.org/journals/psychology/articles/10.3389/fpsyg.2021.638928/full

Weight Regulation in Menopause. Published in *Menopause*, 2021 (Vol. 28, Issue 8), by Knight MG et al. Available at journals.lww.com/menopausejournal/abstract/2021/08000/weight_regulation_in_menopause.17.aspx

Weight, Shape, and Body Composition Changes at Menopause. Published in *Journal of Midlife Health*, 2021 (Vol. 12, Issue 3), by Fenton A. Available at journals.lww.com/jomh/fulltext/2021/12030/weight,_shape,_and_body_composition_changes_at.2.aspx

Chapter 15: Bone Health

After the Initial Fracture in Postmenopausal Women, Where Do Subsequent Fractures Occur? Published in *eClinicalMedicine*, 2021 (Vol. 35), by Crandall CJ et al. Available at thelancet.com/journals/eclinm/article/PIIS2589-5370(21)00106-1/fulltext

Mortality in Older Adults Following a Fragility Fracture: Real-World Retrospective Matched-Cohort Study in Ontario. Published in *BMC Musculoskeletal Disorders*, 2021 (Vol. 22), by Brown JP et al. Available at bmcmusculoskeletdisord.biomedcentral.com/articles/10.1186/s12891-021-03960-z

The Use of Antidepressants Is Linked to Bone Loss: A Systematic Review and Metanalysis. Published in *Orthopaedic Reviews (Pavia)*, 2022 (Vol. 14, Issue 6), by Mercurio M et al. Available at orthopedicreviews.openmedicalpublishing.org/article/38564-the-use-of-antidepressants-is-linked-to-bone-loss-a-systematic-review-and-metanalysis

Chapter 16: Lifestyle Changes and Alternative Approaches

A Cross-Sectional Study of Smoking and Depression Among US Adults: NHANES (2005–2018). Published in *Frontiers in Public Health*, 2023 (Vol. 11), by Wu Z et al. Available at frontiersin.org/journals/public-health/articles/10.3389/fpubh.2023.1081706/full

A Survey of Medical Cannabis Use During Perimenopause and Postmenopause. Published in *Menopause*, 2022 (Vol. 29, Issue 9), by Dahlgren MK et al. Available at journals.lww.com/menopausejournal/Fulltext/2022/09000/A_survey_of_medical_cannabis_use_during.6.aspx

Alcohol, Drinking Pattern, and Chronic Disease. Published in *Nutrients*, 2022 (Vol. 14, Issue 9), by Barberia-Latasa M. Available at mdpi.com/2072-6643/14/9/1954

Association Between Physical Activity and Risk of Depression: A Systematic Review and Meta-analysis. Published in *JAMA Psychiatry*, 2022 (Vol. 79, Issue 6), by Pearce M et al. Available at jamanetwork.com/journals/jamapsychiatry/fullarticle/2790780

Association of Habitual Alcohol Intake With Risk of Cardiovascular Disease. Published in *JAMA Network Open*, 2022 (Vol. 5, Issue 3), by Biddinger KJ et al. Available at jamanetwork.com/journals/jamanetworkopen/fullarticle/2790520

Caffeine Intake and Anxiety: A Meta-analysis. Published in *Frontiers in Psychology*, 2024 (Vol. 15), by Liu C et al. Available at frontiersin.org/journals/psychology/articles/10.3389/fpsyg.2024.1270246/full

Cognitive-Behavioral Group Therapy for Women With Hypoactive Sexual Desire: A Pilot Randomized Study. Published in *Clinics*, 2022 (Vol. 77), by Lerner T et al. Available at sciencedirect.com/science/article/pii/S1807593222007967

E-Cigarettes—a Review of the Evidence—Harm Versus Harm Reduction. Published in *Tobacco Use Insights*, 2022 (Vol. 15), by Feeney S et al. Available at journals.sagepub.com/doi/10.1177/1179173X221087524

Effectiveness of Physical Activity Interventions for Improving Depression, Anxiety and Distress: An Overview of Systematic Reviews. Published in *British Journal of Sports Medicine*, 2023 (Vol. 57, Issue 18), by Singh B et al. Available at bjsm.bmj.com/content/57/18/1203

Effects of Exercise on Sleep in Perimenopausal Women: A Meta-analysis of Randomized Controlled Trials. Published in *Explore*, 2023 (Vol. 19, Issue 5), by Zhao M et al. Available at sciencedirect.com/science/article/pii/S1550830723000307

Improving Sleep Quality Leads to Better Mental Health: A Meta-analysis of Randomised Controlled Trials. Published in *Sleep Medicine Reviews*, 2021 (Vol. 60), by Scott AJ et al. Available at sciencedirect.com/science/article/pii/S1087079221001416

Smoke at Night and Sleep Worse? The Associations Between Cigarette Smoking With Insomnia Severity and Sleep Duration. Published in *Sleep Health*, 2021 (Vol. 7, Issue 2), by Nuñez A et al. Available at sleephealthjournal.org/article/S2352-7218(20)30270-9/abstract

Smoking and Risk of Sleep-Related Issues: A Systematic Review and Meta-analysis of Prospective Studies. Published in *Canadian Journal of Public Health*, 2020 (Vol. 111), by Amiri S and Behnezhad S. Available at link.springer.com/article/10.17269/s41997-020-00308-3

The Association Between Smoking Status and Post-operative Complications in Pelvic Organ Prolapse Corrective Surgeries. Published in *International Urogynecology Journal*, 2023 (Vol. 34), by Lababidi S et al. Available at link.springer.com/article/10.1007/s00192-022-05255-w

The Effect of Exercise Intervention on Improving Sleep in Menopausal Women: A Systematic Review and Meta-analysis. Published in *Frontiers in Medicine (Lausanne)*, 2023 (Vol. 10), by Qian J et al. Available at frontiersin.org/journals/medicine/articles/10.3389/fmed.2023.1092294/full

The Impact of Caffeine Intake on Mental Health Symptoms in Postmenopausal Females With Overactive Bladder Symptoms: A Randomized, Double-Blind, Placebo-Controlled Trial. Published in *Journal of Women's Health (Larchmont)*, 2022 (Vol. 31, Issue 6), by Staack A et al. Available at liebertpub.com/doi/10.1089/jwh.2021.0467

The Risk of Sexual Dysfunction Associated With Alcohol Consumption in Women: A Systematic Review and Meta-analysis. Published in *BMC Women's Health*, 2023 (Vol. 23), by Salari N et al. Available at bmcwomenshealth.biomedcentral.com/articles/10.1186/s12905-023-02400-5

Use of Moisturizers and Lubricants for Vulvovaginal Atrophy. Published in *Frontiers in Reproductive Health*, 2021 (Vol. 3), by Sarmento ACA et al. Available at frontiersin.org/journals/reproductive-health/articles/10.3389/frph.2021.781353/full

Chapter 17: Hormone Therapies

Compounded Bioidentical Menopausal Hormone Therapy. ACOG Clinical Consensus No. 6. Published in 2023. Available at acog.org/clinical/clinical-guidance/clinical-consensus/articles/2023/11/compounded-bioidentical-menopausal-hormone-therapy

Different Regimens of Menopausal Hormone Therapy for Improving Sleep Quality: A Systematic Review and Meta-analysis. Published in *Menopause*, 2022 (Vol. 29, Issue 5), by Pan Z et al. Available at journals.lww.com/menopausejournal/fulltext/2022/05000/different_regimens_of_menopausal_hormone_therapy.17.aspx

Menopausal Hormone Therapy for the Management of Osteoporosis. Published in *Best Practice & Research Clinical Endocrinology & Metabolism*, 2021 (Vol. 35, Issue 6), by Gosset A et al. Available at sciencedirect.com/science/article/abs/pii/S1521690X21000683

Systemic Estradiol Levels With Low-Dose Vaginal Estrogens. Published in *Menopause*, 2020 (Vol. 27, Issue 3), by Santen RJ. Available at journals.lww.com/menopausejournal/fulltext/2020/03000/systemic_estradiol_levels_with_low_dose_vaginal.15.aspx

Chapter 18: Estrogen-Free Medical Therapies

A Systematic Review of Neurocognitive Dysfunction With Overactive Bladder Medications. Published in *International Urogynecology Journal*, 2021 (Vol. 32, Issue 10), by Duong V et al. Available at link.springer.com/article/10.1007/s00192-021-04909-5

Anticholinergic Drug Exposure and the Risk of Dementia: A Nested Case-Control Study. Published in *JAMA Internal Medicine*, 2019 (Vol. 179, Issue 8), by Coupland CAC et al. Available at jamanetwork.com/journals/jamainternalmedicine/fullarticle/2736353

Oxybutynin vs Placebo for Hot Flashes in Women With or Without Breast Cancer: A Randomized, Double-Blind Clinical Trial (ACCRU SC-1603). Published in *JNCI Cancer Spectrum*, 2020 (Vol. 4, Issue 1), by Leon-Ferre RA et al. Available at academic.oup.com/jncics/article/4/1/pkz088/5601603

The Effectiveness and Value of Fezolinetant for Moderate-to-Severe Vasomotor Symptoms Associated With Menopause: A Summary From the Institute for Clinical and Economic Review's Midwest Public Advisory Council. Published in *Journal of Managed Care & Specialty Pharmacy*, 2023 (Vol. 29, Issue 6), by Wright AC et al. Available at jmcp.org/doi/10.18553/jmcp.2023.29.6.692

Chapter 19: Heart Disease and Diabetes

Association Between Daily Alcohol Intake and Risk of All-Cause Mortality. Published in *JAMA*, 2023 (Vol. 6, Issue 3), by Zhao J et al. Available at jamanetwork.com/journals/jamanetworkopen/fullarticle/2802963

Menopause Transition and Cardiovascular Disease Risk: Implications for Timing of Early Prevention: A Scientific Statement From the American Heart Association. Published in *Circulation*, 2020 (Vol. 142), by El Khoudary SR et al. Available at ahajournals.org/doi/10.1161/CIR.0000000000000912

Obesity, Type 2 Diabetes, and Cancer Risk. Published in *Frontiers in Oncology*, 2020 (Vol. 10), by Scully T et al. Available at frontiersin.org/journals/oncology/articles/10.3389/fonc.2020.615375/full

Rising Prediabetes, Undiagnosed Diabetes, and Risk Factors in Young Women. Published in *American Journal of Preventive Medicine*, 2023 (Vol. 64, Issue 3), by Yoshida Y et al. Available at ajpmonline.org/article/S0749-3797(22)00500-1/fulltext

Supplemental Vitamins and Minerals for Cardiovascular Disease Prevention and Treatment. Published in *Journal of the American College of Cardiology*, 2021 (Vol. 77, Issue 4), by Jenkins DJA et al. Available at jacc.org/doi/10.1016/j.jacc.2020.09.619

Chapter 20: Managing Stress

Celebrating National Family Caregivers Month With BLS Data. Published in 2023 by the U.S. Bureau of Labor Statistics. Available at bls.gov/blog/2023/celebrating-national-family-caregivers-month-with-bls-data.htm

Cognitive-Behavioral Treatments for Anxiety and Stress-Related Disorders. Published in *Focus (American Psychiatric Publishing)*, 2021 (Vol. 19), by Curtiss JE et al. Available at psychiatryonline.org/doi/10.1176/appi.focus.20200045

Cognitive–Behavioral Therapy for Management of Mental Health and Stress-Related Disorders: Recent Advances in Techniques and Technologies. Published in *BioPsychoSocial Medicine*, 2021 (Vol. 15), by Nakao M. Available at bpsmedicine.biomedcentral.com/articles/10.1186/s13030-021-00219-w

Mind and Body Approaches for Stress and Anxiety: What the Science Says. Published in *NCCIH Clinical Digest*, 2024 (January), by the National Center for Complementary and Integrative Health. Available at nccih.nih.gov/health/providers/digest/mind-and-body-approaches-for-stress-science

Mindfulness-Based Stress Reduction vs Escitalopram for the Treatment of Adults With Anxiety Disorders: A Randomized Clinical Trial. Published in *JAMA Psychiatry*, 2023 (Vol. 80, Issue 1), by Hoge EA et al. Available at jamanetwork.com/journals/jamapsychiatry/fullarticle/2798510

Social Role Stress, Reward, and the American Heart Association Life's Simple 7 in Midlife Women: The Study of Women's Health Across the Nation. Published in *Journal of the American Heart Association*, 2020 (Vol. 9), by Stewart AL et al. Available at ahajournals.org/doi/full/10.1161/JAHA.120.017489

Stressful Life Events During the Perimenopause: Longitudinal Observations From the Seattle Midlife Women's Health Study. Published in *Women's Midlife Health*, 2023 (Vol. 9), by Thomas AJ et al. Available at womensmidlifehealthjournal.biomedcentral.com/articles/10.1186/s40695-023-00089-y

Chapter 21: Screenings and Vaccinations After Menopause

Association Between Dental Diseases and Oral Hygiene Care and the Risk of Dementia: A Retrospective Cohort Study. Published in *Journal of the American Medical Directors Association*, 2023 (Vol. 24, Issue 12), by Yoo JE et al. Available at jamda.com/article/S1525-8610(23)00721-1/abstract

Charting the Path to Health in Midlife and Beyond: The Biology and Practice of Wellness. Published in *Menopause*, 2022 (Vol. 29, Issue 5), by Santoro NF et al. Available at journals.lww.com/menopausejournal/abstract/2022/05000/nams_2021_utian_translational_science.3.aspx

Recommended Vaccinations for Adults. Published in 2024 by the Centers for Disease Control and Prevention. Available at cdc.gov/vaccines/imz-schedules/adult-easyread.html

Updated Cervical Cancer Screening Guidelines. ACOG Practice Advisory. Published April 2021. Reaffirmed April 2024. Available at acog.org/clinical/clinical-guidance/practice-advisory/articles/2021/04/updated-cervical-cancer-screening-guidelines

TERMS YOU SHOULD KNOW

A

Abnormal Uterine Bleeding Bleeding from the uterus that is different from normal menstrual bleeding. This bleeding may be longer or heavier or may happen between periods.

Abscess A collection of pus found in tissue or an organ.

Accidental Bowel Leakage Loss of control of the bowels. This condition can lead to leakage of solid stool, liquid stool, mucus, or gas. Also called fecal incontinence.

Acquired Immunodeficiency Syndrome (AIDS) A group of signs and symptoms, usually of severe infections, in a person who has human immunodeficiency virus (HIV).

Adenomyosis A condition that causes the tissue lining the uterus to grow into the muscle wall of the uterus.

Androgens Hormones made by the body that causes masculine physical characteristics, such as facial hair and a deepening voice.

Anemia Abnormally low levels of red blood cells in the bloodstream.

Anesthesia Relief of pain by loss of sensation.

Anesthetic A medication used to prevent pain.

Anterior Vaginal Wall Prolapse Bulging of the bladder into the vagina. Also called a cystocele.

Antibiotics Medications that treat or decrease the risk of certain infections caused by bacteria.

Antibodies Proteins in the blood that the body makes in reaction to foreign substances, such as bacteria and viruses.

Antidepressants Medications that are used to treat depression.

Anti-Müllerian Hormone (AMH) A hormone made by follicles in the ovaries. It plays a role in the development and functioning of the reproductive system.

Anus The opening of the digestive tract through which bowel movements and gas leave the body.

Aromatase Inhibitors	Medications that lower the level of estrogen in the body. They can be used to treat breast cancer and infertility.
Arteries	Blood vessels that carry oxygen-rich blood from the heart to the rest of the body.
Atherosclerosis	Narrowing and clogging of the arteries caused by a buildup of plaque. Also called hardening of the arteries.
Autoimmune Disorders	Conditions that cause the body to attack its own tissues.

B

Bacteria	One-celled organisms that can cause infections in the human body.
Bacterial Vaginosis	A condition caused by an overgrowth of certain bacteria in the vagina. Symptoms may include vaginal discharge, fishy odor, pain, itching, and burning.
Bariatric Surgery	Surgical procedures that change the digestive system to help with weight loss. Also called weight-loss surgery.
Bartholin Glands	Two glands located on either side of the vaginal opening that make a fluid during sexual activity.
Benign	Not cancer.
Biofeedback	A technique used by physical therapists to help a person control body functions, such as heartbeat or blood pressure.
Biopsy	A minor surgical procedure to remove a small piece of tissue. This tissue is examined under a microscope in a laboratory.
Birth Control	Devices or medications used to prevent pregnancy. Also called contraception.
Bladder	A hollow, muscular organ that holds urine.
Bladder Neck	The narrow part of the bladder above the urethra, the tube that empties urine from the bladder.
Blood Pressure	A measure of how hard blood is pressing against artery walls.
Body Mass Index (BMI)	A number calculated from height and weight. BMI may be used to determine whether a person is underweight, normal weight, overweight, or obese.
Bone Loss	The gradual loss of calcium and protein from bone, making it more likely to break.
Bowels	The small and large intestines.

BRCA1 and *BRCA2*	Genes that keep cells from growing too rapidly. Changes in these genes have been linked to an increased risk of cancer in the breasts, ovaries, and other parts of the body.

C

Cardiovascular Disease	Disease of the heart and blood vessels.
Cervix	The lower, narrow end of the uterus at the top of the vagina.
Cesarean Birth	Birth of a fetus from the uterus through an incision (cut) made in the abdomen.
Chemotherapy	Treatment of cancer with medications.
Chlamydia	A sexually transmitted infection caused by bacteria. This infection can lead to pelvic inflammatory disease, pelvic pain, and infertility.
Cholesterol	A natural substance that is a building block for cells and hormones. This substance helps carry fat through the blood vessels for use or storage in other parts of the body.
Chronic Fatigue Syndrome (CFS)	A condition that causes severe fatigue lasting for at least 6 months. The fatigue from this syndrome is not helped by rest.
Clitoris	A female sex organ found at the top of the vulva.
Cognitive Behavioral Therapy (CBT)	A type of psychotherapy. During CBT, you learn specific skills that help you change the way you think about and cope with problems.
Collagen	Proteins in bone and cartilage that serve as connective tissue between cells.
Colon	The large intestine.
Colonoscopy	An exam of the large intestine using a small, lighted instrument.
Colporrhaphy	Surgery done through the vagina to repair a bulge using the person's own tissue.
Colposuspension	A type of surgery to lift the urethra back into its normal position after it has dropped. The surgery uses stitches placed on either side of the bladder neck.
Complete Blood Count (CBC)	A blood test that measures and describes different cell types in the blood.
Complications	Diseases or conditions that happen as a result of another disease or condition. An example is pneumonia that develops with the flu. An example of a pregnancy complication is preterm labor.

Computed Tomography (CT)	A type of X-ray that shows internal organs and structures in cross section.
Condom	A thin cover for the penis used during sex to prevent sexually transmitted infections.
Corticosteroids	Medications given for arthritis or other medical conditions. These medications are also given to help fetal lungs mature before birth.
Crohn's Disease	A chronic inflammatory bowel disease that can cause abdominal pain, diarrhea, weight loss, and fever.
Cyst	A sac or pouch filled with fluid.
Cystitis	Inflammation of the bladder often caused by infection.
Cystoscopy	A procedure that looks at the inside of the urethra and bladder.

D

Dental Dam	A thin piece of latex or polyurethane used between the mouth and the vagina or anus during oral sex. Using a dental dam can help protect against sexually transmitted infections (STIs).
Depression	Feelings of sadness that last for at least 2 weeks.
Diabetes	A condition that causes high levels of sugar in the blood.
Diastolic Blood Pressure	The force of the blood in the arteries when the heart is relaxed. It is the lower reading when blood pressure is taken.
Diphtheria	A bacterial infection that causes a membrane to form in the throat and block air flow. A toxin made by the bacteria can also damage the heart and nerves.
Diuretic	A medication or substance that increases the production of urine.
Diverticulum	An abnormal pouch or sac in an internal organ or structure.
Dyspareunia	Pain with vaginal sex.

E

Egg	A reproductive cell made in and released from the ovaries. Also called the ovum.
Endometrial Ablation	A minor surgical procedure that destroys the lining of the uterus to stop or reduce menstrual bleeding.
Endometrial Biopsy	A procedure that removes a small amount of the tissue lining the uterus so it can be examined under a microscope.

Endometrial Cancer	Cancer of the lining of the uterus.
Endometrial Hyperplasia	A condition that causes the lining of the uterus to grow too thick.
Endometriosis	A condition that causes tissue that lines the uterus to grow outside of the uterus, usually on the ovaries, fallopian tubes, and other parts of the pelvis.
Endometrium	The lining of the uterus.
Estrogen	A sex hormone made in the ovaries.

F

Factor V Leiden	A genetic disorder that can increase the chance of developing blood clots.
Fallopian Tubes	Tubes through which an egg travels from the ovary to the uterus.
Fecal Incontinence	Loss of control of the bowels. This condition can lead to leakage of solid stool, liquid stool, mucus, or gas. Also called accidental bowel leakage.
Fertility	The ability to get pregnant.
Fibroids	Growths that form in the muscle of the uterus. Fibroids are usually noncancerous. Also called leiomyomas.
Fistula	An abnormal opening or passage between two organs.
Follicles	The fluid-filled sacs that holds eggs. Follicles develop inside the ovaries.
Follicle-Stimulating Hormone (FSH)	A hormone made by the pituitary gland in the brain that helps an egg to mature.

G

Gene	A segment of DNA that contains instructions for the development of a person's physical traits and control of the processes in the body. The gene is the basic unit of heredity and can be passed from parent to child.
General Anesthesia	The use of medications that create a sleep-like state to prevent pain during surgery.
Genitals	The sexual or reproductive organs on the outside of the body.
Genito–Pelvic Pain and Penetration Disorder (GPPPD)	A condition that causes difficulty or pain with vaginal penetration, or fear of penetration.

Genitourinary Syndrome of Menopause (GSM)	A collection of signs and symptoms caused by a decrease in estrogen and other sex hormones. Signs and symptoms can include vaginal dryness, pain with sex, bladder symptoms, frequent urinary tract infections (UTIs), burning, itching, and irritation.
Gestational Diabetes	Diabetes that starts during pregnancy.
Gingivitis	Inflammation of the gums.
GLP-1 Receptor Agonists	Medications used to treat type 2 diabetes and obesity. In the body, they act like the hormone GLP-1, which helps regulate blood sugar levels and appetite.
Glucose	A sugar in the blood that is the body's main source of fuel.
Gonadotropin-Releasing Hormone (GnRH) Agonists	Medical therapy used to block the effects of certain hormones.
Gonorrhea	A sexually transmitted infection that can lead to pelvic inflammatory disease, infertility, and arthritis.

H

Hepatitis B	An infection caused by a virus that can be spread through blood, semen, or other body fluid infected with the virus.
High Blood Pressure	Blood pressure above the normal level. Also called hypertension.
Hormone	A substance made in the body that controls the function of cells or organs.
Hormone Therapy	Treatment with hormones, such as estrogen and progestin, to help treat the symptoms of menopause.
Hot Flashes	Sensations of heat in the skin that occur when estrogen levels are low. Also called hot flushes.
Human Immunodeficiency Virus (HIV)	A virus that attacks certain cells of the body's immune system. If left untreated, HIV can cause acquired immunodeficiency syndrome (AIDS).
Human Papillomavirus (HPV)	The name for a group of related viruses, some of which cause genital warts and some of which are linked to cancer of the cervix, vulva, vagina, penis, anus, mouth, and throat.
Hypertension	High blood pressure.
Hyperthyroidism	A condition that causes the thyroid gland to make too much thyroid hormone.

Hypothyroidism	A condition that causes the thyroid gland to make too little thyroid hormone.
Hysterectomy	Surgery to remove the uterus.
Hysteroscope	A thin, lighted telescope that is used to look inside the uterus and do procedures.
Hysteroscopy	A procedure to view the inside of or perform surgery in the uterus. The procedure uses a lighted telescope inserted through the cervix and into the uterus.

I

Immune System	The body's natural defense system against viruses and bacteria that cause disease.
In Vitro Fertilization (IVF)	A procedure to help achieve a pregnancy. An egg is removed from an ovary, fertilized in a laboratory with sperm, and then transferred to the uterus.
Infertility	The inability to get pregnant after 1 year of having regular vaginal sex without the use of birth control, or after less than 1 year based on factors like medical history, age, or test results.
Inflammation	Pain, swelling, redness, and irritation of tissues in the body.
Inflammatory Bowel Disease (IBD)	The name for a group of diseases that cause inflammation of the intestines. Examples include Crohn's disease and ulcerative colitis.
Insomnia	A common sleep disorder that makes it hard to fall or stay asleep. Insomnia leads to poor sleep quality, daytime fatigue, difficulty concentrating, and irritability.
Insulin	A hormone that lowers the levels of glucose (sugar) in the blood.
Intimate Partner Violence	The use of physical, sexual, or emotional threats or actions against a current or former romantic partner. This type of violence is aimed at establishing control over the other person.
Intrauterine Device (IUD)	A small device that is inserted and left inside the uterus to prevent pregnancy, lighten or stop periods, or reduce the risk of endometrial cancer.
Intravenous (IV) Fluids	Fluids given through a tube inserted into a vein.
Irritable Bowel Syndrome (IBS)	A digestive disorder that can cause gas, diarrhea, constipation, and belly pain.

K

Kegel Exercises	Pelvic muscle exercises. Doing these exercises can help with bladder and bowel control as well as sexual function.
Kidney	An organ that filters the blood to remove waste that becomes urine.
Kidney Disease	A general term for any disease that affects how the kidneys function.

L

Labia Majora	The outer, larger folds of tissue of the female genital area.
Labia Minora	The inner, smaller folds of tissue of the female genital area.
Laparoscope	A thin, lighted telescope that is inserted through a small incision (cut) in the abdomen to view internal organs or perform surgery.
Laparoscopy	A surgical procedure using a thin, lighted telescope called a laparoscope. The laparoscope is inserted through a small incision (cut) in the abdomen and used to view the pelvic organs. Other long, thin instruments can be used with it to perform surgery.
Leiomyomas	Growths that form in the muscle of the uterus. Leiomyomas are usually noncancerous. Commonly called fibroids.
Ligaments	Bands of tissue that connect bones or support large internal organs.
Lupus	An autoimmune disorder that affects the connective tissues in the body. The disorder can cause arthritis, kidney disease, heart disease, blood disorders, and complications during pregnancy. Also called systemic lupus erythematosus or SLE.
Lynch Syndrome	A genetic condition that increases a person's risk of cancer of the colon, rectum, ovary, uterus, pancreas, and bile duct.

M

Magnetic Resonance Imaging (MRI)	A test to view internal organs and structures by using a strong magnetic field and sound waves.
Mammogram	An X-ray image used to show breast cancer or other breast problems.
Mammography	X-rays of the breast that are used to find breast cancer or other breast problems.
Melanocortin Receptor Agonists	Medications used to treat low sex drive. In the body, they act like melanocortins, a group of hormones needed for sexual response. They also have effects on metabolism and pigmentation.

Menopause	The last menstrual period, often happening around age 51. Menopause can only be confirmed after 1 year of no periods.
Menopause Transition	The stage of life that begins with the first symptoms of perimenopause and ends a few years after the last period.
Menstrual Cycle	The monthly changes that prepare the body for a possible pregnancy. A menstrual cycle is defined as the first day of menstrual bleeding of one cycle to the first day of menstrual bleeding of the next cycle.
Menstrual Period	The monthly shedding of blood and tissue from the uterus. Also called menstruation.
Menstruation	The shedding of blood and tissue from the uterus that happens monthly except during pregnancy. Also called menstrual periods.
Metabolic Syndrome	A combination of factors that can lead to diabetes and heart disease. These factors include high blood pressure, too much weight in the abdomen, high blood sugar level, low levels of "good" cholesterol, and high levels of fats in the blood (triglycerides).
Metabolism	The physical and chemical processes in the body that maintain life.
Mixed Urinary Incontinence	Involuntary loss of urine when there is urgency to urinate and when there is physical exertion, sneezing, or coughing.
Multiple Sclerosis	A disease of the nervous system that leads to loss of muscle control.
Mumps	A viral infection that affects the salivary glands. It causes painful swelling of the cheeks and jaw and can cause infertility in men.
Myomectomy	Surgery to remove uterine fibroids that leaves the uterus in place.

N

Nicotine	An addictive drug found in tobacco.
Nocturia	Waking up more than once each night to urinate.
Nonsteroidal Anti-Inflammatory Drugs (NSAIDs)	Medications that relieve pain by reducing inflammation. Many types are available over the counter, including ibuprofen and naproxen.

O

Obesity	A condition characterized by excessive body fat.
Obliterative Surgery	A type of surgery that narrows or closes off the vagina to create support for organs that have dropped down.

Obstetrician–Gynecologist (Ob-Gyn)	A doctor with medical and surgical training and education in the female reproductive system.
Obstructive Sleep Apnea	A serious sleep disorder that causes a person to have brief pauses in breathing during sleep.
Oocyte Cryopreservation	A procedure that removes and freezes eggs for later use with in vitro fertilization (IVF). Also called egg freezing.
Orgasm	The feelings of physical pleasure that can happen during sexual activity.
Osteopenia	A loss of bone mineral density that makes bones weaker than they should be.
Osteoporosis	A condition of thin bones that could allow them to break more easily.
Ovarian Cancer	Cancer that develops in the ovaries or fallopian tubes.
Ovaries	Organs that contain the eggs necessary to get pregnant. Ovaries also make important hormones, such as estrogen, progesterone, and testosterone.
Overactive Bladder (OAB)	The sudden urge to urinate, usually with frequent visits to the bathroom, including at night. OAB is about feeling an urgent need to urinate, while incontinence involves the loss of urine.
Ovulate	The act of an ovary releasing an egg.
Ovulation	The time when an ovary releases an egg.
Oxygen	An element that people breathe in to sustain life.

P

Pelvic Exam	A physical examination of the pelvic organs, including the vagina, cervix, uterus, and ovaries.
Pelvic Floor	A muscular area connected to the back muscles and abdominal muscles that supports the pelvic organs.
Pelvic Floor Disorders	Any disorder of the muscles and tissues that support the pelvic organs.
Pelvic Inflammatory Disease	An infection of the uterus, fallopian tubes, or ovaries.

Pelvic Organ Prolapse	A condition that causes one or more pelvic organs to drop down. This condition is caused by weakening of the muscles and tissues that support the organs in the pelvis, including the vagina, uterus, and bladder.
Pelvis	The lower portion of the trunk of the body.
Penetration	The act of inserting a penis, finger, or other object into the vagina or anus, or inserting a sex organ into the mouth.
Perimenopause	The time period leading up to menopause.
Perineum	The area between the vagina and the anus.
Pessary	A device that can be inserted into the vagina. It is typically used to support organs that have dropped down from their normal position or to help control urine leakage.
Pituitary Gland	A gland located near the brain that controls growth and other changes in the body.
Plaque	A waxy substance made up of cholesterol and different types of cells. Plaque can form within the walls of arteries and causes atherosclerosis.
Pneumonia	An infection of the lungs.
Polycystic Ovary Syndrome (PCOS)	A condition that leads to a hormone imbalance that affects menstrual periods, ovulation, fertility, hair growth, metabolism, and body size.
Polyps	Abnormal tissue growths that can develop on the inside of an organ. Polyps usually are not cancerous.
Posterior Vaginal Wall Prolapse	Bulging of the rectum or the small intestine into the back wall of the vagina. Also called a rectocele.
Postmenopausal	Being in postmenopause, the stage of life that comes after menopause.
Postmenopause	The stage of life that comes after menopause, which is confirmed after 1 year of no periods.
Post-Traumatic Stress Disorder (PTSD)	A mental health disorder that some people develop after experiencing or witnessing one or more frightening, dangerous, or shocking events.
Prediabetes	A condition that leads to higher-than-normal blood sugar but not high enough to be type 2 diabetes.

Preeclampsia	A disorder during pregnancy or after childbirth that causes high blood pressure and other signs of organ injury. These signs include an abnormal amount of protein in the urine, a low number of platelets, abnormal kidney or liver function, pain over the upper abdomen, fluid in the lungs, a severe headache, or vision changes.
Premature Menopause	Menopause that happens before age 40.
Premenstrual Syndrome (PMS)	A term used to describe a group of physical and behavioral changes that may happen before menstrual period.
Primary Ovarian Insufficiency	A condition that causes the ovaries to stop working normally before age 40.
Progesterone	A sex hormone that is made in the ovaries and prepares the lining of the uterus for pregnancy.
Progestin	A synthetic form of progesterone that is similar to the hormone made naturally by the body.
Prostaglandins	Chemicals that are made by the body that have many effects, including causing the muscles of the uterus to contract, usually causing cramps.
Psychotherapy	Talking with a licensed mental health care professional to find ways to cope with or change troubling emotions, thoughts, and behaviors.
Puberty	The stage of life that leads to sexual maturity. It includes change in the external genitals, the appearance of pubic hair, and growth spurts.

R

Radiation	A type of energy that is transmitted in the form of rays, waves, or particles.
Radiation Therapy	A type of cancer treatment that uses radiation.
Radiologist	A doctor who specializes in interpreting images taken with various medical imaging techniques.
Reconstructive Surgery	Surgery to repair or restore a part of the body that is injured or damaged.
Rectum	The last part of the digestive tract.
Regional Anesthesia	The use of medications to block sensation in a region of the body.

Rheumatoid Arthritis (RA)	A chronic disease that causes pain, swelling, redness, and irritation of the joints and changes in the muscles and bones. The condition can become more severe with time.

S

Sacrocolpopexy	A type of surgery to repair vaginal vault prolapse. The surgery attaches the vaginal vault to the sacrum with surgical mesh.
Sacrohysteropexy	A type of surgery to repair uterine prolapse. The surgery attaches the cervix to the sacrum with surgical mesh.
Seizure Disorders	Any condition that causes seizures, which cause changes in movement, consciousness, mood, or emotions. Epilepsy is one kind of seizure disorder.
Selective Estrogen Receptor Modulators (SERMs)	Medications that stimulate certain tissues that respond to estrogen while not stimulating other tissues that respond to estrogen.
Selective Serotonin–Norepinephrine Reuptake Inhibitors (SNRIs)	A type of medication used to treat mental health conditions like depression, anxiety, panic disorders, and chronic pain. They work by increasing the levels of serotonin and norepinephrine in the brain.
Selective Serotonin Reuptake Inhibitors (SSRIs)	A type of medication used to treat depression and other mental health conditions. They work by increasing the levels of serotonin in the brain. They also block the brain from reabsorbing serotonin.
Sepsis	A life-threatening condition caused by a buildup of infectious toxins (usually from bacteria) in the blood. Symptoms include fever, rapid heart rate, breathing difficulty, and mental confusion.
Serotonin Receptor Agonist/Antagonists	Medications that affect serotonin levels in the brain and body.
Sexual Abuse	Sex acts that are forced on one person by another without consent.
Sexual Intercourse	The act of the penis entering the vagina. Also called vaginal sex.
Sexual Interest/Arousal Disorder	A condition that causes a lack of interest in sexual activity, arousal, or both.
Sexually Transmitted Infections (STIs)	Infections that are spread by sexual contact. Infections include chlamydia, gonorrhea, trichomoniasis, human papillomavirus (HPV), herpes, syphilis, and human immunodeficiency virus (HIV).

Shingles	A viral infection that causes a painful, blistering rash on one side of the body or face.
Sleep Apnea	A disorder that causes interruptions of breathing during sleep.
Sonohysterography	A procedure that injects sterile fluid into the uterus through the cervix while ultrasound images are taken of the inside of the uterus.
Sperm	A cell made in the testicles that can fertilize an egg.
Sphincter Muscle	A muscle that can close a bodily opening, such as the sphincter muscle of the anus.
Stress Urinary Incontinence	Involuntary loss of urine with physical exertion, sneezing, or coughing.
Stroke	A sudden interruption of blood flow to all or part of the brain, caused by blockage or bursting of a blood vessel in the brain. A stroke often results in problems with speaking, learning, and movement. In some cases one side of the body may be paralyzed.
Syphilis	A sexually transmitted infection (STI) caused by an organism called Treponema pallidum. This infection may cause major health problems or death in its later stages.
Systolic Blood Pressure	The force of the blood in the arteries when the heart is contracting. It is the top reading when blood pressure is taken.

T

Tamoxifen	An estrogen-blocking medication sometimes used to treat breast cancer.
Testosterone	A hormone made by the testes and in smaller amounts by the ovaries. This hormone is responsible for masculine characteristics such as hair growth, muscle development, and a lower voice.
Tetanus	A disease caused by bacteria that can enter the body through a puncture wound, such as from a metal nail, wood splinter, or insect bite. The bacteria make a toxin that can paralyze the breathing muscles.
Thyroid Gland	A butterfly-shaped gland located at the base of the neck in front of the windpipe. This gland makes, stores, and releases thyroid hormone, which controls the body's metabolism and regulates how parts of the body work.
Tranexamic Acid	A medication to treat or prevent heavy bleeding.
Transducer	A device that sends out sound waves and translates the echoes into electrical signals.

Transfusion	Giving the body blood, plasma, or platelets to replace what has been lost through heavy bleeding or an illness.
Transgender	A term used to describe a person whose gender identity is different from the sex they were assigned at birth.
Transvaginal Ultrasound Exam	A type of ultrasound where the device is placed in the vagina.
Trichomoniasis	A type of vaginal infection caused by a parasite. This infection is passed through sex.
Triglycerides	A form of body fat found in the blood and tissues. High levels can cause heart disease.
Tuberculosis (TB)	A disease that affects the lungs and other organs in the body. TB is caused by bacteria.

U

Ultrasound Exam	A test that uses sound waves to examine inner parts of the body. During pregnancy, ultrasound can be used to check the fetus. Also called ultrasonography or sonography.
Urethra	A tube-like structure. Urine flows through this tube when it leaves the body.
Urgency Urinary Incontinence	The involuntary loss of urine that comes with a sudden, strong urge to urinate.
Urinary Incontinence	Involuntary loss of urine.
Urinary Tract	The group of organs that make, store, and remove urine. It includes the kidneys, bladder, and urethra.
Urinary Tract Infection (UTI)	An infection in any part of the urinary system, including the kidneys, bladder, or urethra.
Uterine Artery Embolization	A procedure to block the blood vessels to the uterus. This procedure is used to stop bleeding after delivery. It is also used to stop other causes of bleeding from the uterus.
Uterine Prolapse	A condition where the uterus drops into or out of the vagina.
Uterus	A muscular organ in the female pelvis. During pregnancy, this organ holds and nourishes the fetus. Also called the womb.

V-Y

Vaccine — A substance that trains the immune system to respond to and fight disease. Many vaccines are made from very small amounts of weak or dead agents that cause disease (bacteria, toxins, and viruses). Other vaccines use proteins or pieces of proteins to teach the body to fight disease (like mRNA vaccines).

Vagina — A tube-like structure surrounded by muscles. The vagina leads from the uterus to the outside of the body.

Vaginal Vault Prolapse — Descent of the vagina after a hysterectomy (removal of the uterus).

Vulva — The external female genital area.

Veins — Blood vessels that carry blood from various parts of the body back to the heart.

Vulvodynia — Pain in the vulva that does not go away or keeps coming back and does not have a specific cause.

Yeast Infection — An infection caused by an overgrowth of a fungus. Symptoms may include itching, burning, and irritation of the vulva or vagina and a thick, white discharge.

INDEX

Page numbers followed by italicized letters *b*, *f*, and *t* indicate boxes, figures, and tables, respectively.

abaloparatide, 168*t*
abdominal issues, pelvic organ prolapse surgery and, 147
Abnormal Bleeding Diary, 14, 22, 78
abnormal uterine bleeding
   before and after your procedure for, 76
   definition, 261
   evaluation, 68–69
   low-dose estrogen cream and, 201–202
   medications, 72–74
   menopause transition and, 35
   other causes of, 19–21
   overview, 67
   perimenopause and, 14–15
   REIs and treatment of, 45
   resources, 78
   testing for, 70–72
   treatment procedures, 74–76
abscess, 120, 261
accidental bowel leakage, 37, 44, 50, 125, 134–135
ACE. *See* angiotensin-converting enzyme inhibitors
acne, 49
acquired immunodeficiency syndrome (AIDS), 25–26, 165, 261
acupuncture, sleep and, 93*b*
acute abnormal uterine bleeding, 15, 68
adenomyosis, 20, 28, 70, 261
ADHD. *See* attention-deficit/hyperactivity disorder
adrenaline, 222
advanced practice registered nurse (APRN), 47
AIDS. *See* acquired immunodeficiency syndrome
alcohol drinking
   CVD risk and, 210
   heart disease and diabetes risk and, 216
   hot flashes and, 59
   menopause symptoms and, 179
   mood, anxiety, and brain self-care and, 83*b*
   sleep quality and, 92
   urinary incontinence and, 128
allergic reactions, compounded medications and, 195*b*
Alzheimer disease, 39–40
AMH. *See* anti-müllerian hormone
anal plugs, accidental bowel leakage and, 135

androgens, 108, 118, 202, 261
anemia, 70, 261
anesthesia, urethral bulking under, 133
anesthetics, 71, 106, 121, 261
angiotensin-converting enzyme inhibitors (ACE inhibitors), 218
angiotensin II receptor blockers (ARBs), 218
anorexia nervosa, 165
anterior vaginal wall prolapse, 139, 140*f*, 261
antibiotics, 73, 121, 132, 261
antibodies, thyroid disorders and, 240
antidepressants
   bone loss and, 164
   counseling and, 83–84
   definition, 261
   estrogen and, 190
   as estrogen-free medical therapies, 199
   hot flashes and, 58
   lichen simplex chronicus and, 120
   ob-gyn management of, 44
   for sleep disorders, 98
   sleep quality and, 90
   for vulvodynia, 119
antifungal medications, 121
antihistamines, 95*b*, 121–122
anti-müllerian hormone (AMH), 29, 261
antiseizure medications, 164
anus, 102–103, 120–121, 135, 261
anxiety. *See also* mental health
   alcohol drinking and, 179
   caffeine and, 178
   diagnosing, 81–82
   hot flashes and, 58, 60
   managing risk for, 10
   menopause transition and, 38–39
   mind–body practices and, 180
   perimenopause and, 18–19
   physical activity and, 176
   premature menopause and, 9
   resources, 87–88
   self-care for, 82–83*b*
   sleep and, 181
   sleep quality and, 16
   smoking and, 177
   supplements for, 84*b*
   treatment for, 82–84
   weight distribution and, 151
APRN. *See* advanced practice registered nurse

ARBs. *See* angiotensin II receptor blockers
aromatase inhibitors, 27, 57, 262
arousal, problems with, 102
arrhythmia, 209
arteries, 208, 208*f*, 210–211, 262. *See also* blood vessels
arthritis, sleep quality and, 16
ashwagandha, 183
Asian American women, 6*b*, 91, 164, 165
atherosclerosis, 208, 208*f*, 212, 262
attention-deficit/hyperactivity disorder (ADHD), 85
attitudes, on menopause, 34
autoimmune disorders, 31, 90, 210, 223, 262

bacteria, 114, 126, 127, 184, 262
bacterial vaginosis, 115
bariatric surgery, 157–158, 219, 262
Bartholin gland cysts, 120
Bartholin glands, 262
bazedoxifene and estrogen, 62, 189
benign growths or cysts, 28, 67, 262. *See also* cysts; polyps
beta-blockers, 218
biofeedback, 93*b*, 106, 135
bioidentical hormone therapy, 195*b*. *See also* compounded bioidentical hormones
biopsy
    definition, 262
    high-risk breast, cancer and, 237
    hysteroscopy and, 71, 71*f*
    sexual problems and, 104, 115
    squamous intraepithelial lesion and, 120–121
BI-RADS system, of mammogram results, 236
birth control
    abnormal bleeding and, 70
    definition, 262
    menopause transition and, 5
    pills, 21
    pregnancy during perimenopause and, 19
    premature and early menopause and, 30
    primary ovarian insufficiency and, 31
bisphosphonates, 167*t*
Black Americans. *See also* race and ethnicity
    breast density and, 238*b*
    fracture rates among, 164
    FRAX calculation for, 165
    hot flashes and, 36, 58
    hysterectomy and, 28
    menopause symptoms and, 5, 6*b*
    sleep problems and, 91
    stress and, 222
    uterine cancer and, 77
black cohosh, 182–183
bladder
    definition, 262
    empty, testing for abnormal bleeding and, 70, 71

bladder *(continued)*
    estrogen level and, 18
    injury, pelvic organ prolapse surgery and, 147
    menopause transition and, 37
    overactive, urogynecologist treatment of, 44
    pain during sex and, 102–103
    pelvic floor and, 37, 137
    pelvic organ prolapse surgery and, 144
    support devices, 130
    training, 129–130
    urgency urinary incontinence and, 126*f*
    urinary incontinence and, 125–126
bladder diary, 128, 129*b*, 136, 148
bladder neck, 133, 262
bladder stones, 127
bladder training, 129–130, 143
bleeding disorders, 20–21, 22, 70, 74. *See also* abnormal uterine bleeding; menstrual periods
bloating, systemic hormone therapy and, 191
blood clots, 15, 118, 188, 192, 202, 223
blood pressure, 64, 152, 211*b*, 222, 262. *See also* heart disease; high blood pressure
blood sugar testing, 214*b*
blood vessels, 209, 211, 223. *See also* arteries; veins
BMI. *See* body mass index
body mass index (BMI), 150, 164, 238*b*, 262
body temperature regulation, hot flashes and, 57
body weight, hot flashes and, 58
bone density, 161
bone health, 161–163, 162*f*, 171, 190. *See also* bone loss; osteopenia; osteoporosis
bone loss. *See also* osteopenia; osteoporosis
    definition, 262
    diagnosing, 165–166, 165*t*
    HIV/AIDS and, 26
    lifestyle and, 169–171
    managing risk for, 9
    menopause transition and, 4
    premature and early menopause and, 29
    risk factors, 164–165
    treatment, 62, 166–169, 167–168*t*
bone mineral density test, 165. *See also* DEXA scans
bone resorption, 162
booster shots, keeping track of, 10
Botox, 131
bowel training, 135
bowels, 18, 144, 147, 262. *See also* accidental bowel leakage
brain fog, 4, 39–40, 79, 85, 86–87, 86–87*t*. *See also* dementia; memory changes
brain health, 63*b*, 82–83*b*, 84*b*, 183–184, 227
BRCA1 and *BRCA2* genetic mutations, 237, 263
breast biopsy, 237, 238
breast cancer
    estrogen-free medical therapies and, 197

breast cancer *(continued)*
　　gynecologic oncologist treatment of, 44
　　screenings for, 10, 236–238
　　systemic hormone therapy and, 191, 192
　　treatment, hot flashes and, 57
　　WHI on hormone therapy and risk of, 188
breast density, 236, 237*f*, 238*b*
breast exams, 235
breast soreness, 191
breast ultrasound, 238
breathing, stress and, 224
bremelanotide, 106
bruising, menopause transition and, 41

caffeine, 59, 92, 128, 178–179
calcitonin, 168*t*
calcium, in bones, 161, 170
calcium channel blockers, 218
calorie intake, 154–155
cancer, 30, 49, 52, 103, 182. *See also specific types*
cancer medications, 27. *See also* chemotherapy
cannabinoids, 95*b*
cannabis, 183
capsaicin, 59
cardiovascular disease (CVD), 208, 208*f*, 209, 210, 212, 263
caregiving, stress in, 225–226
CBC. *See* complete blood count
CBD, menopause symptoms and, 183
CBT. *See* cognitive behavioral therapy
CBT-I. *See* cognitive behavioral therapy for insomnia
cervical cancer, 10, 44, 234–235
cervix, 19, 28, 120–121, 263
cesarean birth, 28, 263
CFS. *See* chronic fatigue syndrome
chamomile, as sleep aid, 95*b*
chemical exposure, premature and early menopause and, 24–25
chemotherapy, 26–27, 57, 58, 197, 210, 263
childbirth, urinary incontinence and, 127, 128
childhood neglect or abuse, hot flashes and, 58
chlamydia, 110, 263
cholesterol
　　brain health and, 87
　　chronic disease and, 9
　　CVD risk and, 210
　　definition, 263
　　diabetes risk and, 215
　　guide to, 212
　　heart disease and stroke and, 207
　　limiting intake of, 218
　　ospemifene and, 108, 118, 202
　　resources, 219
　　reviewing test results for, 213*b*
chronic fatigue syndrome (CFS), 25, 80, 263
chronic stress, 221–224. *See also* stress
clitoris, 102, 119, 263

clonidine, 64, 200, 201*t*
clotting factors, bleeding disorders and, 20–21
cognitive behavioral therapy (CBT)
　　definition, 263
　　for hot flashes or night sweats, 61, 180
　　pelvic pain and, 123
　　for sexual problems, 105
　　for stress management, 229
　　for vulvodynia, 119
cognitive behavioral therapy for insomnia (CBT-I), 97, 99, 180
collagen, 40–41, 161
colon, 263
colon cancer, 10, 238–239, 244
colonoscopy, 239, 263
colporrhaphy, 144–145, 263
colposuspension, 133, 263
combination bariatric surgery, 157–158. *See also* bariatric surgery
combined hormonal birth control, 72
combined hormone therapy, 98
community beliefs, menopause transition and, 6–7
compact bone, 161, 162*f*
complete blood count (CBC), 70, 263
complications, surgery and, 132, 158, 177, 263
compounded bioidentical hormones, 184–185, 194–195, 195*b*
computed tomography (CT), 239, 264
condoms, 71, 105*b*, 110, 184, 264
constipation, 138
contact dermatitis, 119–120
continuous positive airway pressure machines (CPAP machines), 97
corticosteroids, 90, 164, 264
cortisol, 222
cotton swabs, identifying vaginal or vulvar discomfort areas and, 115, 116*f*
cough stress test, 129
coughing, 128, 138
counseling, for depression, 83–84
counselors, 49, 229–230
COVID-19 vaccination, 243*t*
CPAP. *See* continuous positive airway pressure machines
Crohn's disease, 123, 223, 239, 264
cross-training, 153
CT. *See* computed tomography
CVD. *See* cardiovascular disease
cystitis, 123, 264
cystoscopy, 147, 148, 264
cysts, 25, 28, 264. *See also* benign growths or cysts

dementia. *See also* brain fog; memory changes
　　early, brain fog compared with, 86–87, 86–87*t*
　　gum disease and, 241

dementia *(continued)*
    inadequate sleep and, 90
    managing risk for, 9
    risk, hot flashes and, 63*b*
    UTIs and, 126
    women and, 39–40
denosumab, 167*t*
dental checkups, 241, 245
dental dams, 110, 184, 264
depression
    definition, 264
    diabetes risk and, 215
    diagnosing, 80–81
    early menopause and, 29
    genito-pelvic pain and penetration disorder and, 123
    hot flashes and, 58
    insomnia and, 89
    managing risk for, 10
    menopause transition and, 38–39, 79
    mid-life, CVD risk and, 210
    perimenopause and, 18–19
    premature menopause and, 9, 29
    resources, 87–88
    sexual desire and, 102
    sleep quality and, 16
    stress and, 223
    supplements for, 84*b*
    systemic hormone therapy and, 190
    treatment for, 82–84
    urinary incontinence compared with, 128
    weight gain and, 150
dermatologists, 49, 51
DES, cervical cancer screening and, 234
desire, sexual, problems with, 102
desvenlafaxine, 199, 200*t*
DEXA scans, 165, 168–169, 171
diabetes
    blood sugar testing and, 214*b*
    bone loss and, 165
    brain health and, 87
    endocrinologist treatment of, 47–48
    eye exams and, 241
    inadequate sleep and, 90
    lifestyle changes and risk reduction, 215–218
    light exposure during sleep and, 93
    managing risk for, 10
    medications, 198, 218–219
    nerve and muscle problems with, 127
    obesity and, 150
    ospemifene and, 118, 202
    overview, 207
    pelvic organ prolapse and, 141
    premature and early menopause and, 25, 29
    resources, 219–220
    risk factors, 215
    sexual health and, 103
    stress and, 223

diabetes *(continued)*
    vaccinations and, 243
    what to know about, 212–215
diastolic blood pressure, 211, 264
diet. *See* nutrition
dietary changes, accidental bowel leakage and, 135
dietary supplements. *See* supplements
dietitians, registered, 49, 51
digestion, stress and, 223–224
diphtheria, 264
disabilities, people with, 46*b*, 222
discrimination, health care and, 46*b*, 222
diuretics, 128, 179, 218, 264
diverticulum, 127, 264
dong quai, 183
dual energy X-ray absorptiometry (DXA), 165
dyspareunia, 103, 264

early life stressors, menopause transition and, 4
early menopause. *See also* premature menopause; primary ovarian insufficiency
    estrogen-free medical therapies and, 197
    fertility and, 29
    medical and surgical causes, 26–28
    other concerns with, 29–30
    premature menopause compared with, 23
    resources, 31–32
    symptoms, 8–9
    systemic hormone therapy and, 193
    treatment for, 30
eating. *See* nutrition
eczema, dermatologist treatment of, 49
EDCs. *See* endocrine-disrupting chemicals
eggs, 7, 8*b*, 23, 29, 264. *See also* oocyte cryopreservation
eldercare, agencies providing in-home, 226
electrical stimulation therapy, 135
electronics, unplugging from, sleep quality and, 94
EMDR. *See* eye movement desensitization and reprocessing
emotions, 6–7, 9, 16, 150. *See also* mental health; mood swings
endocrine-disrupting chemicals (EDCs), 24–25
endocrinologists, 47–48, 51
endometrial ablation, 74–75, 264
endometrial atrophy, 20
endometrial biopsy, 72, 264
endometrial cancer
    abnormal bleeding and, 20, 70
    definition, 265
    estrogen alone and, 189
    local hormone therapy and, 194
    low-dose estrogen cream and risk of, 117, 201–202

endometrial cancer *(continued)*
   resources, 78
   systemic hormone therapy and, 192
endometrial hyperplasia, 20, 70, 265
endometriosis
   chronic fatigue syndrome and, 25
   definition, 265
   estrogen-free medical therapies and, 203
   genito–pelvic pain and penetration disorder and, 123
   medications, bone loss and, 164
   outside the endometrium, 20
   REIs and treatment of, 45
   surgery for, 28
   toolkit on, 78
endometrium, 8*b*, 20, 28, 265
endurance exercises, 152
escitalopram, 199, 200*t*
estrogen
   blood vessels and heart and, 209
   bone density and, 162
   brain function and, 79, 85
   chronic fatigue syndrome and, 25
   collagen levels and, 40–41
   in combined hormonal birth control, 72
   cream, pessaries and, 143
   definition, 265
   function of, 7, 8*b*
   hot flashes and night sweats and, 56–57, 62
   menopause transition and, 4
   menstrual cycle and, 67–68
   metabolism and, 150
   mood and memory and, 18
   oral compared with patches, 191
   pain during sex and, 107
   perimenopause and, 14
   prasterone and, 108
   primary ovarian insufficiency and, 31
   sleep quality and, 90
   stress and, 223
   urinary incontinence and, 127
   vaginal, urinary incontinence and, 131
   vaginal and vulvar changes and, 36, 117
   vaginal dryness and, 102, 184
estrogen-free medical therapies
   hot flashes and, 198–200
   for hot flashes or night sweats, 200–201*t*
   overview, 197
   resources, 203–204
   talking with your ob-gyn about, 203
   for vaginal symptoms, 200–202
   when to talk about, 202–203
eszopiclone, 98
ethnicity. *See* race and ethnicity; *specific ethnic groups*
exercise. *See also* weight management
   aging, hormones and, 151
   bone health and, 161

exercise *(continued)*
   endurance, 152
   heart disease and diabetes risk and, 216
   increasing, in midlife, 152–153, 176
   Kegel, 106, 107*b*, 130, 142, 268
   lack of, CVD risk and, 210
   lack of, urinary incontinence and, 128
   midlife, 152*b*
   mood, anxiety, and brain self-care and, 82–83*b*
   non-weight-bearing, bone density and, 169–170
   sleep quality and, 92
   stress and, 226–227
eye exams, 241, 245
eye movement desensitization and reprocessing (EMDR), 229–230, 231
eyes, high blood pressure and blood vessels in, 211

factor V Leiden, 192, 265
fallopian tubes, 8*b*, 28, 44, 57, 71, 71*f*, 265
falls, avoiding, 166*b*
family, talking about menopause with, 34
family beliefs, menopause transition and, 6–7
family caregivers resource, 230
family history, 4, 24, 138, 210, 215, 237, 239
family nurse practitioner (FNP), 47
fasting, intermittent, 154*b*
fats, choosing healthy sources of, 217
fecal incontinence, 37, 129*b*, 265. *See also* accidental bowel leakage
feeling, stress and, 223
female pattern hair loss, 49
fertility, 26, 29, 44–45, 265
fezolinetant, 64, 198, 200*t*
fibroids
   abnormal bleeding and, 20, 69
   chronic fatigue syndrome and, 25
   combined hormonal birth control for, 72
   definition, 265
   depiction of, 69*f*
   genito–pelvic pain and penetration disorder and, 123
   REIs and treatment of, 45
   toolkit on, 78
   treatment procedures, 74
   uterine surgery and, 28
fibromyalgia, 25
financial stress, 80, 82
fish oil, abnormal bleeding and, 21
fistula, 127–128, 265
fitness, 151–155. *See also* exercise
flibanserin, 107
flu vaccination, 243*t*
fluid intake, urinary incontinence and, 129
fluoxetine, 199, 200*t*
FNP. *See* family nurse practitioner

follicle-stimulating hormone (FSH), 29, 56–57, 265
follicles, ovarian, 8*b*, 14, 31, 265
folliculitis, 119
food diary, accidental bowel leakage and, 135
forgetfulness. *See* memory changes
fractures, bone loss and, 163
friends, talking with, 34, 227
fruits, eating, 217
FSH. *See* follicle-stimulating hormone

gabapentin, 64, 98, 199
gallbladder disease, 192–193
Gellhorn pessary, 142, 142*f*
gender-affirming care, 59
general anesthesia, 71, 265
genes or genetics
    breast cancer and, 237
    colon cancer and, 239
    definition, 265
    lichen sclerosus and, 119
    menopause transition and, 4
    premature and early menopause and, 24
    primary ovarian insufficiency and, 31
genitals or genital area, 113, 124, 265
genito–pelvic pain and penetration disorder (GPPPD), 103, 122–123, 265
genitourinary syndrome of menopause (GSM), 37, 103, 114–115, 118–119, 203, 266
geography, hysterectomy rate and, 28
gestational diabetes, 210, 215, 266
gingivitis, 241
ginkgo, 21
ginseng, 21, 183
GLP-1 receptor agonists, 156–157, 198, 219
glucose, diabetes and, 25
GnRH. *See* gonadotropin-releasing hormone medications
gonadotropin-releasing hormone medications (GnRH medications), 73, 266
gonorrhea, 110, 266
GPPPD. *See* genito–pelvic pain and penetration disorder
Graves disease, 240
GSM. *See* genitourinary syndrome of menopause
gynecologic oncologists, 44, 52

hair, 4, 40–41, 49, 119, 191
hair follicles, 119
Hashimoto disease, 240
HDL. *See* high-density lipoprotein
headaches, 191
health care, menopause and openness to, 34
hearing, 87, 242, 245
heart attack, 9, 209
heart disease. *See also* blood pressure
    HIV/AIDS and, 26

heart disease *(continued)*
    inadequate sleep and, 90
    managing risk for, 10
    medications, 218
    menopause transition and, 4
    ospemifene and, 202
    overview, 207
    premature and early menopause and, 29
    resources, 219–220
    risk, hot flashes and, 63*b*
    stress and, 223
    systemic hormone therapy and, 192
    what to know about, 208–209
heart failure, 208
heart valve problems, 209
heated spaces, hot flashes and, 59
hemoglobin A1C test, 214*b*
hepatitis B, 266
hepatitis B vaccination, 243*t*
herbal remedies, 184
herpes zoster vaccination, 244*t*
high blood pressure. *See also* blood pressure
    brain health and, 87
    chronic disease and, 9
    definition, 266
    eye exams and, 241
    guide, 210–212, 211*b*
    heart disease and stroke and, 207
    inadequate sleep and, 90
    light exposure during sleep and, 93
    mind–body practices and, 180
    obesity and, 150
    ospemifene and, 118, 202
    during pregnancy, CVD risk and, 210
    sexual health and, 103
    stress and, 223
    systemic hormone therapy and, 193
    urinary incontinence compared with, 128
high-density lipoprotein (HDL), 212, 213*b*
Hispanic Americans
    fracture rates among, 164
    FRAX calculation for, 165
    hot flashes and night sweats and, 36, 58
    hysterectomies and, 28
    menopause symptoms and, 6*b*
    osteoporosis and, 164
    sleep problems and, 91
    stress and, 222
    type 2 diabetes and, 215
HIV. *See* human immunodeficiency virus
home, stress at, 225
hormone therapies
    for abnormal bleeding, 72–73
    breast density and, 238*b*
    definition, 266
    fracture risk and, 168
    history and controversy, 188
    hot flashes or night sweats and, 36, 57, 62

hormone therapies *(continued)*
    local, side effects of, 194–195
    local, use and benefits of, 193–194
    low-dose estrogen cream, 117
    menopause transition and, 8
    ob-gyn management of, 44
    for osteoporosis, 167t
    ovarian surgery and, 28
    overview, 187
    premature and early menopause and, 9, 30
    resources, 196
    for sexual problems, 104
    systemic, benefits of, 190–191
    systemic, delivery and action of, 188–189
    systemic, side effects and risks, 191–193
    systemic, use of, 117–118
    talking with your ob-gyn about, 196
    for urinary incontinence, 131
    weight management and, 152b
    when to stop, 193
hormones. *See also* androgens; anti-müllerian hormone; estrogen; follicle-stimulating hormone; insulin; progesterone; testosterone
    bleeding changes and, 67–68
    changing levels of, 113–115, 114f
    compounded bioidentical, 184–185
    hot flashes and, 55
    menopause and, 7–8
    menopause transition attitudes and, 34
    regulation by, 8b
    sexual desire and, 102
    sleep quality and, 16, 90
    smoking and levels of, 24
    stress and, 223
    treating disorders related to, 44–45
    vaginal and vulvar changes and, 17
    weight gain and, 150
hot drinks, hot flashes and, 59
hot flashes. *See also* night sweats
    alcohol drinking and, 179
    anxiety and depression and, 39, 79, 80
    basics of, 55–57
    caffeine and, 178
    causes, 57–59
    cultural variations, 6b
    daily life and, 33
    definition, 266
    early menopause and, 29
    estrogen-free medical therapies and, 198–200
    future heart and brain health and, 63b
    heart disease and, 209
    hormone therapy for, 72, 117–118, 187
    insomnia and, 89
    management, 41
    managing, 60–62
    medical treatment for, 62, 64

hot flashes *(continued)*
    menopause transition and, 4, 35–36
    mind–body practices and, 180
    obesity and, 150
    overview, 55
    perimenopause and, 5, 14, 16
    physical activity and, 176
    premature menopause and, 23, 29
    resources, 65, 203
    sleep and, 180–181
    smoking and, 177
    supplements for, 182–183
    systemic hormone therapy and, 190
    triggers, 59–60
    uterus or ovary removal and, 57
HPV. *See* human papillomavirus
HPV vaccine, 234
human immunodeficiency virus (HIV), 25–26, 110, 165, 234, 243, 266
human papillomavirus (HPV), 120–121, 234, 266
hunger, sleep quality and, 94
hyaluronic acid, 116–117, 184
hydrocortisone cream, 121
hypertension, 210–211, 211b, 266
hyperthyroidism, 240, 266
hypnotherapy, 61
hypnotic relaxation therapy, 180
hypothyroidism, 240, 267
hysterectomy
    ACOG video on, 78
    cervical cancer screening and, 234–235
    chronic fatigue syndrome and, 25
    CVD risk and, 210
    definition, 267
    hot flashes and, 57
    pelvic organ prolapse and, 138, 146
    race and ethnicity and, 5
    reasons for and process of, 75
    total or partial, 28
hysteroscope, 71, 71f, 76, 267
hysteroscopy, 71, 71f, 74, 267

IBD. *See* inflammatory bowel disease
IBS. *See* irritable bowel syndrome
immune system, 25–26, 119, 212, 223, 234, 267
immunization resources, 245
in vitro fertilization (IVF), 29, 267
incontinence, patient guides to, 148
infections, 25, 70, 223
infertility, 27, 45, 47–48, 267
inflammation, 63b, 212, 267
inflammatory bowel disease (IBD), 21, 223–224, 239, 267
influenza vaccination, 243t
insomnia. *See also* sleep problems
    antidepressants and, 84
    cognitive behavioral therapy for, 180

insomnia *(continued)*
   definition, 267
   fezolinetant and, 64
   perimenopause and, 16, 89
   physical activity and, 176
   symptoms, 96
   treatment specialists, 48
insulin, 25, 267
intermittent fasting, 154*b*
intimate partner violence, 4, 58, 110, 123, 128, 267
intrauterine device (IUD), 19, 31, 72, 189, 267
intravenous fluids (IV fluids), 68–69, 267
irritable bowel syndrome (IBS), 122–123, 224, 267
IUD. *See* intrauterine device
IV. *See* intravenous fluids
IVF. *See* in vitro fertilization

joint pain, 191

kava, 95*b*, 183
Kegel exercises, 106, 107*b*, 130, 142, 268
kidney disease, 49, 165, 268
kidney failure, 21
kidneys, 211, 268

labia majora, 119, 268
labia minora, 119, 268
laparoscope, 76, 268
laparoscopy, 133, 144, 157–158, 268
laser therapy, vaginal, FDA warnings on, 119
latex, oils dissolving, 105*b*, 116, 184
LDL. *See* low-density lipoprotein
learning changes, menopause transition and, 39–40
leiomyomas, 69, 268
LGBTQ community, 46*b*, 51, 222
lichen planus, 120
lichen sclerosus, 119
lichen simplex chronicus, 120
lifestyle changes
   evaluating product claims and, 185
   nonprescription products and supplements and, 181–185
   overview, 175
   pelvic organ prolapse and, 143
   resources, 186
   self-care and, 175–181
   when what you're trying isn't working, 185–186
ligaments, 103, 137, 268
light exposure, sleep quality and, 93
liver disease, 192, 243
loneliness, combating, 227
low-density lipoprotein (LDL), 212, 213*b*
lubricants, 105*b*, 116–117, 124, 184–185
lung disease, 243

lupus
   CVD risk and, 210
   definition, 268
   estrogen-free medical therapies and, 203
   ospemifene and, 108, 118, 202
   pelvic organ prolapse and, 138
   stress and, 223
Lynch syndrome, 239, 268

magnesium, 95*b*
magnetic resonance imaging (MRI), 75–76, 268
malabsorptive bariatric surgery, 157. *See also* bariatric surgery
mammography and mammograms, 236–237, 245, 268
masturbation, 105*b*
medications
   abnormal bleeding, 21, 72–74
   accidental bowel leakage and, 134, 135
   bone loss and, 164
   estrogen-free, for hot flashes, 64
   fall risks and, 166*b*
   heart disease and diabetes, 218–219
   hormonal, for hot flashes, 62
   osteoporosis, 167–168*t*
   pelvic pain, 123
   sexual problems and, 103, 106–108
   sleep problems and, 16, 17, 98
   urinary incontinence, 128, 131–132
   weight loss, 156–157
meditation, sleep and, 93*b*
Mediterranean diet, 159
melanocortin receptor agonists, 106, 268
melatonin, 95*b*
melatonin agonists, 98
memory changes, 18, 39–40. *See also* brain fog
meningioma, 192
menopause (menopause transition). *See also* early menopause; postmenopause or postmenopausal; premature menopause
   abnormal bleeding, 67–78
   bleeding and, 35, 77
   bone health, 161–171
   controlling signs and symptoms of, 33–34
   cultural variations in, 6–7*b*
   definition, 269
   emotions and, 6–7, 79–88
   estrogen-free medical therapies, 197–204
   experience of, 3
   fibromyalgia and, 25
   healthy lifestyle and, 9–10
   hormone therapies, 187–196
   hot flashes and night sweats, 35–36, 55–65
   learning about, 34
   learning and memory changes, 39–40
   lifestyle changes, 175–186
   medical and surgical, 26–28

menopause *(continued)*
    mood and anxiety issues, 38–39
    mood and memory, 79–88
    obesity and, 150
    ovulation during, 68
    pelvic organ prolapse and, 138
    perimenopause and, 13
    predicting signs and symptoms, 33
    resources, 41–42
    screenings and vaccinations, 233–245
    sexual health, 38, 101–111
    signs and symptoms overview, 33
    skin and hair changes, 40–41
    sleep problems, 40, 89–100
    symptom tracker, 42
    talking with your ob-gyn about, 41
    timing, 3–5
    urinary and pelvic floor symptoms, 37–38, 125–136
    vaginal and vulvar changes, 36–37, 113–124
menopause care team
    choosing, 43
    dermatologists, 49
    endocrinologists, 47–48
    finding an ob-gyn, 45–46
    finding care that's right for you, 46*b*
    gynecologic oncologists, 44
    mental health specialists, 48–49
    ob-gyns, 43–44
    primary care doctor, 47
    registered dietitians, 49
    REI specialists, 44–45
    resources, 51–52
    sleep specialists, 48
    taking charge of your care, 50
    urogynecologists, 44
menopause workplace resource guide, 230
menstrual cycle, 4, 5, 67–68, 269. *See also* menstrual periods
menstrual periods (bleeding). *See also* abnormal uterine bleeding
    definition, 269
    final, brain fog and, 85
    genitourinary syndrome of menopause after, 115
    hot flashes and, 56
    menopause and changes in, 3, 35
    perimenopause and, 5–6, 13
    premature menopause and, 23
    progestin-only hormonal birth control and, 72
menstruation, 7, 269
mental health. *See also* mood swings
    finding practitioners for, 52
    healthy lifestyle and, 9
    premature and early menopause and, 30
    resources, 87–88
    sexual health and, 103–104

mental health *(continued)*
    stress, adult friendships and, 227
    treatment specialists, 48–49
    weight distribution and, 151
mental health nurses, 48–49
mesh, surgical, 132, 133, 145, 147
metabolic disorders, 47–48
metabolic syndrome, 16, 269
metabolism, 150–151, 181, 239, 269
metformin, 156
midlife health problems, sexual health and, 103
mind–body practices, 92–93*b*, 180, 228
Mindfulness Coach, 230
mindfulness therapies, 83*b*, 93*b*, 105, 229
mindfulness-based stress reduction, 61–62
mixed urinary incontinence, 126, 269
mood swings. *See also* depression; mental health
    alcohol drinking and, 179
    caffeine and, 178
    menopause transition and, 4, 38–39, 79
    mind–body practices and, 180
    perimenopause and, 14, 18
    physical activity and, 176
    self-care for, 82–83*b*
    sleep and, 181
    smoking and, 177
MRI. *See* magnetic resonance imaging
MRI-guided ultrasound surgery, 75–76
multiple sclerosis, 127, 269
mumps, 26, 269
muscles, 150–151, 224
music, sleep and, 93*b*
myomectomy, 74, 269

naps, daytime, 94
narcolepsy treatment specialists, 48
Native American women, 164
native tissue repair, for pelvic organ prolapse, 144
nature, visiting, stress and, 227
nervous system, stress and, 222
neurologists, 48
nicotine, 60, 92, 177–178, 269. *See also* smoking
night sweats. *See also* hot flashes
    cognitive performance and, 85
    managing, 60–62
    menopause transition and, 36
    perimenopause and, 14, 16
    premature menopause and, 23
    resources, 65
    vasomotor symptoms of, 55, 56
nocturia, 37, 269
noise at night, sleep quality and, 93
nonbinary people, hot flashes and, 59
nonhormonal treatments for menopause, 204. *See also* estrogen-free medical therapies

nonsteroidal anti-inflammatory drugs (NSAIDs), 21, 73, 269
nurse practitioners (NPs), 47, 48–49
nurses, 48
nutrition
    bladder irritants and, 130
    healthful, stress reduction and, 227
    heart disease and diabetes risk and, 216–217
    midlife focus and tips on, 153–155, 154b
    mood, anxiety, and brain self-care and, 83b
    sleep quality and, 94
nutrition experts, 49, 51

OAB. *See* overactive bladder
obesity. *See also* overweight; weight gain
    BMI and, 150
    CVD risk and, 210
    definition, 269
    diabetes risk and, 215
    heart disease and stroke and, 207
    hot flashes and, 16, 58
    light exposure during sleep and, 93
    mind–body practices and, 180
    pelvic floor and, 107b
    pelvic organ prolapse and, 138
    stress and, 223
    systemic hormone therapy and, 192
    treatment for, 49
    urinary incontinence and, 128
obliterative surgery, 144, 146, 269
obstetrician–gynecologist (ob-gyn)
    accidental bowel leakage and, 134
    annual checkup with, 9–10
    annual wellness visits after menopause, 233–235
    bleeding changes and, 14, 67
    definition, 270
    finding, 42, 45–46, 46b, 51
    hormone therapy and, 8, 187
    hot flashes treatment and, 59
    menopause symptoms management and, 41
    menopause transition research and, 33
    mood and memory changes and, 79
    postmenopausal bleeding and, 77b
    premature menopause and, 23
    protecting long-term health and, 207
    sexual health and, 101
    sexual problem treatments and, 104
    sleep problems and, 99
    stress and, 222, 228–229
    types of, for menopause care, 43–44
    urinary incontinence and, 128–129
    vaginal and vulvar changes and, 115
    weight management and, 149–150
obstructive sleep apnea (OSA), 16, 40, 48, 90, 96–97, 270
off-label medications, 198, 204
oils, food-grade, vaginal dryness and, 116, 184

oocyte cryopreservation, 29, 270. *See also* eggs
oral sex, 105b, 110
orexin receptor antagonists, 98
orgasm, 38, 84, 102, 179, 270
OSA. *See* obstructive sleep apnea
ospemifene, 108, 118, 201t, 202
osteopenia, 162, 163, 270
osteoporosis, 10, 48, 162, 162f, 163, 270. *See also* bone loss
outdoor activities, mood, anxiety, and brain self-care and, 83b
ovarian cancer, 28, 44, 237, 270
ovarian torsion surgery, 28
ovaries
    aging, smoking and, 24
    annual wellness checks of, 234
    definition, 270
    endometrial hyperplasia and, 70
    menopause transition and, 4
    radiation therapy and, 26–27
    removal, CVD risk and, 210
    removal, genitourinary syndrome of menopause and, 115
    removal, hot flashes and, 57
    surgery to remove, menopause and, 27–28
overactive bladder (OAB), 126, 270
over-the-counter medicines, 95b, 185, 186
overweight, 215. *See also* obesity; weight gain
ovulate, 270
ovulation, 27, 31, 67–68, 72, 270
oxybutynin, 64, 199–200, 201t
oxygen, 209, 270

pain during sex, 62, 102–103, 113, 117, 147, 179
Pap tests, 234
Parkinson's disease, 127
paroxetine mesylate, 64, 199, 200t
partners, sexual, 94, 105b
PCOS. *See* polycystic ovary syndrome
pelvic exams, 21, 70, 104, 120–121, 234–235, 270
pelvic floor, 18, 37, 103, 127, 270
pelvic floor disorders, 44, 50, 136, 270
pelvic floor physical therapy
    menopause care and, 50
    for pelvic pain, 123
    resources, 111, 136
    sexual health and, 106
    for urinary incontinence, 130–131
    for vulvodynia, 119
pelvic inflammatory disease, 28, 103, 270
pelvic masses, 44
pelvic organ prolapse
    causes, 138
    definition, 271
    menopause transition and, 37
    nonsurgical treatments, 142–143, 142f

pelvic organ prolapse *(continued)*
  overview, 137
  pain during sex and, 103
  physical therapy for, 50
  repeat surgery for, 146–147
  resources, 148
  smoking and, 177
  stress urinary incontinence and, 134
  surgery, 143–144
  symptoms, 138
  talking with your ob-gyn about, 141
  types, 139–140, 140*f*
  urinary incontinence and, 127
  urogynecologist treatment of, 44
  weight loss and, 176
pelvic pain, 25, 50, 122–123, 123–124, 233
pelvis, 20, 26–27, 71, 128, 137, 271
penetration
  aging and, 101
  alternatives, 105*b*
  definition, 271
  difficulty with, 110
  genito–pelvic pain and penetration disorder and, 122–123, 265
  pain with, 103
  pelvic floor weakness and, 106
percutaneous tibial nerve stimulation (PTNS), 132
perimenopause. *See also* abnormal uterine bleeding
  absence of periods and, 21
  attitudes and, 34
  birth control and, 19
  bleeding changes in, 14–15, 67–68
  bleeding disorders and, 20–21
  body and mind and, 15
  definition, 13, 271
  estrogen declines during, 79
  fertility issues during, 45
  heart disease signs and symptoms and, 211
  hot flashes and, 16, 55–56
  medications and, 21
  mood and memory changes and, 18–19
  pregnancy and, 19
  sleep changes and, 16–17, 89–91
  symptoms, 5–6
  talking with your ob-gyn about, 21–22
  tracking early signs of, 13–14
  urinary changes and, 18
  uterine conditions and, 19–20
  vaginal and vulvar changes and, 17, 113
perineum, 102–103, 271
peripheral artery disease, 209
pessaries, 130, 142–143, 142*f*, 148, 271
pets, sleep quality and, 94
phosphate, in bones, 161
physical activity. *See* exercise
physical therapists, 49–50, 51, 111, 136, 148

pituitary gland, 21, 271
plant-based eating, 154
plaque, arterial, 208, 208*f*, 210–211, 271
platelets, bleeding disorders and, 20–21
PMS. *See* premenstrual syndrome
pneumonia, 27, 271
POI. *See* primary ovarian insufficiency
polycystic ovary syndrome (PCOS), 21, 45, 72, 215, 271
polypectomy, 74
polyps, 19, 69, 69*f*, 239, 271. *See also* benign growths or cysts
porphyria cutanea tarda, 193
positive self-talk, 34
posterior vaginal wall prolapse, 139, 140*f*, 271
postmenopausal bleeding, 75, 77
postmenopause or postmenopausal. *See also* menopause; screening tests
  definition, 4, 271
  hormone therapies and, 188
  sexual desire during, 106
  urgency urinary incontinence in, 126
  vaginal and vulvar changes and, 17
  women on, as positive, 34
  yoga and sleep in, 93*b*
post-traumatic stress disorder (PTSD), 59, 229–230, 271
potassium, bone health and, 171
prasterone, 108, 118, 201*t*, 202
prediabetes, 214–215, 214*b*, 241, 271
preeclampsia, 210, 272
pregabalin, 200
pregnancy, 19, 29, 31, 76, 127, 193
premature menopause. *See also* early menopause; primary ovarian insufficiency
  bone loss and, 164
  causal factors, 23–26
  CVD risk and, 210
  definition, 272
  early menopause compared with, 23
  fertility and, 29
  medical and surgical causes, 26–28
  other concerns with, 29–30
  resources, 31–32
  symptoms, 8–9
  systemic hormone therapy and, 193
  treatment for, 30
premenstrual syndrome (PMS), 18, 80, 272
primary care doctors, 43, 47, 51, 77*b*
primary ovarian insufficiency (POI), 21, 23, 31, 165, 210, 272
product research, evaluating claims of, 185, 186
progesterone
  chronic fatigue syndrome and, 25
  definition, 272
  function of, 7, 8*b*
  menstrual cycle and, 67–68

progesterone *(continued)*
  metabolism and, 150
  perimenopause and, 14
  primary ovarian insufficiency and, 31
  sleep quality and, 90
progestin
  in combined hormonal birth control, 72
  definition, 272
  for hot flashes or night sweats, 62
  systemic hormone therapy and, 118, 188, 189
  urinary incontinence and, 131
progestin-only hormonal birth control, 72
prostaglandins, 73, 272
protein, 161, 171, 217
psychiatric nurses and nurse practitioners, 48–49
psychiatric pharmacists, 49
psychiatrists, 48
psychologists, 48
psychotherapy, 84
PTNS. *See* percutaneous tibial nerve stimulation
PTSD. *See* post-traumatic stress disorder
puberty, 27, 272
pubic hair, 115

RA. *See* rheumatoid arthritis
race and ethnicity
  bone loss and, 164
  diabetes risk and, 215
  hot flashes and, 16, 36, 58
  menopause transition and, 5
  sleep problems in menopause transition and, 91
  uterine cancer disparities and, 77*b*
  uterine surgery and, 38
radiation, definition of, 272
radiation therapy, 26–27, 128, 210, 239, 272
radiofrequency ablation, 76
radiologists, 236, 272
raloxifene, 167*t*
ramelteon, 98
reconstructive surgery, 144, 272
rectovaginal exams, 235
rectum, 37, 103, 130, 137, 272
red clover, 182
regional anesthesia, 272
REI. *See* reproductive endocrinology and infertility specialists
relaxation techniques, 65, 93*b*
reproductive endocrinology and infertility specialists (REI specialists), 44–45
respiratory syncytial virus (RSV), 244*t*
respiratory therapists, 48
respite care, agencies providing, 226
restless leg syndrome, 48, 97
restrictive bariatric surgery, 157. *See also* bariatric surgery

rheumatoid arthritis (RA), 138, 165, 210, 223, 273
ring pessary with knob, 142, 142*f*
ring pessary with support, 142, 142*f*
romosozumab, 168*t*
Roux-en-Y gastric bypass, 157–158
RSV. *See* respiratory syncytial virus

sacral neuromodulation, 132, 135
sacrocolpopexy, 145, 273
sacrohysteropexy, 145, 273
sadness, 80–81
safer sex, talking about, 110–111
saline infusion sonography (SIS), 71–72
scientific research, evaluating claims of, 185, 186
screening tests
  after menopause, 233–235
  breast cancer, 235–236, 236*f*
  cancer, 10
  cervical cancer, 234–235
  colon cancer, 238–239
  depression, 81
  eye exams, 241
  hearing tests, 242
  overview, 233
  resources, 244–245
  skin cancer, 242
  thyroid gland, 239–240, 240*f*
seizure disorder medications, 90
seizure disorders, 273
selective estrogen receptor modulators (SERMs), 108, 118, 189, 202, 273
selective serotonin reuptake inhibitors (SSRIs), 164, 199, 200*t*, 273
selective serotonin–norepinephrine reuptake inhibitors (SNRIs), 199, 200*t*, 273
sepsis, 126, 273
SERMs. *See* selective estrogen receptor modulators
serotonin receptor agonist/antagonists, 107, 273
sex drive, low, 44
sex therapists, 109–110, 111
sex therapy, 124
sexual assault or abuse, 46*b*, 110, 273
sexual function disorders, 44
sexual health
  alcohol drinking and, 179
  changes, physical therapy for, 50
  finding practitioners for, 52
  menopause transition and, 38
  in midlife, 102–104
  mind–body practices and, 180
  new partners and, 110–111
  obesity and, 150
  overview, 101
  physical activity and, 176

sexual health *(continued)*
  problems, treatments for, 104–108
  resources, 111
  self-care, 105*b*
  sexual skills training, 106
  sleep and, 181
  systemic hormone therapy and, 190
  talking with your ob-gyn about, 233
  when to talk with your ob-gyn, 108–109
  when to talk with your partner, 109–110
sexual intercourse. *See also* pain during sex
  Bartholin glands and, 120
  bleeding or spotting after, 15, 38, 68, 115
  definition, 273
  pelvic organ prolapse surgery and, 146
  perimenopause and, 17
  vaginal and vulvar changes and, 36
sexual interest/arousal disorder, 102
sexual relationship changes, 104
sexually transmitted infections (STIs), 70, 103, 110–111, 115, 233, 273
shingles, 274
shingles vaccination, 244*t*
SIL. *See* squamous intraepithelial lesion
SIS. *See* saline infusion sonography
sitting, urinary incontinence and, 128
skeleton. *See also* bone health
  stress and, 224
skin, 4, 40–41, 49, 191
skin cancer self-checks, 242, 245
sleep
  alcohol drinking and, 179
  caffeine and, 178–179
  exercise and, 92, 176
  menopause symptoms and, 180–181
  mind–body connection and, 92–93*b*
  practicing good hygiene with, 227–228
  setting hours for, 91
  smoking and, 177
  stress management and, 92
  substance use and, 92
  systemic hormone therapy and, 190
sleep aids, 95*b*
sleep apnea, 99, 150, 274. *See also* obstructive sleep apnea
sleep problems. *See also* insomnia
  brain fog and, 39, 85
  diabetes risk and, 215
  finding practitioners for, 52
  impact on daily life, 33
  key steps in resolving, 91–95
  menopause transition and, 4, 40, 89
  mid-life, CVD risk and, 210
  perimenopause and, 16–17, 89–91
  premature and early menopause and, 29
  resources, 99–100
  sleep disorders, 96–97
  treatment for, 62, 97–98

sleep problems *(continued)*
  weight gain and, 151
  when to talk with your doctor, 98–99
sling, traditional, 133
smoking. *See also* nicotine; race and ethnicity
  CVD risk and, 210
  depression during menopause transition and, 80
  heart disease and diabetes risk and, 215, 216
  hot flashes and, 16, 58, 60
  menopause transition and, 5
  mood, anxiety, and brain self-care and, 83*b*
  pelvic organ prolapse and, 141
  premature and early menopause and, 24
  quitting, menopausal symptoms and, 177–178
  urinary incontinence and, 128
  vaccinations and, 243
SNRIs. *See* selective serotonin–norepinephrine reuptake inhibitors
social workers, 49
sodium intake, limiting, 218
sonohysterography, 71–72, 274
soy and soy products, 182, 184
sperm, 8*b*, 29, 274
sphincter muscles, 127, 274
spicy foods, hot flashes and, 59
spinal cord damage, 127
spine, osteoporosis of, 163, 163*f*
spongy bone, 161, 162*f*
sports nutrition, 49
squamous intraepithelial lesion (SIL), 120–121
SSRIs. *See* selective serotonin reuptake inhibitors
St. John's wort, 184
stamina exercises, 152
steroid cream or ointment, 121
STIs. *See* sexually transmitted infections
strength training, 152, 153, 170
stress
  alcohol drinking and, 179
  caffeine and, 178
  in caregiving, 225–226
  chronic, absence of periods and, 21
  early life, menopause transition and, 4
  as health issue, 222–224
  at home, 225
  management resources, 88
  managing, overview, 221–222
  mind–body practices and, 180
  physical activity and, 176
  resources, 230–231
  science-based self-care strategies, 226–228
  sleep and, 90, 92, 181
  smoking and, 177
  therapy for managing, 229–230
  weight distribution and, 151
  at work, 224–225

Stress in America survey, 227, 230
stress urinary incontinence
   about, 125–126
   menopause transition and, 37
   pelvic organ prolapse and, 134, 144
   pelvic organ prolapse surgery and, 147
   smoking and, 177
   urethra and, 126f
stroke. *See also* blood pressure
   blood clots and, 208
   definition, 274
   depression during menopause transition and, 80
   managing risk for, 9
   nerve and muscle problems with, 127
   obesity and, 150
   ospemifene and, 118, 202
   osteoporosis medications and, 167
   overview, 207
   premature and early menopause and, 29
   risk, hot flashes and, 63b
   sexual health and, 103
   systemic hormone therapy and, 192
   WHI on hormone therapy and risk of, 188
substance abuse, 88
sugars, cutting down on, 217
supplements, 84b, 181–183, 185, 186
surgery
   accidental bowel leakage and, 135
   pelvic organ prolapse, 143–144
   pelvic pain and, 124
   types, for pelvic organ prolapse, 144–146, 148
   urinary incontinence, 128, 132–134
   weight management, 157–158
suvorexant, 98
syphilis, 110, 274
systolic blood pressure, 211, 274

T_3. *See* triiodothyronine
T_4. *See* thyroxine
tai chi, 93b
talk therapy. *See* cognitive behavioral therapy
tamoxifen, 27, 57, 274
TB. *See* tuberculosis
Td. *See* tetanus and diphtheria vaccination
Tdap. *See* tetanus, diphtheria, whooping cough vaccination
testosterone, 59, 108, 274
tetanus, 274
tetanus, diphtheria, whooping cough vaccination (Tdap vaccination), 244t
tetanus and diphtheria vaccination (Td vaccination), 244t
THC, sleep and, 95b
therapists, 49
thinking, stress and, 223
throat, squamous intraepithelial lesion and, 120–121

thyroid cancer, 240
thyroid disease, 70, 239–240
thyroid gland, 21, 48, 240f, 274
thyroid medication, 164
thyroxine (T_4), 239
tranexamic acid, 73, 274
transducer, 71, 274
transfusion, blood, 68–69, 275
transgender men or women, 59, 275
transvaginal ultrasound exams, 71, 275
trauma, 46b, 80, 103
travel outside the United States, vaccinations and, 243
trichomoniasis, 275
trigger-point injections or therapy, 106, 119, 124
triglycerides, 210, 212, 213b, 275
triiodothyronine (T_3), 239
T-scores, DEXA scan, 165–166, 165t
tuberculosis (TB), 26, 275
tumors, ultrasound of, 238

ulcerative colitis, 239
ultra-processed foods, intake of, 218
ultrasound exams, 21, 71, 275
ultrasound surgery, MRI-guided, 75–76
underweight, 21
urethra
   definition, 275
   pelvic floor muscles and, 137
   pelvic organ prolapse and, 103
   perimenopause and, 18
   synthetic midurethral sling for, 132
   urinary incontinence and, 126f, 127
urethral bulking, 133
urgency urinary incontinence, 37, 50, 126, 126f, 179, 275
urinary changes, 18, 113
urinary incontinence
   alcohol drinking and, 179
   caffeine and, 179
   definition, 275
   devices and physical therapy, 130–131
   factors in, 127–128
   first approaches, 129–130
   medications, 131–132
   menopause transition and, 37
   nerve stimulation, 132
   ob-gyn management of, 128–129
   overview, 125
   perimenopause and, 18
   resources, 136
   sexual health and, 103
   surgical treatments, 132–134
   talking with your ob-gyn about, 135, 233
   types, 125–126, 126f
   urogynecologist treatment of, 44
urinary tract, 113, 144, 147, 193–194, 275

urinary tract infections (UTIs)
    definition, 275
    genito–pelvic pain and penetration disorder and, 123
    menopause transition and, 37, 114
    pelvic organ prolapse surgery and, 146
    perimenopause and, 18
    talking with your ob-gyn about, 233
    urinary incontinence and, 126
    vaginal estrogen and, 194
urinating, sleep disruption and, 16
urogynecologists, 44, 51, 104
uterine artery embolization, 74, 275
uterine cancer, 20, 28, 44, 77b, 78
uterine prolapse, 28, 139, 140f, 275
uterus
    abnormal bleeding conditions of, 19–20
    annual wellness checks of, 234
    definition, 275
    hormones and, 7
    hysteroscopy and, 71, 71f
    pain during sex and, 102–103
    pelvic floor and, 37, 137
    perimenopause and, 13
    removal, hot flashes and, 57
    removal, menopause and, 28
    systemic hormone therapy and, 189
UTIs. See urinary tract infections

vaccinations, 242–244, 243t
vaccines, 10, 245, 276
vagina. See also pain during sex; sexual intercourse
    annual wellness checks of, 234
    changing hormone levels and, 113–115, 114f
    definition, 276
    estrogen and, 8b
    hysteroscopy and, 71, 71f
    identifying areas of discomfort, 115, 116f
    irritation of, 14
    local hormone therapy and, 193–194
    lubricants, moisturizers, and dilators, 124
    menopause transition and, 17, 36–37
    obliterative surgery and, 144
    pelvic floor and, 37, 137
    reduced sensation in, 102
    squamous intraepithelial lesion and, 120–121
    systemic hormone therapy and, 189
    transvaginal ultrasound exam and, 71
    uterine cancer surgery and, 28
    vaginal pain, 50
vaginal balloon devices, 135
vaginal cancer, 44
vaginal closure surgery, 144, 146
vaginal dryness
    hormone therapy for, 72
    menopause transition and, 4, 38
    ob-gyn management of, 44

vaginal dryness *(continued)*
    ospemifene for, 118
    systemic hormone therapy and, 190
    treatments for, 62, 116–118, 202
vaginal estrogen, 194
vaginal moisturizers, 116, 184
vaginal penetration. *See* penetration
vaginal ring, 19
vaginal spotting or bleeding, 191
vaginal vault prolapse, 140, 140f, 276
valerian, 95b
vaping, smoking compared with, 177–178
vasomotor symptoms. *See* hot flashes
vegetables, eating, 217
veins, 210–211, 276
venlafaxine, 199, 200t
vertebrae, weakening of, 163
violence. *See* intimate partner violence
virtual colonoscopy, 239
vitamin B_{12} deficiency, 82
vitamin D, 161, 170–171
vitamin E, 21, 183
vulva
    definition, 276
    identifying areas of discomfort, 115, 116f
    irritation of, perimenopause and, 14
    local hormone therapy and, 193–194
    menopause transition and, 17, 36–37, 115
    other disorders of, 118–121
    reduced sensation in, 102
    self-care, 121–122
    self-examination guide, 124
    sexual health and, 105b
    skin care, 122b
vulvar cancer, 44
vulvodynia, 118–119, 276

warming, sleep quality and, 94
weigh-ins, 155
weight gain, 128, 150–151, 181. *See also* obesity; overweight
weight loss, rapid, 21
weight management
    heart disease and diabetes risk and, 216
    hormone therapy and, 152
    intermittent fasting and, 154b
    managing midlife fitness and, 151–155
    medications, 156–157
    overview, 149–150
    physical activity and, 176
    resources, 158–159
    sleep and, 181
    surgery, 157–158
    urinary incontinence and, 129
    when to talk with your ob-gyn, 155–156
weight-bearing activities, 169
WHI. *See* Women's Health Initiative, National Institutes of Health

whole grains, eating, 217
Women's Health Initiative (WHI), National Institutes of Health, 188
work, stress at, 224–225
World Health Organization, 179

yam, wild, 184
yeast infections, 113, 276
yoga, 93*b*

zaleplon, 98
zolpidem, 98

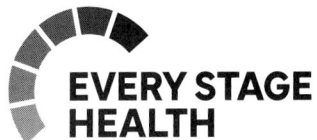

From the American College of Obstetricians & Gynecologists

Trusted ob-gyn guidance for every body.

everystagehealth.org

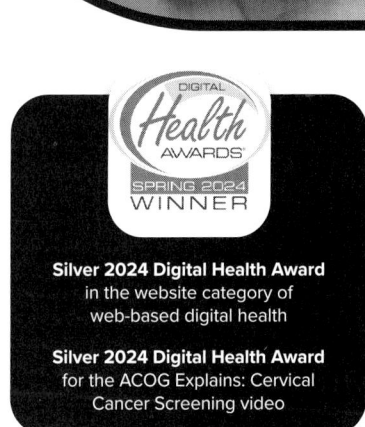

Powered by ACOG guidance, Every Stage Health offers evidence-based resources for every stage of life.

You'll find these features and more:

- ❯ Frequently updated health topic FAQs
- ❯ Videos that explain complex topics
- ❯ Real stories from women and ob-gyns
- ❯ A dictionary of medical terms
- ❯ Printable visual aids—explore the library at acog.org/infographics
- ❯ Health tools, such as a menopause symptom tracker
- ❯ Health quizzes

Silver 2024 Digital Health Award in the website category of web-based digital health

Silver 2024 Digital Health Award for the ACOG Explains: Cervical Cancer Screening video

Find in-depth info on ACOG books at everystagehealth.org

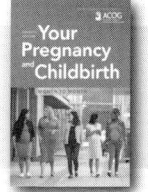 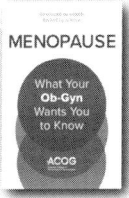

everystagehealth.org